C000048392

Irish women in medicine, c.1880s–1920s

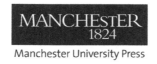

MANCHESTER
1824

Manchester University Press

Irish women in medicine, c.1880s–1920s

Origins, education and careers

Laura Kelly

Manchester University Press

Copyright © Laura Kelly 2012

The right of Laura Kelly to be identified as the author of this work has been asserted
by her in accordance with the Copyright, Designs and Patents Act 1988.

Published by Manchester University Press
Altrincham Street, Manchester M1 7JA, UK
www.manchesteruniversitypress.co.uk

British Library Cataloguing-in-Publication Data is available

Library of Congress Cataloging-in-Publication Data is available

ISBN 978 0 7190 9740 9 *paperback*

First published by Manchester University Press in hardback 2012

This paperback edition first published 2015

The publisher has no responsibility for the persistence or accuracy of URLs for any external or third-party internet websites referred to in this book, and does not guarantee that any content on such websites is, or will remain, accurate or appropriate.

Printed by Lightning Source

To my parents,
John and Angela

Contents

Plates, figures and tables

Plates

Figures

Tables

Acknowledgements

THIS BOOK is based on my doctoral thesis which I undertook under the supervision of Dr Aileen Fyfe at NUI Galway from 2007 to 2010. My greatest debt of thanks therefore is to Aileen for her unending support and encouragement. Without her, this book would not have been possible.

I am thankful to several archivists and librarians who helped me with my research. My utmost thanks are to Robert Mills, librarian at the Royal College of Physicians, who was always accommodating with research visits and extremely helpful in answering the many queries I had relating to the KQCPI. Thanks are also due to Harriet Wheelock, archivist at the Royal College of Physicians, who alerted me to several other useful sources and photographs. I am grateful also to Mary O'Doherty, archivist at the Royal College of Surgeons, who was similarly accommodating and helpful. Mary also alerted me to the *Medical Students' Register*, which proved vital in tracing students who had not attended the Queen's Colleges, for which I am very grateful. Thanks also to the other archivists and librarians I encountered during my many research trips, in particular, Professor Richard Clarke (Royal Victoria Hospital), John Foley (NUI Archives), Dr Kieran Hoare (NUI Galway Special Collections), Ursula Mitchell (QUB Special Collections), Estelle Gittins (Manuscripts Department of TCD), Catriona Mulcahy (UCC University Archives), Victoria Rea (Royal Free Hospital Archives) and the staff of the Presbyterian Women's Association in Belfast. A special thanks to Professor Seamus MacMathuna, the registrar of NUI Galway, who gave me access to the matriculation albums of Queen's College Galway and who was very generous in answering my queries.

I am thankful also to the staff at Manchester University Press for their advice during the publication process. I would also like to thank Ralph Footring for his excellent and most appreciated work in copy-editing this book. Acknowledgement is also owed to the journals *Women's History Review* and *Medical History*, which gave me permission to reprint material from them.

I am very grateful to the relatives of the women doctors who were the focus of Chapter 7. In particular, I owe a huge debt of thanks to Niall Martin, whose grandmother Emily Winifred Dickson was one of the first Irish women doctors and an important focus of this book. Niall was extremely generous in allowing me access to his collection of papers and photographs relating to his grandmother and he and his wife Jenny were very hospitable to me when I visited Edinburgh. Niall and his family were also very patient in answering my many email queries. I would also like to thank Mary Mullaney, who kindly agreed to an oral history interview about her mother, Dr Mary McGivern, and who was very hospitable when I went to Sligo to visit her. Thank you also to Dr Maura Dowling, who kindly lent me the equipment to record the interview. I am thankful to Brian O'Connor also, who sent me an article written by his mother, Dr Jane D. Fulton, and who answered many email queries I sent him.

Thank you also to the many correspondents who replied to my requests for information in the Irish press, in particular, Brian McEnroy, who spoke to me about his aunt, Margaret, Dr Sheena Scanlon, who spoke to me about her experiences as a female doctor from the 1950s on, Joyce Darling, who wrote to me about her mother, Olive Pedlow, and Dr Joe Conway, who wrote to me about his mother, Dr Josephine Benedicte Conway. I am grateful to Professor Barbara Wright, who sent me information relating to her mother, Dr Rosaleen Hoskin. Thank you also to Professor Leslie Clarkson, who took the time to send me information to aid my research.

I also greatly appreciate the comments of Professor Greta Jones and Professor Gearoid O'Tuathaigh, who examined my thesis. Both offered extremely helpful ideas which have aided the development of the thesis to book. I also very much appreciate the comments and feedback of the two anonymous referees, which have greatly improved the book.

I was very fortunate to hold an Irish Research Council for the Humanities and Social Sciences postgraduate fellowship from 2008 to 2010, which allowed me to undertake the research upon which this book is based. I am grateful also to the Department of History of NUI Galway, which provided me with a fellowship in the first year of my PhD study, and to the Arts Faculty, for two travel grants. I am also thankful to the Wellcome Trust for a travel expenses grant which supported research trips in my first year of study.

I am grateful also to many mentors over the years. Professor Steven Ellis, head of the History Department at NUI Galway, really sparked my interest in history during my undergraduate degree and has always been helpful and generous with his time and advice. I am grateful also to Dr Enda Leaney, who really got me interested in the history of science and medicine when I took his courses as an undergraduate. I am thankful to Professor Marguerite Dupree, who supervised my masters dissertation at the University of Glasgow and who encouraged my interest in the history of medicine, medical education and students. I am grateful to colleagues at the Centre for the History of Science, Technology and Medicine at the University of Manchester who provided me with useful feedback on my work while I was a visiting student at the Centre in 2009, in particular, Dr Ian Burney, Dr Michael Brown, Professor John Pickstone and Professor Michael Worboys. Thanks also to my colleagues at the Department of History, NUI Galway, and to many friends in the history of medicine community for support and advice.

I am grateful to my friends who supported me throughout the writing of the thesis and book, in particular, Sarah, Sarah, Maeve, Lucy, Claire and Kate. A special thanks are also due to Jack Nea for his love, support and many fun times during the writing of the thesis and book.

Finally, I owe a huge debt of thanks to my parents, John and Angela, and my brothers, Seán and Ciarán. Thanks to Dad for help with the graphs and statistics in the book and for proof-reading it. My parents have always been extremely supportive and encouraging of me and my work and I could not have achieved this without their love and support. To them this book is dedicated.

Laura Kelly

Abbreviations

Medical institutions

CU	Catholic University
GMC	General Medical Council
KQCPI	King and Queen's College of Physicians of Ireland (later Royal College of Physicians of Ireland)
LSMW	London School of Medicine for Women
NUI	National University of Ireland
QCB	Queen's College Belfast
QCC	Queen's College Cork
QCG	Queen's College Galway
RCPI	Royal College of Physicians of Ireland
RCSci	Royal College of Science
RCSI	Royal College of Surgeons in Ireland
RUI	Royal University of Ireland
TCD	Trinity College Dublin
UCD	University College Dublin

Medical degrees

FRCSI	Fellow of the Royal College of Surgeons in Ireland
LRCP LRCS Edin, LFPS Glas	Conjoint Licence of the Scottish Colleges of Physicians and Surgeons in Edinburgh and Glasgow

LRCPI & LM, LRCSI & LM	Conjoint Licence of the Irish Colleges of Physicians and Surgeons
MB BCh BAO	Bachelor of Medicine and Surgery
MD	Doctor of Medicine

Commonly cited works

BMJ   *British Medical Journal*
DMP   *Dublin Medical Press*
ODNB   *Oxford Dictionary of National Biography*

Introduction

My mother had serious illnesses for nearly a year and I nursed her and when she recovered to some extent (always an invalid) I decided to take up medicine – the school of the College of Surgeons was just opened to women when I began medicine in the autumn of 1887 (Victoria's 50 year Jubilee) at the (mixed) school and the College and qualified in 1891....

Emily Winifred Dickson[1]

EMILY WINIFRED DICKSON, from Dungannon, Co. Tyrone, enrolled at the Royal College of Surgeons in Ireland at the age of twenty-one. With her father's encouragement, she had decided that she wanted to pursue a medical education. She had originally faced discouragement in her pursuit of admission to university. An application to Trinity College Dublin had been accepted with the support of the medical faculty, but was ultimately rejected due to opposition from the theologians of the university. Dickson was one of the earliest of 759 women who matriculated in medicine at Irish institutions between 1885 and 1922. Of these 759 women, 452 went on to qualify with medical degrees or licences. Certainly, Dickson was one of the pioneering women doctors of her generation and exceptional in terms of her ability and university career. However, she was typical of the women medical graduates of her generation and the next, in terms of the challenges she faced. In spite of these challenges, Dickson seems to have found herself readily accepted in the Irish medical profession in her early career and gained support from the medical hierarchy, in a surprising contrast to the received view of the Irish medical profession in the period as depicted by F. O. C. Meenan, in his history of the Catholic University School of Medicine:

There is no reason to suppose that aspiring women doctors found conditions more favourable in Ireland. They met the same determined opposition and prejudice from the medical establishment.[2]

1

Likewise, more recently, Irene Finn has argued that the Irish medical profession, with the exception of the King and Queen's College of Physicians of Ireland (KQCPI), held a hostile view towards women in medicine.[3] I will argue against these ideas by showing that Irish university authorities and members of the medical hierarchy in Ireland possessed a positive attitude towards women in the medical profession. Moreover, I consider the history of women in the medical profession in Ireland as being crucial to understanding the history of women in the medical profession in Britain. Up until 1886, the KQCPI played a virtually unique role in the qualification of women doctors in Britain and Ireland, with forty-eight of the first fifty women who were registered in Britain as qualified medical practitioners before this year taking their examinations at the KQCPI.[4] It is notable that Irish universities and hospitals opened their doors to women medical students earlier than their British counterparts, which is somewhat surprising considering that Ireland was at this time part of the United Kingdom and one might have expected similar trends.

The social, cultural and political context

THE PERIOD within which this book is set was one of vast social, cultural and political change in Ireland. The beginning of the nineteenth century opened with the Act of Union, passed in 1800 and coming into effect in January 1801. The act united Ireland with Britain under one parliament, with all Irish MPs now sitting in Westminster. Up until 1922, with the passing of the Anglo-Irish Treaty which followed the Irish War of Independence, Ireland was ruled by Britain. The 1840s to 1850s witnessed increasing agitation from Catholics, with the Repeal of the Union movement led by Daniel O'Connell in the 1830s and 1840s, and the establishment of the Irish Republican Brotherhood in 1858, which staged a failed rising in 1867. In 1873 Isaac Butt's Home Rule Party was established to seek the restoration of the Irish parliament. What followed was a politically turbulent fifty years. Charles Stewart Parnell assumed leadership of the Home Rule Party in 1880 and there were two failed attempts to pass Home Rule Bills in 1886 and 1893, under Prime Minister William Gladstone. The year 1886 also saw the establishment of the Unionist Party, which organised itself against Home Rule from the mid-1880s and into the early twentieth century. From the 1880s until 1922, successive British governments implemented a policy of 'constructive Unionism', for instance through the establishment of the Congested Districts Board in 1891, which poured money and expertise into 'congested' and poor areas in the west of Ireland, while the Department of Agriculture and Technical Instruction was set up in order to improve agricultural performance and profits.[5]

Meanwhile, the 1880s and 1890s witnessed the birth of the Gaelic revival through the establishment of the Gaelic Athletic Association (GAA), which revived interest in Irish sports, and the Gaelic League, which promoted the Irish language. The Irish Literary Revival, which began in the 1890s, led by Anglo-Irish writers such as W. B. Yeats and Lady Gregory, also fostered nationalism and Irish identity. The Home Rule Party split in 1890 after the scandal over the divorce case of its leader, Parnell. In 1898 the Local Government Act set up county councils and urban district councils, and women's representation increased at local level. In 1900, the Home Rule Party reunited under the leadership of John Redmond, and Home Rule was passed by the British parliament in 1914 but its implementation was postponed until after the First World War. Cumann na nGaedheal, a nationalist non-violent organisation, was founded by Arthur Griffith in 1900, with women accepted as equal members.[6]

The decade from 1912 to 1922 was increasingly turbulent. The year 1912 saw the establishment of the Ulster Volunteers, a militia to support the Ulster Unionists, led by Edward Carson. The Irish Labour Party (full title Irish Trade Union Congress and Labour Party) was also established in this year; the famous Dublin Lock-Out, where members of the Irish Transport and General Workers Union were locked out of their workplaces, occurred the following year. The Irish Citizen Army was founded following the Lock-Out and in 1914 the Irish Volunteers, with its female auxiliary group Cumann na mBan, was formed. The outbreak of the First World War caused huge divisions in Irish nationalism, with the majority of Volunteers, calling themselves the National Volunteers, supporting John Redmond's call to fight with Britain, while a minority, retaining the name Irish Volunteers, under the leadership of Eoin MacNeill, refused to fight.[7]

The Easter Rising took place in 1916, with three groups involved, the Irish Volunteers, Irish Citizen Army and Irish Republican Brotherhood. The leaders of the Rising were court-martialled and executed, sparking a wave of popular support for nationalism and a victory for the nationalist Sinn Féin party in the general election of December 1918. The Sinn Féin MPs refused to take up their seats at Westminster, instead establishing their own parliament, Dáil Éireann, in Dublin on 21 January 1919, with the War of Independence, which lasted until July 1921, beginning the same day. In 1920, the British government introduced the Government of Ireland Act, which established Northern Ireland as part of the United Kingdom, while the Anglo-Irish Treaty, which established the Irish Free State, was accepted in 1921. In 1922, the Irish Free State, consisting of twenty-six counties was established, while the status of the North was to be agreed upon by the Boundary Commission. Women over twenty-one years of age in the Free State possessed citizenship on equal terms with men; in the United Kingdom (including Northern Ireland), they had to wait until 1928.[8]

The historiography of women in medicine in Ireland

IN THE PERIOD in which this book is set, there were six medical colleges in Ireland open to students wishing to undertake medical studies: Trinity College in Dublin, which had been founded in 1592; the Royal College of Surgeons, founded in 1784; the three non-denominational Queen's Colleges, at Cork, Galway and Belfast, which had been established in 1845 and opened in 1849; and the Catholic University (later University College Dublin), founded in 1851, which opened for lectures in 1854. The medical corporation, the KQCPI (later the Royal College of Physicians of Ireland), founded in 1654, and the Apothecaries' Hall of Ireland (founded in 1791), offered registerable licences to students who had undertaken their medical education elsewhere.[9]

Evidently, there have been important changes relating to medical education in Ireland since women were first admitted to the medical schools in the 1880s. At that point women medical students were viewed as a rare species, with their achievements frequently heralded in the student press and Irish newspapers. By 1898, for example, women made up approximately 0.8 per cent of medical students matriculating at Irish universities. In 2008, 110 years later, 75 per cent of Irish medical students were female, in comparison with 59 per cent of females across the university sector.[10] In August 2009, the Health Professionals Admissions Test (HPat) was introduced to the Irish university medical admissions system. One reason for the introduction of the test, along with attempting to ensure that the most suitable students were being admitted to Irish medical schools, was to restore a balanced gender ratio of medical students at Irish universities.[11] Professor Finucane, head of the graduate entry for the medical school at the University of Limerick commented, 'The pendulum had swung too far in favour of females ... it is important we have a system that doesn't disadvantage males in the way that 40 to 50 years ago it disadvantaged females.'[12] Comments such as this tend to imply that the Irish system of medical education of the early to mid-twentieth century discriminated against women medical students.

Research on the history of women in medicine in Britain has pointed to unfavourable attitudes towards co-education in British medical schools.[13] However, as I will suggest, this was not necessarily the case in Ireland. Not only did Irish medical schools in the late nineteenth and early twentieth centuries adopt a surprisingly liberal attitude towards women's admission to study medicine, but women were treated favourably while they attended these colleges and universities.

This book also sheds important new light on the experiences of medical students, an area within the history of medicine which has often been neglected, in favour of a focus on the stories of men and women in the profession.[14] Keir Waddington has commented that in the historiography of medical education, 'students are largely absent or silent consumers'.[15] However, it is not just historians of medicine who have been guilty of neglecting the history of students. There has been little research into the experiences of students more generally.[16] Histories of Irish medical schools tend to focus on the background to the founding of the schools, the main events in the schools' histories and the historical actors involved in these events.[17] Likewise, the professors of these schools have been considered more worthy of historical attention.[18] Consequently, we know little about the experiences of medical students and graduates of either gender, although there has recently been some literature about the experiences of women medical students and graduates.[19] Such studies have focused on Britain, however, and some tend to over-rely on statistics rather than on a combination of methods as this study does in order to paint a fuller picture of the history of women in medicine.

In addition to its emphasis on student experience, this book contributes to the Irish social history of medicine more generally. Historians of medicine in Ireland have tended to focus on studies of institutions or famous doctors, in the same way that historians of medicine in Britain did prior to the 1980s.[20] This has been at the expense of wider themes within the social history of medicine in Ireland. In 1993, Ludmilla Jordanova claimed that the social history of medicine in Britain had not yet come of age but, rather, was experiencing growing pains.[21] The same words could be applied to the Irish social history of medicine in its current state.

As has been recently pointed out, the most common type of literature in the Irish history of medicine has tended to be histories of institutions, often written by past employees. These types of studies tend to ignore the experiences of the individuals who gained most from the institutions in question (the patients and medical students gaining their experience there). Rather, they tend to focus on the financing, administration and medical staffing of the institution in the form of chronological narratives.[22] Medical biographies of 'great men' represent a large bulk of the scholarship within the Irish history of medicine and have been joined more recently by the occasional 'great woman'.[23] I will avoid employing the techniques of these types of narratives. Instead, I will contribute to the new way of doing the history of medicine in Ireland, through drawing on less commonly used sources to give a deeper insight into the experiences of women medical students and graduates in Ireland in the period.

There have been works on women medical students at the University of Glasgow and, more recently, of medical students, both male and female, at the University of Glasgow and the University of Edinburgh, and these provide useful case studies for comparison with my own research.[24] Additionally, there has been excellent work done on the history of women in medicine in America.[25] However, the topic of women in medicine in Ireland has not been sufficiently engaged with by historians. Other studies of women doctors have taken the form of medical biographies, which, of their nature, are limited in their examination of women doctors more generally.[26] In terms of autobiographical sources relating to Irish women doctors, especially early doctors, we are also limited.[27] There has been little written on the history of women in the medical profession in Ireland.

This monograph is part of a wider scholarly movement which is interested in the history of women in the professions.[28] Certainly, more has been written about the history of women in higher education in Ireland under the umbrella of Irish women's history.[29] Within this field, the Irish higher education system has been represented as being 'discriminatory' and 'only one part of the overall patriarchal organisation of Irish society'.[30] There has also been a great deal of work done on the topic of women and philanthropy, which intersects with my topic of study.[31] In particular, this study contributes to the history of women in the professions.[32] It differs from previous studies, however, because it uses a combination of both statistical and contemporary material in order to give a more thorough picture of the educational and professional experiences of women medical graduates.

Women's admission to the medical profession in Britain and Ireland

THERE IS EVIDENCE to suggest that Ireland possessed a history of women doctors starting as early as the sixteenth century. Elizabeth I granted a charter to the Dublin guild of barber-surgeons in 1572 that allowed them to practise; the charter stated (in translation from the Latin) that she granted the guild leader permission to 'make a Fraternity or Guild of the Art of Barbers of his City of Dublin to be for ever called or named the Fraternity or Guild of Saint Mary Magdalene to consist of themselves and other persons as well Men and Women and to receive and accept of any other persons whatsoever fit and discreet and freely willing to join them as Brothers and Sisters of the Fraternity or Guild aforesaid'.[33] This suggests that both women and men were allowed to join the guild, although we do not know if many women actually worked as barber-surgeons in Dublin in this period. Similarly, women were entitled to hold the licence of midwifery from the KQCPI, with one woman, 'Mistress Cormack', receiving the licence in 1696.[34] Details concerning women in medicine in Ireland in the eighteenth century are even hazier. In England in this period there is evidence of women 'surgeonesses' until 1841, with English census returns for that year showing no woman described as 'surgeon', 'apothecary' or 'physician', although there were 676 midwives and 12,476 nurses listed.[35] A. L. Wyman argues that the fall of the female practitioner was a result of the rise of the apothecary. Moreover, the reorganisation of the medical profession caused by the Medical Act 1858, which also applied to Ireland, resulted in the exclusion of outsiders. The act did not specifically exclude women but with the emphasis now placed on standardisation of medical qualifications from universities, to which women had no access, it effectively prevented women from making it onto the *Medical Register*.[36]

One constant theme throughout the history of the medical profession 'has been the effort to define who is a member and who is not'.[37] The 1858 act attempted to unify the fractured state of the medical profession and standardise medical education while keeping unqualified 'quacks' out of the profession. The act established the General Medical Council of Medical Registration and Education in order to distinguish qualified practitioners from unqualified ones, in addition to implementing the legal rights of the profession.[38] The act stipulated that in order to appear on the newly established *Medical Register*, listing all registered medical practitioners in the United Kingdom, a doctor had to possess a licence or medical degree from one of the nineteen registered bodies in Britain and Ireland. However, it failed to put an end to the rigid divisions within the medical profession; rather, it replaced the old tripartite structure of the profession with a new type of medical hierarchy, of hospital consultants and general practitioners. In the Victorian years, the various divisions within the medical profession and the competition for patients that went along with these resulted in professional bitterness and tension and an increasingly competitive medical marketplace.[39]

It was in this context in 1859 that Elizabeth Blackwell became the first woman to appear on the *Medical Register*. Blackwell, an important activist for women's rights, was born in Bristol, England, and reared and educated in the United States. She famously qualified with an MD degree from Geneva College, New York, in 1849 and founded the New York Infirmary for Indigent Women and Children. She went to London in 1857 to attend Bedford College for Women and had her name entered on the *Medical Register* in 1859 owing to a clause in the Medical Act that recognised doctors who had practised in the United Kingdom prior to 1858.[40] In 1865, Elizabeth Garrett Anderson gained a medical qualification from the Apothecaries' Hall, London, that enabled her to become the second female physician on the *Medical Register*. The Apothecaries' Hall edited its charter afterwards so that no more women could take its licence examinations, putting an end to the potential of registration of medical women in Britain. At this point, women had no means of taking university degrees at institutions in the United Kingdom.

From the late 1860s, Sophia Jex-Blake (Bern and KQCPI, 1877)[41] campaigned for admission to study medicine. The struggle of Jex-Blake and her cohort has been well documented.[42] After persuading the University of Edinburgh to admit her to study medicine in 1869, and later being joined by six other women medical students, Jex-Blake and her female classmates experienced great discrimination from their lecturers, fellow students and townspeople in Edinburgh. In 1870, there was a riot in Edinburgh, started by the male medical students at the university who disagreed with the female presence in their classes. Undeterred by this action, the 'Edinburgh Seven' continued with their education until 1873, when they lost a legal challenge against the university after it had decided that they could not pursue their medical degrees. The women then sought medical degrees abroad, but these degrees were worthless if women were prohibited from registering in Britain. The Medical Act 1858 had prohibited anyone with foreign medical degrees who had qualified prior to 1858 from registering in the United Kingdom (unless they had practised in the UK prior to 1858).

However, Jex-Blake and her cohort were beginning to gain support from politicians such as Russell Gurney, a British MP whose wife Emelia was a campaigner for women's higher education, and William Francis Cowper-Temple. Cowper-Temple, an English politician, attempted to have a bill passed in 1875 to allow women to enrol as students at Scottish universities but this was withdrawn so as to allow the universities concerned to decide what action to take. He then promoted another bill to allow women with foreign medical degrees achieved since 1858 to be registered in the country. The reason for the gendered focus of this bill was presumably because men already had the option of taking university degrees in the United Kingdom, while women did not. The matter was discussed by the General Medical Council (GMC) and was heavily covered in the *British Medical Journal*. The GMC did not come to a firm conclusion on the matter, stating that they 'were not prepared to say that women ought to be excluded from the profession'.[43] Cowper-Temple then withdrew his bill and Gurney promoted his Enabling Bill, which was a better compromise, since it did not insist that women with foreign degrees should be entitled to register but, rather, it gave the nineteen licensing bodies the option, if they so wished, to allow women with these degrees to take their examinations.

The council of the Royal College of Surgeons of England composed a petition against what the *Medical Times and Gazette* termed 'this petty patchwork attempt at legislation', on the grounds that it was narrow in focus, since it was not open to men with foreign degrees and because it questioned whether people with degrees from foreign universities should be 'allowed the privilege' of registering in Britain.[44] In spite of this backlash, on 11 August 1876, the Enabling Act was passed by the British parliament. According to the *Englishwoman's Review*, the act 'was not passed on behalf of the *few* women who wish to obtain medical degrees but on behalf of the *many* women who wish to place themselves under medical advisers of their own sex'.[45] The act 'enabled' all of the nineteen recognised medical examining bodies to accept women candidates but stated that they were not obliged to do so. With the introduction of this act, the Edinburgh cohort was given some hope. In Ireland, the KQCPI decided to allow women who had taken their medical degrees abroad to take its licence examinations from 1877 and the Queen's Colleges and Royal College of Surgeons in Dublin allowed women to take medical degrees from the mid-1880s.

In contrast, British universities were slower to open up their medical classes to women. The University of London opened its examinations to women from 1878 (although there were no graduates until 1882) but it was not joined by other universities until the 1890s. The University of Bristol opened its classes to women in 1891, the University of Glasgow in 1892 and the University of Durham in 1893. The remaining Irish universities, the Catholic University and Trinity College Dublin opened their doors to women in 1898 and 1904, respectively, whereas the final British universities to open their doors to women, Cambridge and Oxford, did so in 1916 and 1917, respectively.[46]

On 10 January 1877, Eliza Louisa Walker Dunbar (Zurich, 1872, KQCPI, 1877) became the first woman to qualify with a medical licence from a medical institution in the United Kingdom under the new Enabling Act. A qualification from the KQCPI allowed doctors to practise medicine but first they would have had to acquire a medical education. Until British or Irish universities admitted women to study medicine, a woman wishing to take the medical licence examinations of the KQCPI had first to prove that she had attained medical education at a foreign university. Dunbar had received private medical tuition from Elizabeth Garrett Anderson and had hoped, like Garrett Anderson, to take the examinations of the Apothecaries' Hall. However, after the Apothecaries' Hall revised its regulations so that women could not be admitted to its examinations, Dunbar went to the University of Zurich to study and was soon followed by two other British women, Louisa Atkins and Frances Hoggan (Table 0.1). Dunbar spent four years in Zurich before

Irish women in medicine

Table 0.1 First ten female licentiates of the King and Queen's College of
Physicians of Ireland

Year	Name	Previous qualification
1877	Eliza Louisa Walker Dunbar	MD Zurich
1877	Louisa Atkins	MD Zurich
1877	Frances Elizabeth Hoggan	MD Zurich
1877	Mary Edith Pechey	MD Bern
1877	Sophia Jex-Blake	MD Bern
1878	Annie Reay Barker	MD Paris
1878	Ann Elizabeth Clark	MD Paris
1878	Agnes McLaren	MD Montpellier
1878	Anna Dahms	MD Paris
1879	Jane Elizabeth Waterson	MD Brussels

Source: Roll of licentiates of the KQCPI.

qualifying with a distinction in her MD degree in 1872; she then undertook
postgraduate study in Vienna, before returning to England. After qualifying
from the KQCPI, she worked at the Bristol Hospital for Sick Children.[47]

As mentioned earlier, the majority of British universities did not open
to women until the 1890s and 1900s, with the exception of the University of
London, which decided to admit women to take medical degrees from 1878.
Thus, there were no graduates from the university until 1882, when Mary
Ann Scharlieb and Edith Shove graduated through the London School of
Medicine for Women.[48] The women who took their medical degrees at the
University of London had trained at this school, which had been established
by Sophia Jex-Blake in 1874, and they attained their practical experience
at the Royal Free Hospital.[49] Despite the opening up of examinations at
the University of London to women, the KQCPI continued to be the most
important institution for licensing women medical practitioners into the
1880s, as Table 0.2 shows. The role of the KQCPI diminished after the 1880s,
with no women qualifying with licences from 1889 to 1895 and only one
woman qualifying between 1896 and 1900. It is likely that this was because
universities, such as the Royal College of Surgeons, were now opening up
their degree examinations to women and women were more likely to have
been aiming at these superior qualifications, rather than the licences.

As is apparent, the KQCPI was very important for the registration of
women doctors in the United Kingdom. This book will investigate the reasons
why the KQCPI opened its examinations to women, the backgrounds and
experiences of women medical students at Irish institutions and the careers
that they went on to have after graduation.

Table 0.2 Comparison of numbers of female
licentiates of the KQCPI with numbers of female
medical graduates from the University of London[a]

Year	KQCPI	London School of Medicine for Women
1877	5	0
1878	4	0
1879	3	0
1880	7	0
1881	5	0
1882	3	2
1883	7	0
1884	6	1
1885	4	0
1886	2	0
1887	1	0
1888	1	2
1889	0	1
1890	0	5
1891	0	6
1892	0	7
1893	0	1
1894	0	8
1895	0	8
1896	1	7
1897	0	9
1898	0	9
1899	0	13
1900	0	14
Total	*49*	*93*

[a] Via the London School of Medicine for Women/Royal Free Hospital.
Source: Graduation lists of KQCPI and LSMW.

Outline of chapters

CHAPTER 1 will set the scene for the following chapters, examining the arguments for and against women in medicine that proliferated in the late nineteenth and early twentieth centuries, arguing that Ireland possessed a generally liberal attitude towards women in higher education which determined its attitude towards women in the medical profession.

Chapter 2 will suggest that the KQCPI decided to admit women for a combination of reasons. It is likely that the KQCPI viewed the admission of women from a financial point of view, in terms of gaining income from their student fees. However, also important is the context of Dublin society in the late nineteenth century, which was open-minded to the issue of women's higher education, as demonstrated by women's admission to the Museum of Irish Industry and the Royal College of Science from the 1850s and 1860s. This chapter will highlight the distinctiveness of Irish medical education and the Irish context in a period when attitudes towards women in Britain were often hostile and attempts made by women to gain admission to university to study medicine were frequently hindered.

Chapter 3 examines the women who decided to matriculate in medicine in the period 1885–1922. It is largely based on the statistical work I have conducted on women who matriculated in medicine in that period. Other sources used include student guides from the period and contemporary articles from newspapers and medical journals. It will reveal that women medical students tended to come from well-to-do backgrounds and tended to attend the university closest to them, for financial reasons, although their choice of university also hinged on their religious beliefs and on which universities were open to women at the time. I will also discuss the reasons why women (and men) decided to take up medicine in the late nineteenth and early twentieth centuries, and demonstrate that women students took up medicine as a result of personal experience, a sense of vocation and encouragement from their secondary schools.

Chapter 4 continues themes raised in Chapter 2 regarding the apparently egalitarian system of medical education that existed in Ireland in the period. I argue that the authorities of Irish medical schools and hospitals possessed a distinctive attitude towards their women medical students, with women and men being educated together for all subjects, with the exception of anatomy. Women students were nonetheless often identified as a cohort separate from the men, as is particularly evident in the student magazines, where they were figures of fun. In order to reconcile this sense of 'separateness', Irish women medical students established their own unique identity through their social activities and living arrangements. I also examine how Irish hospitals displayed a largely positive and welcoming attitude towards women medical students, in contrast to hospitals in London, where women were debarred from admission for the most part.

Chapter 5 examines the careers of the 452 women medical students who succeeded in qualifying during the study period. It reveals that women did not simply enter the fields that were promoted as suitable for them (as outlined in Chapter 1, these included, for example, women and children's health and the missionary field), but were more likely to work in general hospitals and public health, areas that were typically seen as male-dominated. The chapter also suggests that the sense of separateness that existed between male and female medical students during their medical education, as outlined in Chapter 4, did not necessarily continue after graduation.

Chapter 6 then discusses whether the First World War, which is claimed to have had a huge impact on women's career opportunities more generally, had an effect on the careers of Irish women medical graduates.

Chapter 7 explores how the issues raised in Chapters 4 and 5 played out in the lives of five particular individuals, Emily Winifred Dickson (RCSI, 1891), Emma Crooks (QCB, 1899), Lily Baker (TCD, 1906), Mary McGivern (UCD, 1925) and Jane D. Fulton (TCD, 1925), in order to add a personal dimension to the statistics presented in Chapters 2 and 3. These case studies demonstrate the importance of the personal story, which is sometimes lost in traditional social histories of medicine, yet rather than being traditional narratives of 'great men' and 'great women', they are narratives of ordinary women who trained at Irish institutions in the period and which demonstrate the themes considered in previous chapters.

Chapter 8 will sum up the main findings and conclusions of the book in addition to pointing to avenues for future research.

Methodology

THE ARCHIVAL MATERIAL for Chapter 3 is the databases I have compiled of women matriculating at Irish institutions between the years 1885, when Irish institutions first started admitting female medical students, and 1922, with the establishment of the Irish Free State. One database relates to women who matriculated as medical students at Irish institutions, while the other relates to the women who succeeded in graduating, upon which the 'Biographical index' at the end of the book is based. That index gives for the women medical students who graduated from Irish institutions: the dates of birth and death; geographical, family and religious background; and details of their university education and subsequent career.

I derived my information relating to students' backgrounds from the matriculation albums for the three Queen's Colleges. The registers for the other colleges were unavailable so I have relied on the *Medical Students' Register* (published annually by the General Medical Council, which gives details of students matriculating each year at British and Irish universities) for basic details of students matriculating at the Royal College of Surgeons, Royal College of Science, Catholic University/University College Dublin and Trinity College Dublin. However, it is possible that not all students matriculating at these universities were listed in the *Register*, in which case they are not included in the database. (Women graduates who were discovered by chance in the

General Medical Council's annual *Medical Directory* but who were not listed in the *Medical Students' Register* have been listed in the 'Biographical index'.) This database therefore represents an almost complete record of women who matriculated in medicine at Irish institutions. The matriculation albums of the Queen's Colleges give each student's name, age, birthplace, father's name and, in some cases, father's occupation and the student's religion, while the *Students' Register* simply gives a name and year of matriculation. In the cases of students about whom there was limited detail in the matriculation albums or whose details were found in the *Students' Register*, additional informa-tion could sometimes be gleaned through the matriculation records of the National University of Ireland and the 1911 Irish census.

After graduation, doctors listed their address and post (if any) in the *Medical Directory*. I created a database of women who were successful in graduating and whose careers I then traced through the *Medical Directory*. Tables of data throughout Chapters 5 and 6 illustrate the main points regarding women doctors' careers. The data are based on my own research into the careers of women medical graduates from Irish institutions.[50] Through tracing the careers of these women using the *Medical Directory* to find their entries for five, ten, fifteen, twenty-five and thirty-five years after graduation, it is possible to give a rough map of the careers of these women graduates. Cohort studies, such as this one, enable historians 'to set individual narratives against the experiences of a wider group of contemporaries'.[51] Through doing this, I aimed to give a general picture of the experiences of women graduates from Irish institutions in the period. The limitation of this method is that, occasionally, personal stories can be lost through a reliance on statistics. However, I have attempted to remedy this where possible through the use of obituaries, memoirs, student guides and contemporary articles from news-papers and medical journals. Additionally, Chapter 7 gives a personal insight into the lives of several women doctors through the use of case studies.

It should be pointed out that there are tables in Chapter 5 and Chapter 6 with percentages produced for samples totalling less than 100 women, but this is unavoidable, given the low numbers of women matriculating and graduating. However, the information still remains suggestive but should not be taken as statistically perfect.

Overview

THIS book is important because, up until now, there had been no compre-hensive study of women in the medical profession in Ireland. It portrays Irish medical schools as being liberal-minded with regard to the admission of women to the medical profession. Moreover, it suggests that women were treated fairly by Irish institutions during their time in medical education. The book thus broadens our understanding of women in the medical profession in Ireland and of women's experiences at university more generally.

Importantly, I will highlight the distinctiveness of Irish medical education and suggest that there were important differences between Ireland and Britain: most significant were that Ireland, and in particular Dublin, was seemingly more liberal than Britain with regard to attitudes towards women's medical education and that the Irish system of medical education appears to have been very much inclusive and paternalistic towards women students. At the same time, despite this, women medical students, in common with their British and American sisters, were certainly seen as a separate cohort from the men, with a distinctive social identity, which was crafted both by them and for them.

Pertinently, this is also a study of women's careers within the medical profession in Britain and Ireland. It demonstrates that women doctors did not necessarily enter the careers that had been prescribed for them by advocates of women's medical education in the nineteenth century. In addition, it highlights patterns of migration of women doctors between Britain and Ireland as well as illuminating differences in career trends between the two countries.

Most importantly, the book will change the way we consider the history of women in medicine in Ireland. Previously, women's entry to Irish higher education and the admission of women to medical education had been depicted as a 'struggle' against male patriarchy and a battle against a hostile Irish medical profession. This is in keeping with the historiography of women in higher education in Britain.[52] I will argue against these ideas, suggesting that there existed in Ireland a liberal medical profession in the late nineteenth century which was supportive of women's admission to medicine, and that, in their educational experiences and subsequent careers, women doctors in Ireland were treated fairly and did not experience the same separatism as their counterparts in Britain.

Notes

1 Typed memoirs of Emily Winifred Dickson, private collection of Niall Martin, Edinburgh.
2 F. O. C. Meenan, *Cecilia Street: The Catholic University School of Medicine, 1855–1931* (Dublin: Gill and Macmillan, 1987), p. 81.
3 Irene Finn, 'Women in the medical profession in Ireland, 1876–1919', in Bernadette Whelan (ed.), *Women and Paid Work in Ireland, 1500–1930* (Dublin: Four Courts Press, 2000), pp. 102–19.
4 The other two women doctors, Elizabeth Blackwell and Elizabeth Garrett Anderson, qualified in 1859 and 1865 respectively through the Apothecaries' Hall, London.

5 Caitriona Clear, *Social Change and Everyday Life in Ireland, 1850–1922* (Manchester: Manchester University Press, 2007), p. x.

6 *Ibid.*, p. xi.

7 *Ibid.*, p. xi.

8 *Ibid.*, p. xii.

9 The records of the Apothecaries' Hall were unavailable for consultation at the time of research for this book. They have recently been catalogued by the Royal College of Physicians. Only six women graduated with licences from the Apothecaries' Hall between 1885 and 1922. These were Sarah Louisa Glynn (1899), Alice M. Barry (1906), Alice Mabel Headwards (1910), Marion Louise Bath(s) (1910), Mary E. M. Logan (1913) and Mary Katherine Helena Neary (1918). (Register of licentiates of Apothecaries' Hall, AH/5/5/1/1 and AH/5/5/1/4, Royal College of Physicians Archives, Dublin. With thanks to Harriet Wheelock for kindly finding this information for me.) Glynn and Logan also graduated through other institutions and have been included in the statistics in this book but the others have not.

10 'New gender ratio for medicine defended', *Irish Times*, 21 August 2009.

11 'Welcome for more men doing medicine', *Irish Times*, 18 August 2009.

12 *Ibid.*

13 Thomas Neville Bonner, *To the Ends of the Earth: Women's Search for Education in Medicine* (Cambridge, MA: Harvard University Press, 1992), pp. 120–37.

14 See Thomas Neville Bonner, *Becoming a Physician: Medical Education in Britain, France, Germany and the United States, 1750–1945* (Oxford: Oxford University Press, 1996) for an overview of the history of medical education in Britain, France, Germany and the United States.

15 Keir Waddington, 'Mayhem and medical students: image, conduct and control in the Victorian and Edwardian London teaching hospital', *Social History of Medicine*, 15:1 (2002), pp. 45–64, on p. 45.

16 Anne Macdona, *From Newman to New Woman: The Women of UCD Remember* (Dublin: New Island, 2001); Carol Dyhouse, *Students: A Gendered History* (London: Routledge, 2006).

17 For example: on Queen's College Cork, Denis J. O'Sullivan, *The Cork School of Medicine: A History* (Cork: UCC Medical Alumni Association, University College Cork, 2007) and Ronan O'Rahilly, *A History of the Cork Medical School, 1849–1949* (Cork: Cork University Press, 1949); on Queen's College Galway, James Murray, *Galway: A Medico-Social History* (Galway: Kenny's Bookshop and Art Gallery, 1994); on Queen's College Belfast, Peter Froggatt, 'The distinctiveness of Belfast medicine and its medical school', *Ulster Medical Journal*, 54:2 (1985), pp. 89–108; on the Royal College of Surgeons, J. B. Lyons, *The Irresistible Rise of the RCSI* (Dublin: Royal College of Surgeons, 1984), Eoin O'Brien, *The Royal College of Surgeons in Ireland: 1784–1984* (Dublin: Eason, 1984), J. D. H. Widdess, *The Royal College of Surgeons in Ireland and Its Medical School* (Edinburgh: E. and S. Livingstone, 1967) and Charles A. Cameron, *History of the Royal College of Surgeons in Ireland and of the Irish Schools of Medicine, Including Numerous Biographical Sketches; Also a Medical Bibliography* (Dublin: Fannin, 1886); on the Royal College of Physicians, J. D. H. Widdess, *A History of the Royal College of Physicians of Ireland, 1654–1963* (Edinburgh: E. and S. Livingstone, 1964); on Trinity College Dublin, T. P. C. Kirkpatrick, *History of the Medical Teaching in Trinity College Dublin and of the School of Physic in Ireland* (Dublin: Hanna and Neale, 1912); and on the Catholic University, Meenan, *Cecilia Street*.

18 For example, Ronan O'Rahilly, *Benjamin Alcock: The First Professor of Anatomy and Physiology in Queen's College Cork* (Cork: Cork University Press, 1948).

19 Barbara Brookes, 'A corresponding community: Dr. Agnes Bennett and her friends from the Edinburgh Medical College for Women of the 1890s', *Medical History*, 52:2 (2008), pp. 237–56; C. Dyhouse, 'Driving ambitions: women in pursuit of a medical

education, 1890–1939', in *Students*, pp. 60–78; J. S. Garner, 'The great experiment: the admission of women students to St Mary's Hospital Medical School, 1916–1925', *Medical History*, 42:1 (1998), pp. 68–88.

20 For histories of institutions, see: Aidan Collins, *St Vincent's Hospital, Fairview: Celebrating 150 Years of Service* (Dublin: Albertine Kennedy Publishing, 2007); T. M. Healy, *From Sanatorium to Hospital: A Social and Medical Account of Peamount 1912–1997* (Dublin: A. and A. Farmar, 2002); F. O. C. Meenan, *St Vincent's Hospital, 1834–1994: An Historical and Social Portrait* (Dublin: Gill and MacMillan, 1994); J. B. Lyons, *The Quality of Mercer's: The Story of Mercer's Hospital, 1734–1991* (Dublin: Glendale, 1991); Elizabeth Malcolm, *Swift's Hospital: A History of St Patrick's Hospital, Dublin, 1746–1989* (Dublin: Gill and Macmillan, 1989); Hanora M. Henry, *Our Lady's Hospital, Cork: History of the Mental Hospital Spanning 200 Years* (Cork: Haven Books, 1989). For histories of great men, see: Davis Coakley, *Irish Masters of Medicine* (Dublin: Town House, 1992); Davis Coakley, *The Irish School of Medicine: Outstanding Practitioners of the 19th Century* (Dublin: Town House, 1988); T. G. Wilson, *Victorian Doctor: Being the Life of William Wilde* (London: Methuen, 1946).

21 Ludmilla Jordanova, 'Has the social history of medicine come of age?', *Historical Journal*, 36:2 (1993), pp. 437–49, on p. 448.

22 Greta Jones and Elizabeth Malcolm, 'Introduction: an anatomy of Irish medical history', in Greta Jones and Elizabeth Malcolm (eds), *Medicine, Disease and the State in Ireland, 1650–1940* (Cork: Cork University Press, 1999), p. 1.

23 Coakley, *Irish Masters of Medicine*, is typical of this genre: it consists of forty biographies of Irish medical men with the purpose of highlighting the 'achievements of Irish doctors who have enhanced the knowledge and practice of medicine on an international level' (p. 5). Notably, Coakley excludes famous Irish women doctors from his study. A more recent example is Margaret Ó hÓgartaigh, *Kathleen Lynn: Irishwoman, Patriot, Doctor* (Dublin: Irish Academic Press, 2006).

24 Wendy Alexander, *First Ladies of Medicine: The Origins, Education and Destination of Early Women Medical Graduates of Glasgow University* (Glasgow: Wellcome Unit for the History of Medicine, 1988). And, more recently, Anne Crowther and Marguerite Dupree, *Medical Lives in the Age of Surgical Revolution* (Cambridge: Cambridge University Press, 2007).

25 Regina Markell Morantz-Sanchez, *Conduct Unbecoming a Woman: Medicine on Trial in Turn-of-the-Century Brooklyn* (Oxford: Oxford University Press, 2000) and *Sympathy and Science: Women Physicians in American Medicine* (Chapel Hill, NC: University of North Carolina Press, 1985); Ellen S. More, *Restoring the Balance: Women Physicians and the Practice of Medicine, 1850–1995* (Cambridge, MA: Harvard University Press, 1999).

26 Ó hÓgartaigh, *Kathleen Lynn*; John Cowell, *A Noontide Blazing. Brigid Lyons Thornton: Rebel, Soldier, Doctor* (Dublin: Currach Press, 2005); Irene Finn, 'From case-study to life: Mary Strangman (1872–1943)', in Mary Clancy, Caitriona Clear and Triona Nic Giolla Choille (eds), *Women's Studies Review Vol. 7: Oral History and Biography* (Galway: Women's Studies Centre, NUI Galway, 2000), pp. 81–98; Irene Finn, 'Councillor Mary Strangman and the "health of the city", 1912–20', *Decies: Journal of the Waterford Archaeological and Historical Society*, 56 (2000), pp. 189–203.

27 Joyce Delaney, who qualified in 1949, has written a lively account of her experiences as a medical student and woman doctor in England: *No Starch in My Coat: An Irish Doctor's Progress* (London: P. Davies, 1971). Sidney Croskery, an Irish woman who trained at the University of Edinburgh in the early twentieth century, has also written an autobiography, *Whilst I Remember* (Belfast: Blackstaff Press, 1983). More common, unsurprisingly, are memoirs of male Irish doctors, such as: J. Dowling, *An Irish Doctor Remembers* (Dublin: Clonmore and Reynolds, 1955); Patrick Heffernan, *An Irish Doctor's Memories* (Dublin: Clonmore and Reynolds, 1958); Charles Stewart Parnell

Hamilton, *East, West: An Irish Doctor's Memories* (London: Christopher Johnson, 1955); James Mullin, *The Story of a Toiler's Life* (Dublin: Maunsel and Roberts, 1921); Thomas Garry, *African Doctor* (London: John Gifford, 1939); Bethel Solomons, *One Doctor in His Time* (London: Christopher Johnson, 1956).

28 Bernadette Whelan (ed.), *Women and Work in Ireland, 1500–1930* (Dublin: Four Courts Press, 2000). There has been recent interest in the roles of Irish women in medicine and science. See, for example: Mary Mulvihill (ed.), *Lab Coats and Lace: The Lives and Legacies of Inspiring Irish Women Scientists and Pioneers* (Dublin: Women in Technology and Science, 2009); Mary Cullen (ed.), *Stars, Shells and Bluebells: Women Scientists and Pioneers* (Dublin: Women in Technology and Science, 1997). In contrast, for a history of the shift in Irish women's working roles in the rural economy, see Joanna Bourke, *Husbandry to Housewifery: Women, Economic Change and Housework in Ireland, 1890–1914* (Wotton-under-Edge: Clarendon Press, 1993).

29 See: Judith Harford, *The Opening of University Education to Women in Ireland* (Dublin: Irish Academic Press, 2008) and 'The movement for the higher education of women in Ireland: gender equality or denominational rivalry?', *History of Education*, 34:5 (2005), pp. 497–516; Gillian McClelland, *Pioneering Women: Riddel Hall and Queen's University Belfast* (Belfast: Ulster Historical Foundation, 2005); Susan M. Parkes, *A Danger to the Men: A History of Women in Trinity College Dublin, 1904–2004* (Dublin: Lilliput Press, 2004); Eileen Breathnach, 'Women and higher education in Ireland (1879–1914)', *Crane Bag*, 4:1 (1980), pp. 47–54. The history of the national and secondary school education of Irish girls has also been well documented: Deirdre Raftery, *Female Education in Ireland 1700–1900: Minerva or Madonna* (Dublin: Irish Academic Press, 2007); Mary Cullen (ed.), *Girls Don't Do Honours: Irish Women in Education in the 19th and 20th Centuries* (Dublin: Women's Education Bureau, 1987); Alison Jordan, *Margaret Byers: A Pioneer of Women's Education and Founder of Victoria College, Belfast* (Belfast: Institute of Irish Studies, Queen's University Belfast, 1987).

30 Mary Cullen, 'Introduction', in Cullen (ed.), *Girls Don't Do Honours*, p. 2.

31 Oonagh Walsh, *Anglican Women in Dublin: Philanthropy, Politics and Education in the Early Twentieth Century* (Dublin: University College Dublin Press, 2005); Maria Luddy, *Women and Philanthropy in Nineteenth-Century Ireland* (Cambridge: Cambridge University Press, 1995). For Irish women in the missionary field, see Myrtle Hill, 'Gender, culture and the "spiritual empire": the Irish Protestant female missionary experience', *Women's History Review*, 16:2 (2007), pp. 203–26.

32 See Whelan (ed.), *Women and Paid Work in Ireland.*

33 Cameron, *History of the Royal College of Surgeons in Ireland*, pp. 60–1.

34 *Ibid.*, p. 100.

35 A. L. Wyman, 'The surgeoness: the female practitioner of surgery, 1400–1800', *Medical History*, 28:1 (1984), pp. 22–41, on p. 39.

36 *Ibid.*, p. 41.

37 Toby Gelfand, 'The history of the medical profession', in Roy Porter and W. F. Bynum (eds), *Companion Encyclopedia of the History of Medicine* (London: Routledge, 1993), vol. 2, pp. 1119–50, on p. 1119. For texts on the history of the British medical profession, see: Anne Digby, *Making a Medical Living: Doctors and Patients in the English Market for Medicine, 1720–1911* (Cambridge: Cambridge University Press, 1994); Irvine Loudon, *Medical Care and the General Practitioner, 1750–1850* (Oxford: Oxford University Press, 1986); Jose Parry and Noel Parry, *The Rise of the Medical Profession: A Study of Collective Social Mobility* (London: Croom Helm, 1976); M. Jeanne Peterson, *The Medical Profession in Mid-Victorian London* (Berkeley, CA: University of California Press, 1978).

38 Mark Weatherall, 'Making medicine scientific: empiricism, rationality and quackery in mid-Victorian Britain', *Social History of Medicine*, 9:2 (1996), pp. 175–94, on p. 176.

39 See Peterson, *The Medical Profession*, and Digby, *Making a Medical Living*.

40 M. A. Elston, 'Elizabeth Blackwell', in L. Goldman (ed.), *The Oxford Dictionary of Biography* (online resource, 2010) (henceforth *ODNB*).

41 For women doctors mentioned in this book, I will list in parentheses their graduation date and the institution (see list of abbreviations, p. xv) from which they received their qualification. So, in the case of Sophia Jex-Blake, we know that she received her qualifications from the University of Bern and the KQCPI in 1877.

42 The story of the 'Edinburgh Seven' has been discussed recently by Anne Crowther and Marguerite Dupree, 'Jex-Blake's women: education and careers', in Crowther and Dupree (eds), *Medical Lives*, pp. 152–75. For Sophia Jex-Blake, see S. Roberts, *Sophia Jex-Blake: A Woman Pioneer in Nineteenth Century Medical Reform* (London: Routledge, 1993).

43 Annis Gillie, 'Elizabeth Blackwell and the "Medical Register" from 1858', *British Medical Journal* (henceforth *BMJ*), 22 November 1958, pp. 1253–7, on p. 1256.

44 'Bill for the registration of foreign medical degrees held by women', *Medical Times and Gazette*, 24 April 1875, p. 446.

45 'Women doctors', *Englishwoman's Review*, 15 June 1877, p. 276.

46 Women were first admitted to study medicine at the other main British universities in the following years: 1894, Welsh National School of Medicine, University of Edinburgh; 1895, University of Aberdeen; 1898, University of St Andrews; 1899, University of Manchester; 1900, University of Birmingham; 1903, University of Liverpool; 1908, University of Sheffield; 1911, University of Leeds (see Medical Women's Federation Archives, Wellcome Library, SA/MWF/C.10). The majority of British hospitals opened to women medical students only during the years of the First World War and then many of these were closed to women after the war and remained closed until the 1940s. This will be discussed further in Chapter 4.

47 M. A. Elston, 'Eliza Louisa Walker Dunbar', *ODNB*.

48 List of graduates of the University of London at www.shl.lon.ac.uk/specialcollections/archives/studentrecords.shtml. With thanks to Richard Temple, archivist at Senate House Library, University of London.

49 Negley Harte, *The University of London 1836–1986* (London: Athlone Press, 1986), p. 128.

50 The technique used is modelled on the work of Crowther and Dupree, who traced the careers of medical graduates from the Universities of Glasgow and Edinburgh in the nineteenth century using the *Medical Directory*. See Crowther and Dupree, *Medical Lives*.

51 *Ibid.*, p. 372.

52 Jane McDermid, 'Women and education', in June Purvis (ed.), *Women's History: Britain, 1850–1945* (London: Routledge, 1995), pp. 107–30, on p. 113.

1

Debates surrounding women's admission to the medical profession

Let British degrees continue to be of perfectly definite value; make the conditions as stringent as you please, but let them be such as are attainable by all students, and are clearly understood by the general public; and then, for all that would worthily win and wear the desired honours, 'a fair field and no favour'. Is there not one of the English, Scotch or Irish Universities that will win future laurels by now taking the lead generously, and announcing its willingness to cease, at last, its policy of arbitrary exclusion?

Sophia Jex-Blake, 1872[1]

WRITING IN 1872, Sophia Jex-Blake pleaded for a British university to open its doors to women medical students and allow them to qualify alongside men. Jex-Blake, a leading British campaigner for women's admission to the medical profession, had by this time been attempting to gain access to medical education for ten years. After a visit to America in 1862, where she worked at the New England Hospital for Women and Children in Boston and was inspired by Lucy Sewell, one of America's pioneer female physicians, Jex-Blake applied to study medicine at Harvard in 1867 but was rejected. She returned home to Britain and was accepted, along with six other women, to study medicine at the University of Edinburgh in 1869. As is well known, Jex-Blake and her cohort experienced great difficulties while at Edinburgh, from both their lecturers and their fellow students, and in 1873 were told that they would be unable to qualify with medical degrees from the institution.

The *Irish Times* reported in June 1874 that 'it was an unfortunate day for Edinburgh when that band of would-be "lady doctors" knocked at the College gates for admission'. The writer of the article spoke strongly against the admission of women to study medicine, arguing that undergraduates were unruly enough but that a 'University filled with females who would call names if they did not pass [this being a jibe at one of the Edinburgh cohort who claimed she was treated unfairly by the University of Edinburgh], is a consummation devoutly to be deprecated'.[2] Jex-Blake went on to found the London School of Medicine for Women in 1874 while still campaigning for women to be entitled to qualify as doctors in Britain.

Meanwhile, as we saw in the Introduction, two politicians, Russell Gurney and William Francis Cowper-Temple, supported women's admission to medical schools. In 1876, Gurney's Enabling Act was passed by the British parliament. It 'enabled' all of the nineteen recognised medical examining bodies to accept women candidates but stated that they were not obliged to do so. In 1877, Jex-Blake attained the degree of MD from the University of Bern, which, along with certain other European universities, appears to have been more liberal towards the admission of women than those in Britain. The University of Zurich, for example, admitted women to its medical classes from 1864.[3] Similarly, at the University of Bern the subject of women's admission received wide support from the faculty and educational officials in the 1870s.[4] Russian, American and British women students flocked to these two universities, as well as those at Geneva and Paris, for medical training.[5]

In the same year that Jex-Blake graduated from Bern, the King and Queen's College of Physicians in Dublin allowed women to take its licence examinations, becoming the first institution in the United Kingdom to allow women to do so, and thus offering women a means of qualifying as registered medical practitioners. Jex-Blake called this event 'the turning point in the whole struggle'.[6] Eliza Louisa Walker Dunbar (KQCPI, 1877) became the first female licentiate of an institution in the United Kingdom following the Enabling Act, with Jex-Blake and her cohort following soon after. In the decade after this, the doors of Irish medical schools were formally opened to women, to allow them to receive medical education in addition to qualifying alongside the men. Despite this, the role of Ireland within the history of women in medicine and the admission of women to the medical profession has tended to be excluded or often briefly passed over in histories of the subject. It is evident, however, that Ireland played an important role in the rise of the female medical practitioner in the late nineteenth century.

Arguments in favour of and against women's admission to the medical profession

THERE were several arguments put forward by members of the medical profession against women in medicine. The *British Medical Journal* in 1870 contended that the medical profession was already well supplied in its numbers and that the introduction of women surgeons might displace an equal number of men surgeons.[7] Yet, just a few months earlier, the *Irish Times* had supported the establishment of a medical class for women at any of the Dublin hospitals, especially considering that there were enough hospitals to permit one of them to allow for the instruction of female students. The newspaper admitted doubt as to 'whether there is in Ireland a considerable demand for lady doctors' but noted that 'it seems there is a demand in other places, and there can be no objection to us supplying the necessary professional instruction in a Dublin school. We commend the subject to the attention of the heads and professors of our existing schools.'[8] Nonetheless, more common were articles such as one in 1876 which claimed that the 'wholesale irruption of fascinating lady doctors' would result in 'ruinous competition' for medical practitioners and, concerning lady doctors with foreign qualifications, the writer stated that 'we should tremble to find ourselves in the hands of lady-physicians coming from those districts of the Union where female suffrage reigns supreme'.[9]

Of course, it was not simply a case of male doctors wishing to have a monopoly over the medical marketplace. Medicine was not seen as a proper career for a woman at this time and, considering the Victorian expectation that women should be dutiful wives and mothers, there was great opposition to the entry of women to higher education generally, although especially to professions such as medicine. Charles West, for example, commented in 1876 that 'the special duties of her sex, which can be devolved on no one else, must be left undone or done slightingly by almost every woman who undertakes medicine as a profession and who attains any reasonable success in its pursuit'.[10] Another common argument against women's admission to medical education was that the study of medicine specifically might endanger a woman physically and mentally.[11]

Arguments against women in medicine were based on Victorian beliefs about women's physical, mental and emotional natures, which were rooted in the physiological theories of the late nineteenth century. Medical practitioners, particularly specialists in gynaecology and obstetrics, who were beginning to notice competition from female doctors in these areas, were instrumental in the attack on the women's higher education movement in nineteenth-century Britain.[12] Menstruation was commonly cited as a barrier to women who wished to undertake higher education. The process of menstruation began to be referred to as a curse rather than as a natural process, as may be seen in the words of James McGrigor Allan, a nineteenth-century opponent of women's suffrage. Writing in 1869 against women in education, he claimed that the 'eternal distinction in the physical organisation of the sexes' meant that the average man was the mental superior of the average woman. He argued:

In intellectual labour, man has surpassed, does now, and always will surpass woman, for the obvious reason that nature does not periodically interrupt his thought and application.[13]

Most notably, Henry Maudsley, the British psychiatrist, argued that women were unable to partake in higher education as a result of menstruation.[14] The *Dublin Medical Press*[15] argued against this notion in 1875, in response to the publication of Maudsley's work:

Education of women, in short, like education of men, should be directed towards cultivating the brain and the muscles equally; and if this golden rule of hygiene be observed, we cannot see why women are to be kept in ignorance or how it will in any way benefit posterity to keep one half of the race in the dark upon all the deepest questions which most interest our happiness.[16]

Evidently, the writer of this article for the *Dublin Medical Press* held a more egalitarian view of the admission of women to study medicine, believing that it would negatively affect the progression of the human race to exclude one sex from education. Similar debates were taking place in America at this time. Dr Edward Clarke's publication *Sex in Education; or, A Fair Chance for the Girls* (1873) questioned whether there was a role for women in the professions. Clarke argued that menstrual functions and co-education were incompatible for American girls, with too much education and mental exertion threatening their physical development, especially when this was undertaken during menstruation.[17] In her 1877 paper 'The question of rest for women during menstruation' Mary Putnam Jacobi (Female College of Pennsylvania, 1864), an American physician, argued against Clarke's notions that menstruation made a role for women in the medical profession impossible. Jacobi suggested that menstruation and education were compatible and used both statistical analysis and experimental methods to back up her arguments. Her essay, submitted anonymously, won the Boylston Prize at Harvard University.[18]

We may gain further insight into contemporary attitudes towards women in medicine from a letter entitled 'A lady on lady doctors' which appeared in the *Lancet* in 1870. The writer used the pen-name 'Mater' but it is unclear whether the author was actually female. Mater's letter opens by arguing that 'No woman, in any dangerous crisis calling for calm nerve and prompt action, would trust her self in the hands of a woman'.[19] The idea that women doctors did not possess the 'calm nerve' required in times of crisis was a common argument put forward by those against women in medicine at the time. It was bound up in Victorian ideology that men were more rational-thinking and sensible than women, who were traditionally viewed as being flighty, hysterical and irrational.[20] Women's very physical natures were also attacked, with Mater arguing that, physically, women were not fit to be doctors because they were lacking 'the coolness and strength of nerves' required of a doctor. Mater also remarked that 'the constitutional variations of the female system, at the best are uncertain and not to be relied upon'.[21] Likewise, in October 1873, an article in the *Irish Times* commented on the unsuitability of women for the medical profession on account of their lack of 'firmness, promptness of decision, and muscular strength'. As well as these flaws, the writer argued that women patients would not have confidence in women doctors.[22]

These views were not representative of all members of the public. For supporters of women in the medical profession, it was women's very natures that made them most suitable to work as doctors. Advocates claimed that there was a definite need for women doctors to treat women patients. In 1869, an article in the *Irish Times* made the point that 'if women prefer to be attended by women, it is only fair that they should have their choice'.[23] Likewise, Thomas Haslam wrote to the *Freeman's Journal* in 1871 making a similar case for the medical education of women. Haslam, who, along with his wife, Anna, would found the Dublin Women's Suffrage Association in 1876, argued that women were most suitable for a career in the medical profession because of their 'intense natural sympathy with children'. He claimed that women would be 'peculiarly qualified for the successful treatment of the diseases of childhood, provided only they receive the necessary training, and that therefore their devotion to this branch of the medical profession would be an unqualified boon to humanity'. Haslam also felt that women were much better qualified than men to treat patients of their own sex:

> It is a melancholy fact that sensitive women often lose their health, sometimes even their lives, through an invincible repugnance to confide their ailments to a male physician, and that many valuable lives might be saved to the community if such persons had had skilled practitioners of their own sex to whom they could speak without a breach of their instinctive delicacy.[24]

This was a key argument put forward by those promoting the medical education of women. The Editor, 'F.J.', responded by stating that 'he [Haslam] advances nothing to which we have the least objection' but commented that there existed the issue of the dissecting room and argued that perhaps women should be educated separately from men for anatomy classes.[25] Indeed, the separation of women and men for anatomy classes would be an issue for Irish medical schools, as will be discussed in Chapter 4.

Sophia Jex-Blake, who was arguably the most vocal authority on the medical education of women in the period, argued that women's emotional natures in fact made them very suited to the medical profession. She stated, 'Women have more love of medical work, and are naturally more inclined, and more fitted for it than most men'.[26] Jex-Blake insisted that there was a 'very widespread desire ... among women for the services of doctors of their own sex'.[27] Such arguments continued into the early twentieth century. In 1903, Ethel Lamport, an English female doctor who trained at the London School of Medicine for Women in the 1890s, declared that women were entitled to be treated by a female physician if they so desired.[28] In Ireland, when the Munster branch of the Irish Association of Women Graduates and Candidate Graduates wrote to the Victoria Hospital for Diseases of Women and Children in Cork requesting that a female doctor be appointed to the hospital's staff, they argued that often women patients preferred to be treated by female physicians.[29]

It was claimed, too, that women patients found it easier to tell their problems to a female doctor. Teresa Billington-Greig (1877–1964), a suffragette who established the Women's Freedom League, commented on the fact that women doctors were better qualified to treat women because they could empathise with problems specific to women.[30] As well as this, she argued that it was much easier for a woman to talk about all of her medical problems to a female doctor rather than to a male one and that, in many cases, women refrained from seeing their male doctor because of the dread they had of the consultation and examination involved.[31] Jex-Blake cited the example of the Boston Hospital for Women and Children, where there were women doctors on the staff and where she worked as a student at its dispensary. She stated that there had been several occasions when she had heard women patients from the lower classes stating their relief at being able to tell their problems to a lady doctor.[32]

However, despite claims that women's gender made them considerably more sympathetic as doctors, opponents tended to argue that the feminine brain was less suited to the study of medicine than its male counterpart.[33] The *British Medical Journal* in 1870 questioned whether the female mind was intelligent enough for medical study.[34] Those arguing against women in medicine implied that women were morally unsuited to careers in the medical profession. Mater, for example, argued that, morally, women were unfit to be doctors because 'they cannot (even the best of them) hold their tongues'.[35] An essential part of medical practice in the nineteenth century was medical confidentiality, which refers to the duty of doctors, as bound by the Hippocratic Oath, to keep secret or confidential any information which their patients might dictate while in their care. The Hippocratic Oath laid the foundations of the medical profession as 'a morally self-regulating discipline'.[36] Through the claim that women would be incapable of upholding this confidentiality, the author reinforced age-old stereotypes of women as chatty gossips, unable to keep secrets and, thus, the idea that they were unfit to become members of the medical profession.

Certain members of the Irish medical profession appear to have disagreed with these views. A Dr Stewart, secretary of the Irish Medical Schools and Graduates Association, for example, claimed in 1892 that his organisation had been the first to admit lady members and that he felt, from his experience, that the British Medical Association would benefit from the introduction of ladies.[37] Likewise, four years earlier, the *Freeman's Journal* reported on Dr Thomas More Madden's address at the annual meeting of the British Medical Association in Glasgow. More Madden, an Irishman, was president of the Obstetrics Section of the British Medical Association at the time and supported the admission of women to the medical profession, particularly their admission to the specialty of obstetrics. More Madden is quoted as having said:

> I cannot agree with those who are opposed to the admission of women into the practice of our department of medico-chirurgical science for which their sex should apparently render them so especially adapted. I can see no valid reason why any well qualified practitioner, male or female, should not be welcomed amongst us. Nor if there are any women who prefer the medical attendance of their own sex, does it seem fair that in this age of free trade they should not be afforded every opportunity.[38]

More Madden also argued that there was a distinctive need for women doctors in India and Oriental countries, 'where millions of suffering women and children are fanatically excluded from the possibility of any other skilled professional assistance; and I therefore think that such practitioners are entitled to admission into our ranks in the British Medical Association'.[39] This was a common argument put forward by supporters of women in the medical profession in the period, in particular by members of the medical profession itself who may have had fears about the overcrowding of their profession within the United Kingdom. Even Queen Victoria, who was otherwise opposed to women doctors, expressed in 1883 her support for efforts being made to raise a guarantee fund for the benefit of women doctors willing to go out from Britain to settle and work in India.[40] Jex-Blake, however, was critical of non-university courses that were established for the purpose of training women to provide medical care in the Zenana missions, arguing that such courses could not possibly equip women with the skills and training necessary for the medical profession.[41]

From the 1910s onwards, calls for women doctors to go to India became more frequent in the press, perhaps as fears concerning the overcrowding of the medical marketplace became more resolute. In the 28 January 1910 edition of the *Irish Times*, there was a report on the annual meeting of the Society for the Propagation of the Gospel in which the views of a Reverend J. A. Robertson, secretary to the Medical Missions Department, were published. In Robertson's view, 'the only way to get at the women of India and the women of the Mahommedan world was through women doctors'.[42] Similarly, in February 1914, the *Irish Times* reported on a meeting of another missionary society which encouraged women doctors to go and work in India, and a report in May 1920 commented on a meeting of the Zenana Missionary Society and the great necessity for women doctors in India.[43]

While admitting women a role in the missionary field, opponents of women doctors regularly expressed fears about the consequences that the admission of women to the medical profession might have for women's other roles, particularly within the family. Mater drew attention to problems that might arise for the husbands and children of lady doctors:

> But granting (as we must) the privilege of matrimony to these aspiring ladies, how then? Under certain resulting conditions, what is to become of the patients? Is a 'nursing mother' to suckle her babe in the intervals snatched from an extensive practice? Or is the husband of the 'qualified practitioner' to stay at home and bring up the little one with one of those 'artificial breasts' so kindly invented to save idle and selfish women from fulfilling the sweetest and most healthful duties to maternity?

And:

> A man's home should be to him also a rest. Will it be much of this with his wife in and out all day, called up all night, neglecting the household management and leaving the little ones to the care of servants? I think not.[44]

Similar sentiments were expressed in the pages of the *Irish Times*. In 1895, a letter to the editor from 'Tommie' expressed strong objections to women 'endeavouring to occupy male positions'; the writer feared that the day might come when men would have to 'don the petticoats and take up their position beside the cradle'.[45] In 1897, a similarly anti-feminist article was published in response to a piece by Janet E. Hogarth, an activist for women's rights. The article was extremely critical of Hogarth and echoes the sentiments of Tommie's letter, fearing that the world would not be better for the transformation of the 'modern woman'.[46]

Not only was it suggested that women's work as doctors would endanger their roles as wives and mothers, but it was also believed that mental strain through medical education might cause damage to the female reproductive system.[47] These sentiments reflect Victorian attitudes which placed middle-class women firmly in the home.[48] Deborah Gorham explains this by arguing that, as a result of the tension produced by industrial change, Victorians sought to establish the family as a source of stability, and this resulted in 'a cult of domesticity, an idealised vision of home and family, a vision that perceived the family as both enfolding its members and excluding the outside world'.[49] This 'cult' assisted in relieving the tensions 'that existed between the moral values of Christianity, with its emphasis on love and charity, and the values of capitalism, which asserted that the world of commerce should be pervaded by a spirit of competition and a recognition that only the fittest should survive'.[50] Thus, the Victorian middle classes were able to reconcile the stark differences between the harsh reality of their industrial society and the moral values endorsed by Christianity.

The patriarchal family became regarded as the building block of the civilised Victorian society upon which Britain's stability depended.[51] As a result, arguments concerning women's domestic roles were of great importance to the Victorian middle-class man or woman – what to do with these women doctors if they married and chose to have children as well as a career? Of course, this question was not restricted to the debate concerning women doctors but applied to women wishing to have a career in any profession. The traditionalist attitude of Mater's 1897 article quoted above, in calling the working female doctor 'idle' and 'selfish' and displaying abhorrence at the idea that her husband might have to stay at home to look after the children, is typical of its time. The application of this argument specifically against women in medicine has a long history, such as in the *Morning Chronicle* newspaper in 1858, which stated that, as well as being physically disqualified from careers in medicine, women were also disqualified as a result of their duties as wives and mothers.[52] These ideas were backed up by the Catholic Church in Ireland.[53]

These perceptions of suitable gender roles continued into the twentieth century. An article in the *Irish Times* in 1907 entitled 'Women doctors, dead failures', apparently written by a medical man, alleged that women would not succeed as doctors because they 'are singularly unsuccessful in much that they undertake'.[54] The author believed that women were better off working in 'the modiste than in the mortuary' and closed his article with the sentence 'I am afraid the plain, unvarnished truth is that all the best work of the world has been, and always will be, done by men'.[55]

Unsurprisingly, Jex-Blake was one of those who argued against this, claiming that every intelligent human being had the right to 'choose out his or her own life work and to decide what is and what is not calculated to conduce to his or her personal benefit and happiness'.[56] A career in the profession of her choosing was presented as a fundamental right of a woman by those involved in the women's movement in the late nineteenth and early twentieth centuries. Jex-Blake felt that medicine should be no exception. She even made the argument that there was historical evidence in favour of the medical education of women and that 'those learned in Greek literature will remember that Homer speaks of medical women both in the *Iliad* and in the *Odyssey*' and that Euripides has a nurse remind Queen Phaedra that if her disease 'is such as may not be told to men' there are skilled women at hand to whom she can turn.[57] Ethel Lamport also drew attention to the story of Queen Phaedra and to other medical women in Greek literature as well as mentioning figures from the Middle Ages in various European countries who were successful female doctors.[58] Despite the historical precedence of women healers, opponents of women in medicine claimed that women could have a role in caring for the sick but without becoming doctors. For instance, Mater argued:

> Let women then be nurses, tenders of the sick, free from the very faintest taint of prudery or affectation in anything and everything that comes in their way when helping and sustaining the sufferings of those around them; but let there be a line beyond which they sink from treading.[59]

It may appear to be a paradox that nursing was deemed suitable for women while medicine was not, but nursing was not always seen as a proper career for a middle-class woman in Ireland at the time. In late nineteenth-century Ireland, aside from that done by nuns, nursing was undertaken mostly by poor women without training, who carried out their work in return for maintenance within the hospital.[60] This began to change from the 1890s when nurse training schemes based on the Nightingale model were established in all of the major voluntary hospitals in Dublin.[61] Florence Nightingale herself had argued that there was a separate sphere for women in medicine through the profession of nursing: women should attend to problems of sanitation, hygiene and midwifery, not medicine or surgery, thus alleviating any fears among male doctors concerning competition.[62] Nightingale and her followers had wished to reconstruct nursing into a respectable female occupation through an emphasis on 'Christian vocation, entailing self-sacrifice, devotion and moral certainty'.[63] Dublin in the 1890s thus witnessed the emergence of the 'lady nurse' recruited from the lower-middle-class, better-off artisans and farmers as well as women from the middle and upper-middle classes.[64] In spite of this, medicine remained a more financially lucrative career choice for middle-class women and would have brought with it an upgrade in social status. Medicine was viewed as an elite profession that required a great deal of rigorous training, whereas nursing, though a crucially important occupation, was held in less regard. Jex-Blake, in a pamphlet entitled *Medical Women*, spoke out against the idea of nursing being seen as a suitable career for women while medicine was not:

> It has always struck me as a curious inconsistency that while almost everybody applauds and respects Miss Nightingale and her followers for their brave disregard of conventionalities on behalf of suffering humanity, and while hardly any one

would pretend that there was any want of feminine delicacy in their going among the foulest sights and most painful scenes, to succour, not their own sex, but the other, many people yet profess to be shocked when other women desire to fit themselves to take the medical care of those of their sisters who would gladly welcome their aid. Where is the real difference? If a woman is to be applauded for facing the horrors of an army hospital when she believes that she can there do good work, why is she condemned as indelicate when she professes her willingness to go through an ordeal, certainly no greater to obtain the education necessary for a medical practitioner?[65]

Evidently, there were other issues at play. Occasionally, medicine was viewed as being a profession for 'ladies' while nursing was viewed as a career for 'women'. In 1876, an article by Jonathan Hutchinson, senior surgeon to the London Hospital, appeared in the *British Medical Journal* which claimed that the study of medicine by women might 'lower feminine delicacy'.[66] Emily Davies, a pioneer in the women's higher education movement in Britain, writing in a paper entitled 'Medicine as a profession for women' (1862), claimed that 'the business of a hired nurse cannot be looked upon as a profession for a lady' and that medicine was a far more suitable profession for women of the middle classes.[67] She furthermore pointed out that the salary of a hospital nurse was no better than that of a butler or groom and, for this reason, women of the middle classes should attempt to gain access to medicine instead.

Conclusion

T HOSE ARGUING AGAINST WOMEN in the medical profession in Britain claimed that women's natures made them unsuited to work as doctors. As with arguments concerning women's role in higher education, opponents claimed that medical education would put unnecessary strain on women students and that menstruation would hinder their education. It is evident that not everyone shared these views, with supporters of women's admission to the medical profession arguing that there was a definite demand for women doctors from female patients who would be more comfortable being attended by a woman than by a man. Additionally, it was claimed that there was a need for women doctors in the missionary field. Despite this, opponents claimed that medicine was not a suitable career for women and that women should choose the alternative career path of nursing if they wished to care for the sick. I have suggested that, as with the backlash more generally against middle-class women in higher education and in the workplace at this time, these notions were constructed in order to protect the institution of the family and of the Victorian wife and mother, all of which were seen as crucial for a healthy economy and society.

Notes

1 Sophia Jex-Blake, 'Medicine as a profession for women', in *Medical Women: Two Essays* (Edinburgh: William Oliphant, 1872), p. 68.
2 *Irish Times*, 30 June 1874, p. 5.
3 Cornelie Usborne, 'Women doctors and gender identity in Weimar Germany (1918–1933)', in Laurence Conrad and Anne Hardy (eds), *Women and Modern Medicine*, Clio Medica Series (Amsterdam: Rodopi, 2001), pp. 109–26, on p. 109.
4 Thomas Neville Bonner, *To the Ends of the Earth: Women's Search for Education in Medicine* (Cambridge, MA: Harvard University Press, 1992), p. 64.
5 Bonner, *To the Ends of the Earth*, pp. 57–80.
6 Sophia Jex-Blake, *Medical Women: A Thesis and a History* (Edinburgh: Oliphant, Anderson and Ferrier, 1886), p. 204.
7 'The admission of ladies to the profession', *BMJ*, 7 May 1870, p. 475.
8 Editorial article, *Irish Times*, 8 November 1869, p. 2.
9 Untitled article, *Irish Times*, 15 February 1876, p. 4.
10 Charles West, *Medical Women: A Statement and an Argument* (London: J. and A. Churchill, 1878), p. 30.
11 Joan Burstyn, 'Education and sex: the medical case against higher education for women in England, 1870–1900', *Proceedings of the American Philosophical Society*, 117:2 (1973), pp. 79–89.
12 *Ibid.*, p. 81.
13 James McGrigor Allan, 'On the real differences in the minds of men and women', *Journal of the Anthropological Society of London*, 7:212 (1869), p. 46, cited in Cynthia Eagle Russett, *Sexual Science: The Victorian Construction of Womanhood* (Cambridge, MA: Harvard University Press, 1989), p. 30.
14 Henry Maudsley, 'Sex in mind and education', *Fortnightly Review*, 15 (1874), pp. 466–83.
15 The *Dublin Medical Press* (henceforth *DMP*) was a weekly Irish medical journal issued by the Irish Medical Association. Its editors were members of the Royal College of Surgeons. It ran from 1838 to 1926 and was classed as being 'independent/neutral' in its political stance, although it was generally conservative and middle class in its outlook. It had a circulation of 24,562 in 1850. (Source: *Waterloo Directory of English Periodicals and Newspapers, 1800–1900* and personal communication with Ann Daly.)
16 'Sex in education', *DMP*, 27 January 1875, p. 79.
17 Carla Bittel, *Mary Putnam Jacobi and the Politics of Medicine in Nineteenth-Century America* (Chapel Hill, NC: University of North Carolina Press, 2009), pp. 122–3.
18 *Ibid.*, p. 126.
19 'Mater', 'A lady on lady doctors', *Lancet*, 7 May 1870, p. 680.
20 See, for example, Katharina Rowold's collection of contemporary documents relating to women and higher education *Gender and Science: Late Nineteenth-Century Debates on the Female Mind and Body* (Bristol: Thoemmes Press, 1996) and Elaine Showalter, *The Female Malady: Women, Madness and English Culture, 1830–1980* (London: Virago Press, 1987) for a history of nineteenth- and twentieth-century perceptions of women's natures which influenced their psychiatric treatment.
21 'Mater', 'A lady on lady doctors', p. 680.

22 'Queen's University of Ireland: meeting of convocation', *Irish Times*, 16 October 1873, p. 3.

23 *Irish Times*, 8 November 1869, p. 2.

24 Thomas Haslam, 'Letter to the editor', *Freeman's Journal*, 2 February 1871, p. 3.

25 *Ibid.*

26 Sophia Jex-Blake, 'The medical education of women', a paper read at the Social Science Congress, Norwich, October 1873 (London: no publisher given, 1874), p. 3.

27 *Ibid.*, p. 4.

28 Ethel F. Lamport, 'Medicine as a profession for women', in *Education and Professions*, The Women's Library, vol. 1 (London: Chapman and Hall, 1903), p. 257.

29 Undated letter (from the period 1902–13) from the Munster Branch of the Irish Association of Women Graduates and Candidate Graduates to the Board of Management of Victoria Hospital, Cork, University College Dublin Archives (NUWGA1/3).

30 Teresa Billington-Greig, 'Why we need women doctors', in *Woman's Wider World* – (weekly syndicated article), 28 February 1913, Women's Library, London (7/TBG2/G7).

31 *Ibid.*

32 Jex-Blake, 'The medical education of women', p. 41.

33 Jonathan Hutchinson, 'A review of current topics of medical and social interest', *BMJ*, 19 August 1876, p. 233.

34 'Lady surgeons', *BMJ*, 2 April 1870, p. 338.

35 'Mater', 'A lady on lady doctors', p. 680.

36 Robert Baker, 'The history of medical ethics', in W. F. Bynum and Roy Porter (eds), *Companion Encyclopedia of the History of Medicine* (London: Routledge, 1993), vol. 2, pp. 852–87, on p. 853.

37 'British Medical Association. The admission of lady doctors: interesting discussion', *Freeman's Journal*, 29 July 1892, p. 6.

38 Untitled article, *Freeman's Journal*, 9 August 1888, p. 4.

39 *Ibid.*

40 'The Queen and medical women', *Englishwoman's Review*, 13 January 1883, p. 33.

41 Sophia Jex-Blake, *Medical Education of Women: A Comprehensive Summary of Present Facilities for Education, Examination and Registration* (Edinburgh: National Association for Promoting the Medical Education of Women, 1888), p. 18 (Wellcome Archives, SA/MWF/C3). The Zenana missions refers to the work of women missionaries who converted Indian women to Christianity.

42 'Society for the Propagation of the Gospel: annual meeting', *Irish Times*, 28 January 1910, p. 9.

43 'Dublin University mission to Chota Nagpur: ladies' auxiliary annual meeting', *Irish Times*, 21 February 1914, p. 5; and 'Zenana missionary society: record year's income', *Irish Times*, 21 May 1920, p. 7.

44 'Mater', 'A lady on lady doctors', p. 680.

45 'Tommie', 'The editor's letter box', *Irish Times*, 2 February 1895, p. 1.

46 Untitled article, *Irish Times*, 2 December 1897, p. 6.

47 Burstyn, 'Education and sex', p. 79.

48 Margaret Bryant, *The Unexpected Revolution: A Study in the History of the Education of Women and Girls in the Nineteenth Century* (London: University of London Institute of Education, 1979), p. 28.

49 Deborah Gorham, *The Victorian Girl and the Feminine Ideal* (London: Croom Helm, 1982), p. 4.

50 *Ibid.*

51 Joan Perkin, *Victorian Women* (New York: New York University Press, 1993), p. 74.

52 'Petticoat physic', *Morning Chronicle*, 11 January 1858, p. 6.

53 David Barry, 'Opposition to female suffrage from a Catholic standpoint', *Irish*

Ecclesiastical Record, 27 (September 1909), in Maria Luddy, *Women in Ireland 1800–1918: A Documentary History* (Cork: Cork University Press, 1995), pp. 280–3..

54 'Women doctors, dead failures', *Irish Times*, 2 February 1907, p. 18.
55 *Ibid.*
56 Jex-Blake, 'The medical education of women', p. 6.
57 *Ibid.*, p. 5.
58 Lamport, 'Medicine as a profession for women', pp. 278–86.
59 'Mater', 'A lady on lady doctors', p. 680.
60 Maria Luddy, *Women and Philanthropy in Nineteenth-Century Ireland* (Cambridge: Cambridge University Press, 1995), p. 51.
61 Gerard M. Fealy, *A History of Apprenticeship Nurse Training in Ireland* (London: Routledge, 2006), p. 68.
62 Mary Poovey, *Uneven Developments: The Ideological Work of Gender in Mid-Victorian England* (Chicago, IL: University of Chicago Press, 1986), p. 186.
63 Sue Hawkins, *Nursing and Women's Labour in the Nineteenth Century: The Quest for Independence* (London: Routledge, 2010), p. 23 and p. 27.
64 Fealy, *A History of Apprenticeship Nurse Training*, p. 69.
65 Jex-Blake, *Medical Women*, pp. 35–6.
66 Hutchinson, 'A review of current topics of medical and social interest', p. 233.
67 Emily Davies, 'Medicine as a profession for women' (1862), in Emily Davies, *Thoughts on Some Questions Relating to Women, 1860–1908* (Cambridge: Bowes and Bowes, 1910), p. 37.

2

The admission of women to the
KQCPI and Irish medical schools

IN 1898, a report in the *Freeman's Journal* on the opening to women of the Catholic University Medical School compared the change in the attitude of the general public towards women doctors to the altered outlook towards lady cyclists:

> How a few short years have changed all of this! How thoroughly we have become accustomed to, and how warmly we approve of, the lady cyclist. So it is with other departures.... How many fair and gentle womanly women – as well, no doubt, those of the more stern or manly type – may now be found in these countries among the ranks of the medical profession![1]

In the same year, the *Freeman's Journal* also commented that 'the lady doctor is getting on. She has broken down the barrier of bigotry and exclusiveness and forced her way into the profession. She has now her recognised position and status, and is no longer, except amongst the particularly ill-conditioned, a theme for rude jests and jibes'.[2]

By this time, it had been twenty-one years since the historic decision of the King and Queen's College of Physicians of Ireland (KQCPI) to allow women to take its licence examinations. In March 1878, a year after the admission of women to the KQCPI, the *Lancet* reported on the question of the admission of women to the Royal College of Physicians in London. The fellows of the College were strongly opposed to the admission of women. Sir George Burrows moved that he felt that men and women should not be educated together, while a Dr West argued that women's natures made them unfit to be doctors. A Dr Bucknill stated that allowing women to take the medical examinations of the College would be a retrograde step towards the 'modern desire of making women work'.[3] According to the *Medical Times and Gazette*, the fellows of the Royal College of Physicians believed 'that women are making a grievous mistake in desiring to become practitioners of medicine; that it is a career eminently unsuited for them; and that entering it, besides being of no benefit to themselves generally, will be of no gain to medicine and will be paid for by the public'.[4] In fact, the Royal College of Physicians in London did not allow women to take its licentiate examinations until thirty-three years after the KQCPI, when Dossibhai Rustomji Cowasji Patell became its first female licentiate, in 1910.[5]

Reasons for the liberality of the KQCPI

CONSIDERING THAT the Royal College of Physicians in London held such hostile views towards the admission of women to take its licences, we may wonder why the Irish College differed. I will argue that the decision of the KQCPI to admit women in 1877 was the result of four main factors. Firstly, the early history of women in higher education in Ireland was important. Secondly, the personnel on the council of the KQCPI when the decision was made proved pertinent. Thirdly, there were financial considerations. Finally, the absence of a perceived threat to professional practice may also be viewed as an important factor.

Dublin had an unusual history of liberality in the education of women. The Museum of Irish Industry had admitted both men and women to its public lectures on science and to its courses on scientific subjects from the 1850s.[6] The government Department of Science and Art in London provided an annual grant of £500 to the Museum of Irish Industry for the provision of series of lectures on scientific topics to societies in provincial towns in Ireland and, as in Dublin, these courses were open to both men and women.[7] The Museum of Irish Industry was unusual because, unlike similar institutions in Britain, such as the technical colleges and the mechanics' institutes, it was open to women. Clara Cullen comments that it is difficult to determine precise numbers of women students at the Museum of Irish Industry but, given the large number of female students who appear in the lists of prize-winners, they are likely to have comprised a significant proportion of the student body. The vast majority of these ladies were from the middle classes.[8] The successor of the Museum of Irish Industry, the Royal College of Science, came into existence in 1867 following a Treasury decision in 1865 to convert the Museum and Government School of Science.[9] The Royal College of Science admitted women to its classes from its opening year.[10] The College admitted two types of students: associated students, who attended for three years and who, on the successful completion of the course, received the Diploma of Associateship; and non-associated students, who attended individual courses as they pleased.[11] One writer to the _Freeman's Journal_ in 1870 commented that Dublin had 'achieved honour in other countries by its liberality to ladies in connection with the Royal College of Science' and hoped that the Dublin medical schools would soon follow the example set by Paris and (briefly) Edinburgh.[12] In contrast, women wishing to undertake scientific education in Britain were more limited: they could attend the single-sex colleges of Girton and Newnham at Cambridge from 1869 and 1871, University College London from 1878 and Bedford College from the 1880s. The Royal College of Science in London did not admit women until 1900.[13]

The late nineteenth century witnessed the emergence in Ireland of Catholic and Protestant girls' second-level colleges. Protestant schools for girls had been established in the 1860s in response to the need for academic education for middle-class girls. The most important ones were the Ladies' Collegiate School, Belfast (1859), Victoria College (1887) and Alexandra College (1866). These schools were crucial in spearheading the Irish women's higher education movement.[14] The school magazine of Alexandra College often drew attention to the achievements of former pupils in the medical profession, while also providing articles to educate girls on possibilities for them in the professions.[15] Catholic women's colleges emerged from the 1880s in response to the growing demands of Catholic women for higher education in a Catholic setting. The main teaching orders which promoted higher education for middle-class Catholic women were the Dominican, Loreto and Ursuline orders.[16] These Catholic and Protestant schools fostered a sense of vocation in young women but also encouraged them to pursue educational goals and university education. Judith Harford has argued that it was denominational rivalry with the Protestant schools which resulted in the Catholic hierarchy's commitment to and encouragement of women's higher education in the late nineteenth century.[17] Catholic sisterhoods not only played a vital role in women's education but were also responsible for the management of Irish hospitals. In contrast with Britain, the majority of hospitals in Ireland were founded by Catholic sisterhoods.[18] Within these institutions, the nuns were responsible for the nursing care, hygiene and hospital management.[19] Thus, religious women occupied a semi-separate sphere in the context of hospital management and nursing in Ireland, while male doctors were responsible for the medical care. Given the vital role of nuns in the management of and nursing care within Irish hospitals, it is possible that the Irish medical and religious hierarchy recognised a role for women as doctors and the need for women doctors to tend to women patients.

Also important is the fact that the council of the KQCPI in the 1870s was composed of senior members of the Irish medical profession who happened to be in favour of the admission of women to the medical profession, among them the Reverend Dr Samuel Haughton, Dr Aquilla Smith and Dr Samuel Gordon. Haughton was responsible for the promotion of the School of Physic Amendment Act 1867, which became known as 'Haughton's Act'.[20] Under this act, the professors of the KQCPI 'no longer had to be Protestant, and persons of all nations, whether or not holders of a university medical degree, could be appointed. The election of the professors of the College was placed entirely in the hands of the fellows who no longer had to resign that status in order to become candidates.'[21] Haughton's role in the promotion of the act in 1867 suggests that he was open to the inclusion of all in medical education. The idea that non-Protestants and people from outside the United Kingdom could become professors at the KQCPI would have been ground-breaking for an institution with such strong Protestant roots, but it indicates that the College was willing to introduce reforms in medical teaching.

Haughton was also responsible for the transformation of Sir Patrick Dun's Hospital in Dublin.[22] Under his guidance, the hospital was extended to provide surgical, obstetric and gynaecological services as well as medical services. He also introduced a modern system of trained nursing into the hospital.[23] In his obituary in the *British Medical Journal* in November 1897, Haughton is hailed as a brilliant scientific writer and for having been responsible for bringing about many reforms in medical education in Dublin in the late nineteenth century.[24] In addition to his work in the medical schools, Haughton gave public science lectures in Dublin at Trinity College. One, on a Saturday in March 1876, was attended by a large audience which included a number of ladies.[25] It is possible that it was in this role that he came to recognise that women and men could be educated together.

Another hypothesis might be that Haughton's openness to women medical students was a result of his religiosity.[26] Haughton had been ordained a priest in the Church of Ireland in 1847 and although he was not obliged to undertake pastoral duties, he 'took his orders seriously and preached throughout his life'.[27] It is possible that this religiosity endowed Haughton with the belief that women should be attended by women physicians and thus encouraged his support of the admission of women to medical schools. It is likely that Haughton also viewed medicine as a vocation rather than as a profession. T. D. Spearman has commented that one reason why Haughton entered into medical education at Trinity College Dublin may have been because as a boy he had hoped that he might one day work as a medical missionary in China.[28] A Christian like Haughton might well have felt that a call from God was a real and absolute command that could apply to women as well as men. Medicine and caring for the sick could fall into this category of vocation and, thus, if a woman wanted to pursue this 'call', she ought to be allowed to do so.

Less is known about the other two players in the admission of women to the KQCPI. Dr Aquilla Smith, who had proposed the motion that Edith Pechey be accepted to take the examinations for the medical licence, has a similarly glowing obituary in the *British Medical Journal*. He is called 'one of the best known and most distinguished of the profession in Ireland' and is said, because of his knowledge of educational matters, to have served as the representative of the KQCPI on the General Medical Council (GMC) from 1858 until 1888.[29] Dr Samuel Gordon was president at the time of the admission of women to the KQCPI; he had nine daughters and is heralded in his obituary as having been a brilliant physician and teacher with a 'paternal and kindly' manner.[30] Like Smith and Haughton, his obituary paints the picture of a man who was deeply interested in medical education and its reform.

Consistent with an open attitude towards women medical students, Irish voluntary hospitals had a history of allowing women onto their wards for clinical experience and lectures, and women medical students appear to have been readily accepted. At Dr Steevens' Hospital in Dublin, a female student, Mrs Janthe Legett, had been admitted to the hospital's classes from November 1869 until the summer of 1873, seemingly without question.[31] Legett, who undertook her preliminary examinations to enter the University of Edinburgh in October 1870, conducted her practical experience and lectures at the Dublin hospital. One Edinburgh academic, Professor Handyside, on learning that the candidate had followed the anatomy course at Dr Steevens' Hospital, congratulated the lady on having studied in so excellent a school.[32] Legett herself, writing to Sophia Jex-Blake, commented of her experiences at the hospital:

> I had the unanimous consent of the Board to pursue my medical studies in Steevens' Hospital. As to the medical students, they are always civil. Dr Macnamara, President of the College of Physicians of Ireland, said it was his opinion that the presence of ladies would refine the classes.[33]

Likewise, Dr Hamilton, the medical secretary of Dr Steevens' Hospital, commented that the hospital staff had found the system of mixed classes to work 'very well'.[34] Irish institutions continued to have inclusive attitudes towards women medical students following women's admission, with women and men being educated together for all classes with the exception of anatomy and women medical students reporting positive educational experiences.

As was the case with the admission of women medical students to Irish hospital wards, it is also possible that financial factors were pertinent to the College's decision to admit women students. Fees were a crucial source of income for the KQCPI. In 1874, for example, the total income for the half-year ended 17 October was £801. Of this, £771 came from fees for medical licences.[35] Similarly, for the half-year ended 17 April 1875, the total income was £809 with the sum from fees being £758.[36] By October 1877, it is evident that fees had become an even more important source of revenue for the College: the total revenue for that half-year was £1,201, with the fees totalling £1,048.[37] Not only was income up but, by 1877, the finances of the College were in a healthier state. Whereas in 1875 the College balance at the end of the half-year in October 1875 had been £1,476, two years later the balance had risen to £2,526. It is possible that the council of the College viewed the admission of women to take its medical licences as a means of generating income.

Perhaps also important was the fact that, since the late seventeenth century, women had been entitled to take the midwifery licence at the KQCPI if they so wished, with Mistress Cormack taking a licence in 1696, and Mrs Catherine Banford taking one in 1732, although no further women took the licence in midwifery until 1877.[38] It is possible that the College perceived the admission of women as midwives as a precedent for the subsequent admission of women to take licences in medicine.

More crucial, perhaps, is the fact that the women who were applying to take the licences of the KQCPI were British women who had attained their medical education abroad. These women did not go on to practise in Ireland, nor does it appear that they had any intention of doing so at the time of their applications for admission. It is likely that the Irish medical profession, as represented by the council of the KQCPI, did not feel as threatened by the issue of prospective professional competition as their counterparts in Britain did.

The admission of women to the KQCPI

A S WE SAW in Chapter 1, in January 1877 Eliza Louisa Walker Dunbar became the first female licentiate of the KQCPI, but this was the climax of over three years of petitioning by some other women. In December 1873, Mary Edith Pechey (KQCPI, 1877) had written to the KQCPI requesting to know the power of the College to admit women to examination and to give them a licence in midwifery and whether such a licence would be registerable under the Medical Act 1858.[39] Pechey, born in Colchester, England, was the daughter of a Baptist minister, William Pechey, and his wife, Sarah. Pechey presumably expected that the College would be more likely to award women licences in midwifery than in medicine. In 1874, the council of the KQCPI informed Pechey that 'women have been examined for a Licence in Midwifery by the King and Queen's College of Physicians and that the College will be prepared to examine Women for a Qualification in Midwifery, but are unable to state whether such Qualification is Registerable under the Medical Act'.[40]

Pechey, along with Jex-Blake and Annie Clark, another of the 'Edinburgh Seven', went to the University of Bern in order to undertake further medical study. Pechey and Jex-Blake both qualified with MD degrees from the University of Bern in January 1877, while Clark graduated from Paris in 1878. Pechey's role in the battle for women to attain admission to study medicine in the late nineteenth century appears to have been neglected by historians, who have tended to focus on her fiery counterpart, Sophia Jex-Blake, a name that is far more synonymous with the history of women in medicine. Pechey, however, appears to have been active in petitioning the Irish schools of medicine to admit women (see below). In 1883, she moved to India, where she was heavily involved in medical work among Indian women.[41]

In early 1874, another figure, Louisa Atkins, enters the story. Atkins was a married Englishwoman who had trained for her MD degree at the University of Zurich.[42] Unlike Pechey, however, Atkins requested permission to be examined for a licence in medicine rather than midwifery. A special meeting of the council of the KQCPI was held in January that year at which Haughton proposed an application on behalf of Atkins for admission to be examined for the licence in medicine.[43] The proposal was seconded by Sir Dominic Corrigan, an eminent physician of the Dublin School of Medicine and vice-chancellor of the Queen's University of Ireland.[44] An amendment was proposed by a Dr Lyons and seconded by Aquilla Smith: 'That before deciding the question of the admission, nor non-admission, of Mrs Louisa Atkins to examination for the Licence of the College, the Opinion of the Law Officers of the Crown be taken as to whether, under the Charter and Acts, the College is competent to admit females to the Licence of the College'.[45] The amendment was defeated by sixteen votes to twelve, before a second amendment was proposed by Dr Steele and seconded by Dr Hayden, the vice-president of the College at the time: 'That the College is of opinion that it is inexpedient that Women should be admitted to examination for the Licence to practise Medicine'. Despite the support of Corrigan and Haughton for Atkins' admission, this amendment was passed as a resolution, with twenty-two votes in favour, five votes against, and one fellow declining to vote.[46]

Meanwhile, Pechey was busily writing to Irish institutions requesting that she be admitted. In spite of the fact that she had achieved her degree at Bern, she was in need of a registerable licence from an institution in the United Kingdom so that she could have her name placed on the *Medical Register* and be allowed to practise. Luckily for Pechey and her counterparts, the KQCPI decided to take advantage of the Enabling Act 1876. In October 1876, a letter from Pechey 'petitioning the College to avail themselves of the new power granted by the Act 39 and 40 Vict. Chap. 41 and to admit women to the examination for the Licence of Medicine' was referred to at an ordinary meeting of the KQCPI.[47] The motion 'that Miss Pechey's prayer to be admitted to examination for the Licence in Medicine be complied with, after her papers have been certified by the Committee of Inspection' was proposed by Smith, seconded by Haughton and resolved.[48] Permission was then granted to Pechey to present herself for the First Professional Examination for the licence.

The decision of the College to admit Edith Pechey made headlines in both the *Dublin Medical Press* and the *Medical Times and Gazette*, an English journal, which commented that Pechey had been accepted for admission and that another candidate, Eliza Louisa Walker Dunbar, was expected to present herself for examination the following February.[49] The *Dublin Medical Press* commented that Edith Pechey had been accepted for the medical licence and that a similar application for the admission of women to study medicine at the Queen's Colleges was now underway and that this application had 'the support of very influential members, and also of the Government'.[50]

In spite of being admitted to the KQCPI, Pechey also wrote to Queen's College Galway on 19 October 1876 and to Queen's College Belfast in November. It is possible that she did this because a degree would have been a superior qualification to a licence. In her letter to the council of Queen's College Galway, which was read out at a council meeting on 23 October 1876, Pechey stated that she had been given permission to take the examinations for the MD degree by the senate of the Queen's University and requested permission from the College to allow her to take four of its classes in order to comply with the regulations concerning attendance at the Queen's University.[51] Pechey said in her letter that if it was necessary for these classes to be separately delivered to men and women, then she offered to remunerate the professors of the College 'for the extra time and trouble which such an arrangement must necessarily entail upon them'.[52] As well as this, Pechey offered to guarantee the payment of a maximum fee of £100 for each class so divided and, because the number of female students would presumably be small for a few years, she offered to guarantee the said payment for a further five years.[53] This promise of such a significant payment clearly indicates how much Pechey wanted to attain a medical degree. Likewise, it is possible she wrote to Queen's College Galway before Queen's College Belfast because the Galway College was in a less stable financial condition. Pechey closed her letter to Galway by stating:

> My object being to obtain a legal qualification to practise Medicine, my strong wish would be to accomplish that object in the way most satisfactory to you, and in accordance with the deep sense I shall experience of your liberality in removing from my way those disabilities under which I have laboured so long.[54]

The council of Queen's College Galway had lengthy discussions on the issue and came to the conclusion that women admitted under the Enabling Act 'are precisely on the same footing as Male Students, with regard to Matriculation, Fees, Attendance on Lectures, and Examinations, and in every other respect', but because they could foresee 'such grave difficulties' in admitting women to the College, they 'declined to avail themselves of the Act'.[55] Similarly, the council of Queen's College Belfast had unanimously 'deemed it inexpedient to comply with Miss Pechey's request', according to a letter received by the council of Queen's College Cork.[56]

Despite Pechey's lack of support from the Queen's Colleges, the KQCPI appears to have been growing more favourable towards the admission of women, as is evident from its treatment of Eliza Louisa Walker Dunbar. In January 1877, at the monthly examination meeting of the KQCPI, an attempt was made to prevent the issuing of a licence to Dunbar by rescinding the resolution that allowed her to be admitted.[57] That this proposition was rejected by nine votes to three suggests that the College council was now favourable towards the admission of Dunbar.[58] It was then resolved that the licence to practise medicine be issued to Dunbar, along with three other male candidates, who had been examined separately from her.[59] Thus, Dunbar became the first female licentiate of the KQCPI. She was also awarded a midwifery licence the day after the award of her medical licence.[60] Her success, in contrast to Louisa Atkins three years earlier, must be attributed to the fact that the Enabling Act was now in operation and the KQCPI had a legal entitlement to admit women to take its examinations if it so wished.

Atkins was clearly still keen to practise medicine and on 2 February 1877, at the monthly business meeting of the KQCPI, her case was reconsidered along with that of Frances Hoggan. Hoggan, the daughter of a vicar, had been reared in Wales but educated abroad as a teenager and later, like Dunbar, received private medical tuition from Elizabeth Garrett Anderson.[61] It was decided that both women should be admitted to take the examination for the licence to practise medicine.[62] Hoggan was granted her licence on 14 February 1877, while Atkins was granted hers in May.[63]

However, complications now arose for Edith Pechey, whose licence had not yet been granted. The following month, at a council meeting, it was decided to suspend Pechey's admission to take the licence examinations on account of her having an MD degree from the University of Bern. For some reason, Pechey's papers from Bern were not in accordance with the by-laws of the KQCPI.[64] The council decided to postpone her admission until a committee had decided whether to include qualifications from the University of Bern in the list of foreign degrees recognised by the College.[65] On 9 March 1877, two members of the council, Dr Lyons and Dr Jennings, attempted to have the resolutions to admit Pechey and Dunbar rescinded, but this motion was rejected, which suggests that the majority of council members were still in favour of the admission of women to take the medical examinations. At the examination meeting on 15 March, Pechey's application was reconsidered by the committee, who decided that her papers, bar a certificate in midwifery, were in accordance with the by-laws of the College, and that she would be admitted to take the licence examinations on presenting a certificate in practical midwifery.[66] Pechey was eventually granted her medical licence, along with Sophia Jex-Blake and Louisa Atkins, on 9 May 1877.[67] The following day, Pechey and Jex-Blake were also granted midwifery licences.[68]

Despite the open attitude of the KQCPI, it is clear that not all members of the Irish medical profession were convinced. In May 1877, after the conferring of the KQCPI medical licences to Atkins, Pechey and Jex-Blake, the *Dublin Medical Press* reported that the ladies were exempted from one-half of their examination on account of their Swiss qualifications. The author of the article stated:

> We have already recorded an earnest protest against this laxity with regard to foreign degrees and we repeat that the license of the Irish College of Physicians must lose a step in public estimation, when it is known that a class of candidates are authorised to write L.K.Q.C.P. after their names, without satisfactory evidence of medical competency. We do not suggest that these ladies would have failed to prove their competency, nor are we able to say whether Swiss degrees are or are not reliable evidence of medical knowledge.[69]

Men with degrees from continental universities had been entitled to take the licence examinations of the KQCPI and other British institutions since the early eighteenth century. However, following the Medical Act 1858, this practice was outlawed for anyone who attained their foreign degree after 1858.[70] The opening up of this clause to women following the Enabling Act 1876 caused alarm in the *Dublin Medical Press*. The journal suggested, quite disparagingly, that through allowing the admission of women who had taken foreign degrees, the KQCPI had taken a step towards the granting of absentia diplomas.[71] Similarly, the *Standard* newspaper claimed in March 1877 that women licentiates of the KQCPI took examinations that were 'less stringent than those undergone by men'.[72] This claim was refuted by the *Englishwoman's Review*, which reported that Dunbar had undertaken the same examinations as her male counterparts and that her clinical and viva voce examinations were undertaken at the same time and in the same room as the male students.[73] Similarly, Hoggan wrote to the *Standard* to protest that, in her experience, 'not only was the examination not less stringent than that undergone by men' but that she additionally had had to undergo a clinical examination and a written paper from which, if she had been a man, her six years' practice in the medical profession as a hospital physician and privately would have exempted her.[74] Fears about the professionalism of the female licentiates of the KQCPI continued, with the *Dublin Medical Press* reporting in 1889 on the case of Annie McCall, who had been an early licentiate of the KQCPI and who had reportedly been indulging in the unprofessional practice of dispensing 'an admixture of "Gospel Address, with hymns and prayer", together with medicine, and all for the small charge of 2*d*'.[75]

The admission of women to other Irish medical schools

DESPITE THE CONTROVERSIES in the press and their rejection of Pechey's offer in 1876, the other Irish medical schools soon followed the example of the KQCPI. In November 1879, the question of the admission of female students arose again at a council meeting at Queen's College Galway, where it was decided that 'the educational advantages of the College should, if feasible, be open to all students irrespective of sex',[76] although no female student was actually admitted to study medicine until 1902. It was not until November 1883 that the governing body of Queen's College Cork allowed the admission of women to classes of lectures provided by the arts professors of the College.[77] Belfast's first female medical student was admitted in 1888, while Cork's was admitted in 1890. The Catholic University followed suit in 1898.[78] In 1884, the Royal College of Surgeons met to decide whether they would admit women and the motion was passed by nine votes to three, with several leading members of the Irish medical profession, such as Sir Charles Cameron, voting in favour.[79] The *Dublin Medical Press*, despite its previous negative attitudes towards the admission of women to the profession, reported favourably on the decision:

> We congratulate the fellows on their good sense and liberality. They have saved the College from being branded as obstructive and jealous, from being left behind by the Royal Irish University and other similar institutions, from being compelled by medical legislation to do what they refused, and, most important, from being guilty of a palpable injustice for the perpetration of which no sufficient reason could be argued.[80]

Mary Emily Dowson, an English woman who trained at the London School of Medicine for Women, became the first female to take the examinations of the Royal College of Surgeons in Dublin in 1886, proving, in the words of the *Dublin Medical Press*, that there was no doubt 'as to the propriety or expediency of ladies entering the domain of surgery'.[81] The journal commended the College for its liberalism:

We are also, we believe, justified in congratulating the College upon having shown itself superior to the prejudices which might have been expected to influence the acts of an institution of its years. In this, as in other of its proceedings of the last few years, the College has shown that it will not be precluded by an obstructive medical conservatism from pursuing the progress which accords with the spirit of our age, and we are convinced that even those who dislike the invasion of surgical precincts by ladies will consider that the College has acted properly in sacrificing the feeling which many of its Fellows must entertain for the sake of doing what seems right and just.[82]

Despite the sometimes negative attitude of the *Dublin Medical Press*, other newspapers praised newly qualified female doctors. The *Freeman's Journal*, in particular in 1898, rejected the negative attitude of the *Dublin Medical Press* towards the possible admission of three women candidates to the fellowship of the Royal College of Surgeons, stating: 'Whether they will pass the examination or not is, the *Medical Press* observes, a different question. The observation shows a trace of the old hostile spirit, and is particularly unhappy in face of the brilliant professional success of some of the lady doctors that the College knows'.[83] Although the KQCPI did not admit women to its fellowships until 1924, when Mary Ellis Teresa Hearn became the first fellow, the Royal College of Surgeons in Ireland admitted women as fellows from 1893, when Emily Winifred Dickson became the first female fellow.[84] From 1893 to 1922, there were twenty-six female fellows of that Royal College of Surgeons.[85] Likewise, the Royal Academy of Medicine in Ireland demonstrated the same liberality as other Irish institutions by admitting women doctors to its meetings from its foundation in 1882. Edith Pechey appears to have become the first female member, in 1883.[86] Women students were allowed to become associates of the Academy after passing their third professional examination, which was 'a great boon', in the words of one student, because it enabled them to hear about all of the interesting cases which entered the various Dublin hospitals.[87] In contrast, in Britain, the British Medical Association closed its membership to women in 1878 and did not reopen it until 1892.[88] And, in 1896, there was a campaign to exclude women from English medical societies.[89]

The admission of women to the fellowships of the Royal College of Surgeons and the Royal Academy of Medicine is testament to the ongoing professional esteem and support for women doctors in Ireland. Considering this, it is evident that the open attitude of the KQCPI was not 'anomalous', as has been argued.[90] Similarly, within the Irish press there were some supporters of women in the medical profession. In March 1893, the *Freeman's Journal* applauded Emily Winifred Dickson and Katharine M. Maguire, both graduates from the Royal College of Surgeons. The author referred to the current issue of *Health Record*, in which the articles by Dickson and Maguire were the very best in the publication.[91]

Conclusion

IN A LETTER to Dr Duffey, of the council of the KQCPI, in 1879, Sophia Jex-Blake wrote: 'I am very sensible as are also Dr [Edith] Pechey and Dr [Agnes] McLaren, of the kindness, justice and liberality shown by the Irish College of Physicians in all its relations to the women who have made medicine their profession and I feel proud to owe to it my own admission to the Register'.[92]

Considering the mixed and often hostile attitude towards women in medicine that existed in Britain in the late nineteenth century, the decision of the KQCPI to admit women with foreign qualifications to take its licentiate examinations may seem surprising. The resolution appears to have been the result of a combination of factors: Dublin had already proved its liberality towards women in higher education through the admission of women to the Museum of Irish Industry in the 1850s and the Royal College of Science since the 1860s, and it was likely that this atmosphere was instrumental in the decision. Nuns had occupied a unique sphere in Irish health care, which paved the way for the entrance of lay women to medical care. Likewise, the higher education of women had been supported at secondary level by the Catholic hierarchy, while the Irish medical hierarchy of the KQCPI appear to have been supportive of the decision to admit women.

Financial factors might have also played a role in this decision. The KQCPI, like the Irish teaching hospitals, which had similarly demonstrated a positive attitude towards the admission of women, garnered a considerable income from student fees. The council of the KQCPI may have viewed admitting women to take its licences from a financial perspective, in that it would generate more income. At the same time, because the women who were applying for licences from the KQCPI came from Britain, they posed no competition or threat to the Irish medical marketplace.

Once the KQCPI made the decision to admit women to take these licences, other Irish universities followed suit and from the mid-1880s Irish women began to enrol on medical courses. Between 1885 and 1922, a total of 759 women matriculated in medicine at Irish institutions. In the following chapter, I will examine the social and geographical backgrounds of these first women medical students and discuss their possible reasons for undertaking medical education.

Notes

1 'The medical profession for women', *Freeman's Journal*, 18 August 1898, p. 4.
2 Untitled article, *Freeman's Journal*, 27 January 1898, p. 4.
3 'The Royal College of Physicians: the admission of women', *Lancet*, 23 March 1878, p. 438.
4 'The Royal College of Physicians and medical women', *Medical Times and Gazette*, 25 March 1878, p. 307.
5 Information courtesy of Geraldine O'Driscoll, archivist at the Royal College of Surgeons, London.
6 Clara Cullen, 'The Museum of Irish Industry, Robert Kane and education for all in the Dublin of the 1850s and 1860s', *History of Education*, 38:1 (2009), pp. 99–113, on p. 106.
7 *Ibid.*, p. 107.
8 *Ibid.*, p. 109.
9 Brian B. Kelham, 'The Royal College of Science for Ireland (1867–1926)', *Studies: An Irish Quarterly Review*, 56:223 (1967), pp. 297–309, on p. 300.
10 Clara Cullen, 'The Museum of Irish Industry (1845–1867): research environment, popular museum and community of learning in mid-Victorian Ireland' (PhD thesis, University College Dublin, 2008).
11 Kelham, 'The Royal College of Science for Ireland', p. 302.
12 'Letter to the editor', *Freeman's Journal*, 28 January 1870, p. 4. This was before the University of Edinburgh changed its mind with regard to women medical students.
13 Mary R. S. Creese, 'British women of the nineteenth and early twentieth centuries who contributed to research in the chemical sciences', *British Journal for the History of Science*, 24:3 (1991), pp. 275–305, on p. 278.
14 Judith Harford, 'The movement for the higher education of women in Ireland: gender equality or denominational rivalry?', *History of Education*, 34:5 (2005), pp. 497–516, on pp. 499–500.
15 For example, E. Winifred Dickson, 'Medicine as a profession for women', *Alexandra College Magazine*, 14 (June 1899), pp. 368–75, on pp. 374–5.
16 Judith Harford, *The Opening of University Education to Women in Ireland* (Dublin: Irish Academic Press, 2008), p. 5.
17 Harford, 'The movement for the higher education of women in Ireland', p. 516.
18 For example, the Irish Sisters of Charity founded St Vincent's Hospital in 1833 for the care of the sick poor in Dublin. The Sisters of Mercy founded the Mercy Hospital in Cork in 1857 and the Mater Misericordiae Hospital in Dublin in 1861. See Gerard M. Fealy, *A History of Apprenticeship Nurse Training in Ireland* (London: Routledge, 2006), p. 9.
19 *Ibid.*
20 J. D. H. Widdess, *A History of the Royal College of Physicians of Ireland, 1654–1963* (Edinburgh: E. and S. Livingstone, 1964), p. 214.
21 *Ibid.*
22 T. D. Spearman, 'Rev. Dr. Samuel Haughton', *ODNB*.
23 T. Percy C. Kirkpatrick, *History of the Medical Teaching in Trinity College Dublin and the School of Physic in Ireland* (Dublin: Hanna and Neale, 1912), p. 302.
24 'Obituary: Rev. Samuel Haughton, M.D., D.C.L., LL.D.', *BMJ*, 6 November 1897, pp. 1376–7.
25 'Professor Haughton's lectures', *Irish Times*, 27 March 1876, p. 6.
26 With thanks to Professor Greta Jones for this suggestion.
27 Spearman, 'Rev. Dr. Samuel Haughton'.
28 *Ibid.*
29 'Obituary: Dr. Aquilla Smith, M.D., F.K.Q.C.P.I.', *BMJ*, 5 April 1890, p. 814.

30 'Obituary: Samuel Gordon', *BMJ*, 7 May 1898, pp. 1236–7.
31 T. Percy C. Kirkpatrick, *The History of Doctor Steevens' Hospital Dublin, 1720–1920* (Dublin: Ponsonby and Gibbs, 1924), p. 261.
32 Editorial article, *Irish Times*, 31 October 1870, p. 4.
33 Sophia Jex-Blake, *Medical Women: Two Essays* (Edinburgh: William Oliphant, 1872), p. 143.
34 *Ibid.*
35 'Summary of the income and expenditure of the KQCPI, for half year, ended October 17, 1874', Minutes of the KQCPI, vol. 16, p. 34, Royal College of Physicians, Dublin.
36 'Summary of the income and expenditure of the KQCPI for half year ended April 17, 1875', Minutes of the KQCPI, vol. 16, p. 123, Royal College of Physicians, Dublin.
37 'Summary of the income and expenditure of the KQCPI for half year ended October 17, 1877', Minutes of the KQCPI, vol. 16, p. 402, Royal College of Physicians, Dublin.
38 Information from Robert Mills, librarian at the Royal College of Physicians, Dublin.
39 Ordinary meeting, 2 January 1874, Minutes of the KQCPI, vol. 15, p. 342, Royal College of Physicians, Dublin.
40 *Ibid.*, p. 343.
41 Edythe Lutzker, 'Edith Pechey-Phipson: the untold story', *Medical History*, 11:1 (1967), pp. 41–5, on p. 41.
42 'Obituary: Louisa Atkins MD', *BMJ*, 1 November 1924, pp. 836–7.
43 Special meeting, 7 January 1874, Minutes of the KQCPI, vol. 15, p. 345, Royal College of Physicians, Dublin.
44 L. Perry Curtis jun., 'Sir Dominic John Corrigan', *ODNB*.
45 Special meeting, 7 January 1874, Minutes of the KQCPI, vol. 15, p. 346, Royal College of Physicians, Dublin.
46 *Ibid.*
47 'Ordinary meeting', 6 October 1876, Minutes of the KQCPI, vol. 16, p. 257, Royal College of Physicians, Dublin.
48 *Ibid.*
49 'The admission of women to the profession', *Medical Times and Gazette*, 23 December 1876, p. 709.
50 'Notes on current topics: a registerable qualification for women', *DMP*, 18 October 1876, pp. 321–2.
51 Council meeting, 23 October 1876, Queen's College Galway council minutes, National University of Ireland, Galway (Registrar's Office).
52 *Ibid.*
53 *Ibid.*
54 *Ibid.*
55 *Ibid.*
56 Queen's College Cork governing body minutes, Council meeting, 15 November 1876, p. 265, University College Cork Archives.
57 Monthly examination meeting, 10 January 1877, Minutes of the KQCPI, vol. 16, p. 298, Royal College of Physicians, Dublin.
58 *Ibid.*, p. 299.
59 *Ibid.*, p. 298.
60 Register of midwifery licentiates of the KQCPI, Royal College of Physicians, Dublin (RCPI/365/3).
61 M. A. Elston, 'Frances Elizabeth Hoggan [née Morgan]', *ODNB*.
62 Monthly business meeting, 2 February 1877, Minutes of the KQCPI, vol. 16, p. 308, Royal College of Physicians, Dublin.
63 Roll of licentiates of the KQCPI, 1877–1910, Royal College of Physicians, Dublin.
64 2 March 1877, Minutes of the KQCPI, vol. 16, p. 322, Royal College of Physicians, Dublin.
65 9 March 1877, Minutes of the KQCPI, vol. 16, p. 329, Royal College of Physicians, Dublin.

66 Examination meeting, 15 March 1877, Minutes of the KQCPI, vol. 16, p. 336, Royal College of Physicians, Dublin.
67 Monthly examination meeting, 9 May 1877, Minutes of the KQCPI, vol. 16, p. 350, Royal College of Physicians, Dublin.
68 Register of midwifery licentiates of the KQCPI.
69 'Lady doctors at the Irish College of Physicians', *DMP*, 23 May 1877, p. 417.
70 Jean M. Scott, 'Women and the GMC', *BMJ*, 22–29 December 1984, pp. 1764–7, on p. 1765.
71 *Ibid.*, p. 1765.
72 *Standard*, 5 March 1877. (Scrapbook relating to the Royal Free Hospital and the medical education of women, Royal Free Archives, London.)
73 Untitled article, *Englishwoman's Review*, 13 March 1877, p. 130.
74 'The medical profession for women', *Standard*, 6 March 1877. (Scrapbook relating to the Royal Free Hospital and the medical education of women, Royal Free Archives, London.)
75 'Female practice in south London', *DMP*, 9 October 1889, p. 366.
76 Council meeting, 15 November 1879, Queen's College Galway council minutes, National University of Ireland, Galway (Registrar's Office).
77 Council meeting, 6 November 1883, p. 60, Queen's College Cork governing body minutes, University College Cork University Archives.
78 Annual report of the faculty, 20 May 1898, Catholic University School of Medicine, Governing body minute book, vol. 1, 1892–1911, University College Dublin Archives (CU/14).
79 Special meeting, 23 October 1884, Minutes of council, vol. 7, 1882–84, p. 296, Royal College of Surgeons, Dublin.
80 'Admission of women to the profession', *DMP*, 14 January 1885, pp. 35–6.
81 'The first lady surgeon', *DMP*, 8 June 1886, p. 524.
82 *Ibid.*
83 Untitled article, *Freeman's Journal*, 27 January 1898, p. 4.
84 Register of fellows of the KQCPI 1667–1985, Royal College of Physicians, Dublin (RCPI/365/41); and Roll of fellows of the College, in Royal College of Surgeons in Ireland, *Calendar, October 1923 to September 1924* (Dublin: Dublin University Press, 1923–24), pp. 83–95.
85 Register of fellows of the Royal College of Surgeons in Ireland.
86 Incomplete register of members of the Royal Academy of Medicine in Ireland, Royal College of Physicians Archive, Dublin.
87 Clara L. Williams, 'A short account of the school of medicine for men and women, RCSI', *Magazine of the London School of Medicine for Women and Royal Free Hospital*, no. 3 (January 1896), pp. 91–132, on p. 108.
88 Prior to 1878, only two women, Elizabeth Garrett Anderson and Frances Hoggan, had been successful in achieving membership. See Tara Lamont, 'The Amazons within: women in the BMA 100 years ago', *BMJ*, 19–26 December 1992, pp. 1529–32.
89 Irene Finn, 'Women in the medical profession in Ireland, 1876–1919', in Bernadette Whelan (ed.), *Women and Paid Work in Ireland, 1500–1930* (Dublin: Four Courts Press, 2000), pp. 102–19, on p. 113.
90 *Ibid.*, p. 105.
91 Untitled article, *Freeman's Journal*, 4 March 1893, p. 4.
92 Letter from Sophia Jex-Blake to Dr Duffey, dated 26 March 1879, Royal College of Physicians Archive, Dublin (RCPI/6/3/3). With thanks to Harriet Wheelock for alerting me to this source.

3

Becoming a medical student

IN AUGUST 1898, the *Freeman's Journal* reported:

> Twenty years ago well educated and well-to-do young girls never dreamt of a
> profession, or if they did they were looked upon with amazement by all their
> friends, and worried until the idea was shamed out of their heads. In those days a
> lady doctor was a dreadful anomaly, a thing almost unheard of, and to be avoided.
> Again, how all this, too, is changed![1]

The article was commending the decision of the medical school of the Catholic
University in Dublin to open its doors to women medical students and noted
the striking rapidity with which the public had grown accustomed to the idea
of women in the professions, with the lady medical student at that point being
'nothing to be wondered at'.[2] Likewise, by 1904, women students were so well
established in Irish universities that the student magazine at Queen's College
Galway, *QCG*, reported that the female student was now a recognised part of
college life. The writer commented that the presence of the female student in
the classroom was 'an incentive to the masculine student to work hard and
the sweet smile of a Lady Senior Scholar often compels difficult Mathematical
problems to come right'.[3] Ten years later, the *Quarryman*, the magazine of
Queen's College Cork (QCC), stated that college life would be 'dull' without
lady students and the fact that their numbers were increasing every year was
a positive thing, with the presence of the lady student in Irish universities
representing 'a change for the better'.[4]

Women had first been admitted to Irish universities from the mid-1880s.
Prior to this, following the University Act in 1879 which established the Royal
University of Ireland (RUI), small numbers of women had taken examinations
through Protestant and Catholic women's colleges. The University Act had
specified that the RUI was solely an examining body and that it was up to

students to study at any college they chose, or privately, in order to prepare for its examinations. The first nine Irish female students who graduated through the RUI in 1884 had attended classes at Alexandra College, McIntosh and Tinkler, a 'grind' establishment (i.e. a school that offered private tuition), the Royal College of Surgeons in Ireland and the Rutland School in Mountjoy Square, Dublin.[5] The first Irish university to admit women students was Queen's College Belfast (QCB), in 1882, following an appeal on behalf of the Belfast Ladies Institute. Women students were admitted to lectures in mathematics, Greek and experimental physics. The next university to open to women was QCC, in 1886, when five women students entered. Queen's College Galway (QCG) followed suit two years later, in 1888, with the local Catholic bishop, F. J. McCormack, taking exception and issuing a statement which was read in all the Catholic churches in the diocese and which forbade Catholic girls from attending the institution. In total, fourteen institutions, including the three Queen's Colleges, offered higher education to degree level to women students during the first ten years of the RUI. During that decade, 753 women passed examinations in arts, with 291 of these students having studied at one of the three Queen's colleges. There were also a large number of schools and colleges where female students could prepare for first and sometimes second arts examinations, as well as the matriculation examinations.[6]

Thus, from the mid-1880s, Irish women began to matriculate at medical institutions in Ireland.[7] Numbers of women were initially low but increased during the years of the First World War before decreasing again after 1918. In 1885, just one woman matriculated in medicine but by 1917 this had risen to 112.

In October 1904, seven women matriculated in medicine at Irish institutions. Among them were Harriet MacFaddin (QCG), Amy Florence Nash (RCSI) and Sarah Elizabeth Calwell (QCB), who will be a focus of this chapter. First-year students like MacFaddin, Nash and Calwell were commonly referred to in the student magazines as 'jibs' and often faced ridicule.[8] One writer for *UCG* magazine in 1919 commented that 'the first year Medicos are easily distinguished from the remainder of the "jibs" by that rakish and debonair appearance, characteristic of a budding chronic'.[9]

As for the women we will be following in this chapter, all three had initially taken the matriculation examinations of the RUI, which enabled them to enrol in the universities of their choice. MacFaddin was the daughter of a Church of Ireland clergyman. Medicine ran in Nash's family: her father, William Henry Nash, was a general practitioner, while her younger brother Edgar also went on to medical education. Calwell's father, Robert, was listed as 'builder' in the QCB matriculation records and as 'master carpenter' in the 1911 census. Like Edgar Nash, Sarah Calwell's younger brother David also went on to train as a medical student. Calwell was Presbyterian, while Nash and MacFaddin were both members of the Church of Ireland. These three women were typical in terms of their social backgrounds and their choices of university also reflect their religious persuasions. In this chapter, I will survey the women matriculating in medicine from the 1880s to 1920s, examining their possible reasons for taking up medicine, factors that may have affected their choice of medical school, as well as their social, geographical and religious backgrounds.

Students' backgrounds and reasons for studying medicine

WHAT WERE THE REASONS that might have sustained a woman's decision to take up medicine? Personal experience was often a factor. As we saw in the opening quotation to the Introduction, Emily Winifred Dickson's mother became ill when Dickson was twenty years old and she spent a year nursing her in Dublin. Dickson became deeply interested in medicine during this time and decided, with the encouragement of her father, that she would pursue a medical education.[10] Similarly, Florence Stewart, who studied at QCB in the late 1920s, was also inspired by personal experience. She lived with her aunts in Portrush from the age of eight to fourteen (from 1918 to 1924) and during this time she had her tonsils removed by her doctor and she also remembered her uncle having a perforated ulcer removed by the same doctor.[11] These incidents resulted in a deep interest in becoming a doctor.

Some Irish women may have entered into medical training because they possessed a sense of vocation to take up medicine. Maria Luddy has drawn attention to the involvement of Irish middle-class women in philanthropy in the late nineteenth and early twentieth centuries. She has pointed out how Irish middle-class women, motivated by Christian duty, were heavily involved in charitable work in that period.[12] Certainly, several early Irish women doctors involved themselves in philanthropic work which complemented their medical careers. Ella Ovenden (CU, 1904), Katharine Maguire (RCSci, 1891), Lily Baker (TCD, 1906) and Prudence Gaffikin (QCB but received LRCP LRCS Edin, LFPS Glas, 1900) were all involved in the Women's National Health Association, an organisation aimed at the prevention of tuberculosis. Mabel Crawford (née Dobbin, TCD, 1913) acted as secretary to the Dublin University Mission in addition to playing a leading role in 'Baby Week', an event organised by the Women's National Health Association, the aim of which was to reduce infant mortality rates in Ireland.[13]

For some women, this sense of vocation was what directly inspired them to become doctors. Austrian Anna Dengel (QCC, 1919) was inspired in her schooldays to take up medicine by the story of the Scottish doctor Agnes McLaren. McLaren trained in Montpellier, France, in the 1870s, because British medical schools were not open to women at that time. She then moved to Pakistan, where she founded a hospital for women and children, and spent her life devoted to the missionary cause.[14] Dengel formed a correspondence with McLaren. In her autobiography she wrote:

> Agnes McLaren pleaded for young women to study medicine and then come to the aid of the purdah woman. She even offered to help with their expenses in a small way. Her call came to my ears and kindled a fire in my heart that has not been extinguished to this day. Through her suggestion, I applied for admission to University College, Cork, Ireland, since I needed a British diploma in order to practice medicine in India. Sir Bertram Windle then the president of the medical school, was much interested in Dr. McLaren's ideas. He encouraged me to take up the study of medicine at Queen's College.[15]

Similarly, Sidney Croskery, an Irishwoman who trained at the University of Edinburgh from 1919 onwards, decided to study medicine so that she could work in the missionary field. She stated:

> I remember the day I received my 'call'. I was about seven and a half then. I told Mother with pride on the way home from Fitzroy Avenue church that I was going to be a medical missionary. It had not been a missionary sermon but a travel one. Our minister had just come back from a trip to Australia and he described very vividly immense forests of huge trees all bending the same way. I felt I would have to go and live in some such frightening place but I immediately decided that it would be more bearable if one was a doctor![16]

Unusually, Croskery had been inspired by her mother, who was also a doctor, and her older sister Lilian also decided to take up medical education.[17] Their family environment was clearly a supportive one, with their mother teaching them basic anatomy and showing them how to use a microscope. Although Croskery and Dengel were exceptions to the rule and the number of women medical students who went on to work as missionaries was low, some women medical students might have viewed medicine as a vocation and a pathway into philanthropic work. Anne Digby has pointed out that traditional Victorian upbringing and schooling meant that girls were indoctrinated 'to have high ideals of service to others and these ideals were reinforced by their medical training'.[18]

Students may also have been encouraged to enter the medical profession by teachers in their secondary schools. As discussed in the previous chapter, girls' secondary schools played an important role in the Irish women's higher education movement. Most of the Catholic women students at QCG had been educated at Catholic convent schools such as the Ursuline Convent in

Sligo and Dominican College, Galway, while Protestant girls were likely to have attended the High School, Galway. Protestant students at QCB were most commonly educated at Methodist College and Victoria College, while Catholic students tended to have come from St Dominic's High School. Catholic women medical students at QCC were most likely to have attended neighbouring convent schools, such as the Presentation Convent in Cork and St Angela's College, while Protestant women students had often attended the High School, Cork. It was also common for students of all religions to have been privately educated.[19] It is likely that students at the Dublin colleges would have attended Alexandra College or the Loreto Convent.

Harriet MacFaddin was aged eighteen when she began her medical studies, while Amy Nash was seventeen and Sarah Calwell was sixteen. Writings by medical practitioners suggested the dangers of entering into medical education too young: Isaac Ashe, writing in a prize-winning essay in 1868, stated 'that the mind of a lad of eighteen, even after the best preliminary training, is far from that mature development of the powers of reasoning and judgement'.[20] Comparing the profession of medicine to a career in the Church, for which men were not discharged until the age of twenty-three, he commented that the age of twenty-one was also too young to begin a career in medicine.[21] With regard to age, an 1892 guide for students intending to attend the Catholic University advised that, although a course in medicine could be commenced from the age of fifteen, the best age was between seventeen and twenty-one.[22] Those who intended to join the army or navy were advised to begin their studies early and to enter into service as soon as possible after their twenty-first birthday so that they might retire while still young. The age for entering the services was between twenty-one and twenty-eight, so those aged twenty-four and over when they matriculated in medicine would be unable to join the army or navy.[23]

In the case of the cohort of women medical students, the average age for a student matriculating was twenty-four, although the greatest number of women students were aged eighteen. The youngest in the cohort were aged sixteen (eighteen students) when they matriculated, although there was a small number of women in their late twenties at matriculation, and three women who matriculated in their thirties. Students may have matriculated at a later age either because they had spent a long time saving up in order to attend university or because they had a late vocational call.[24] Frances May Erskine and Marguerite Eveline Moore (both students at QCB), the oldest women in the cohort, started their medical education at the ages of thirty-nine and thirty respectively. Erskine was the daughter of a Presbyterian flax spinner, the eldest of five children, four of whom were unmarried and living at home in 1911, seven years before she matriculated.[25] Moore, who matriculated in 1917, was the eldest daughter of four unmarried children of Samuel Moore, a Presbyterian farmer in Antrim.[26] It is possible that these two women had caring or work responsibilities in the home which meant that they could not attend university until a later age.

Medical student guides from the late nineteenth century advised that anyone wishing to consider undertaking medical education ought to be of average intelligence, with fair pass marks in the Junior Grade Intermediate in the subjects of English, Latin, French (or Greek), arithmetic, algebra, Euclid and natural philosophy.[27] These qualities were specified as being important for the female medical student too. Ethel F. Lamport stated that average intellectual ability, industry and a good general education were necessary.[28] It was also essential that the female student possessed a good scientific and technical knowledge, because this would be tested in the various matriculation examinations.[29] Often, a primary degree in arts was recommended.[30] In addition to a sound preliminary education, fair intellect and good health, it was remarked that women students ought also to possess 'tenacity of purpose, natural good sense, and unwearying industry'.[31] In Elizabeth Garrett Anderson's view, because the standard of professional attainment expected of women was higher than that expected of their male counterparts, there was a distinct sense that women could not afford to be 'second rate', because their professional work would be scrutinised more closely.[32]

Not only were women expected to possess intellectual strengths but certain personality traits were deemed essential. Charles Bell Keetley in his guide for parents of prospective medical students in 1878 stated that the medical student should be kind-hearted and cheery in disposition:

> Who will deny that there is healing in the kindly eye and the cheerful face, encouragement in the manly figure and intellectual aspect, even a soothing balm in the face and form of those on whom fortune has bestowed beauty and grace? And there are sick people who have almost been, like Lazarus, awakened from the dead by a voice.[33]

Although this portrayal of the kindly doctor is aimed specifically at men, other commentators wrote on traits that related specifically to the female doctor. Lamport commented that one problem that hindered women doctors was uncouthness in dress. She drew attention to the public opinion that the medical woman 'must be of necessity an ill-dressed, slovenly, ill-mannered person, if not altogether a strange creature, half man, half woman, with perhaps a touch of "divilry" in her, that it is half-pathetic, half-comic, to hear the expression of surprise when a Woman Doctor is recognised as being a lady first, a Medical Woman after'. She suggested that if a medical woman possessed a soft, refined voice, good manners and was well dressed, she would be more successful in her profession.[34] These types of feminine qualities are similar to those that were expected of the 'angel in the house', the Victorian middle-class wife and mother. Other traits that were deemed necessary included sympathy, insight, the power of inspiring confidence and 'that indescribable, indefinable charm of personality which captivates all, and which is so extremely difficult of attainment for those who do not possess it naturally', a good natural bedside manner.[35]

Ella Ovenden (later Webb, CU, 1904), believed that the one essential qualification was a love of the work, because this was the only thing that would inspire students 'through drudgery, cheer them in disappointment, and give them strength to bear the heavy burden of responsibility which will often threaten to overwhelm them'.[36] Medical education was a serious undertaking and student guides often advised that it should not be entered into lightly, because of the long and severe course of study, which required close attention and confinement to the house, laboratory and classroom, and subsequently long hours in the wards of a hospital gaining clinical experience.[37] Clearly, women medical students needed to possess a great deal of motivation and strength of character to survive this arduous course, and perhaps they required more of this than their male counterparts, who had been an accepted part of student life for centuries. Moreover, women may have put added pressure on themselves to succeed, since career prospects were probably more competitive.[38] Edith Morley, the writer of *Women Workers in Seven Professions* (1914), remarked that enthusiasm was the first and most important qualification.[39] In addition, lady medics ought to possess good health, diligence and steadiness, as well as a 'rich spring of humour and hope'.[40]

After making the decision to undertake medical education, students then had to decide on the type of medical degree they wished to attain. By 1904, with the opening up of Trinity College Dublin (TCD) to women, women wishing to undertake medical education could do so at one of seven institutions in Ireland. Students had two options with regard to the medical qualifications they could attain: the university degree (bachelor of medicine) and the medical licence. Amy Nash aimed for the licence of the Royal College of Surgeons, while Sarah Calwell and Harriet MacFaddin aimed for medical degrees. The Catholic University's *Guide for Medical Students*, published in 1892, advised that every student who could possibly do so should seek a university degree. The difference between the course for the degree and the course for the licence was that, in order to begin the course of medical study for a licence, students needed to pass only a simple preliminary examination (an examination which was said to be easier than the Junior Grade Intermediate), whereas in the case of the RUI degree, which, as we will see later in the chapter, was what most women medical students attained, students first had to pass the matriculation examination, then devote a year to the study of arts (Latin, English, French or Greek, mathematics, physics), before passing the first university examination in arts, and only then were they eligible to begin their medical studies.[41]

The *Irish Medical Student's Guide*, published by the Dublin Medical Press in 1877, argued that if a student aspired to make a good fortune and have a successful career as a city practitioner, and if money and education were plenty, he should take the university degrees in both arts and medicine. If the student aspired to have 'good professional rank on moderate terms', he could acquire the conjoint licence from the College of Surgeons and the College of Physicians in Dublin. With regard to the university degree, the author of the guide pointed out that the student would have to undertake the prolonged study of classics and science as well as his medical studies afterwards, which would take a considerable time and cost a considerable amount of money.[42] However, if the student was content to meet the labour and expense necessary for a university education, he would begin his career as a doctor 'with all the prestige of an educated gentleman'. The guide recommended Trinity as the best university for a medical education for a student for whom money and time were no object. However, it stated that the Queen's Colleges were adequate (in spite of the fact that they did not hold the same prestige as the 'time-revered University of Dublin') because they offered students cheap university degrees; the only disadvantage, according to the guide, was that students would have to be resident for a time at Galway, Cork or Belfast.[43] Notably, there was no mention of the Catholic University in the guide, which had been in existence for over twenty-five years at the time the guide was published. The College of Surgeons and the College of Physicians, on the other hand, were thought to confer qualifications which stood well besides any in the United Kingdom, and those institutions did not require students to reside near the College or to have any qualification bar a single arts examination.[44]

The Catholic University guide, published fifteen years later, shared these sentiments, anecdotally stating that the writer knew many men who qualified with a medical licence and regretted not having attained a university degree. Emily Winifred Dickson is one graduate who did this: she initially qualified with a medical licence from the Royal College of Surgeons in 1891, but 'finding to my surprise I was apparently capable of passing examinations easily (I had the knack) I regretted not aiming at a proper degree and so matriculated at Royal University Dublin'.[45] The university degree was thought to have a higher value in the professional world than a licence and was said to be a more favourable asset than a licence when seeking appointments.[46] This explains why the majority of Irishwomen seeking to enter the medical profession sought a medical degree in preference to a medical licence. In the highly competitive medical marketplace, women doctors with degrees would have had a better chance of career success than those with a licence.

Once students had decided on the type of degree they wished to pursue, they then had to decide which medical school to attend. Keetley specified some of the reasons why a student might select one medical school over another:

> A youth usually goes to some particular place for one or more of these reasons:–
> 1. His father or the surgeon with whom he has been pupil went there before him.
> 2. He knows, or can get an introduction to, some members or member of the staff.
> 3 As a moth flies to the candle, though luckily without the same serious consequence, he is attracted by the glitter of names on the list of medical officers.[47]

In the Irish context, these factors would also have been relevant.

Some students may have chosen a career in medicine because, like Amy Nash, their fathers were doctors, and they may have decided to go to the same medical school as their fathers, as she did. Religious and economic factors would also have been relevant to Irish students of both genders. Students often went to their local universities. It was likely that this was for economic reasons, in that students could save money by living at home while at university, or for personal reasons, for example so that they could be close to their families. Sarah Calwell economised by living at home while studying at university.[48] Likewise, Amy Nash, whose parents lived on Circular Road, Dublin, was able to live at home while attending the Royal College of Surgeons.[49] Harriet MacFaddin boarded at 14 Palmyra Park, Galway, during her first year at university at QCG, which was the address of James Burke, a retired constable in the Royal Irish Constabulary, and his wife Ellie.[50]

Religious beliefs also played an important role in a student's decision regarding which university to attend. Broadly speaking, the majority of students at TCD were of Church of Ireland background, those who attended the Catholic University (later renamed University College Dublin) were Catholic, while attendees at the non-denominational or 'godless' Queen's Colleges came from different religious backgrounds, although Presbyterian students were in the majority at QCB.[51] However, prior to the opening up of TCD to women students, Protestant women would have attended one of the other universities. As Table 3.1 demonstrates, it is difficult to ascertain the religious persuasion of a large number of the students who matriculated because student registers did not always record this. Thus, we do not know the religions of 44.6 per cent of the cohort.

In his evidence before the Royal Commission on University Education in Ireland in 1901, the Reverend Monsignor Gerald Molloy, the president of the medical faculty of the Catholic University, was asked if he knew how many

Table 3.1 Religious persuasions of women medical students matriculating at Irish institutions, 1885–1922

	Catholic	Church of Ireland	Presbyterian	Methodist	Other Christians[a]	Jewish	Unknown/ not given
CU/UCD	65	0	0	0	0	0	78
TCD	7	40	16	4	2	1	53
QCB	13	20	62	13	5	2	128
QCC	104	10	1	5	2	0	2
QCG	14	3	1	0	0	0	16
RCSI	7	15	2	2	1	0	55
Other	1	2	0	0	1	0	6
Total	*211*	*90*	*82*	*24*	*11*	*3*	*338*

[a] Other Christians' may refer to: Baptist, Brethren, Church of England, Congregationalist, Episcopal, Quakers, Unitarian.
Source: Student matriculation records, 1911 census records.

of the medical students were Catholics and how many were Protestants. One might assume that all students attending the university were Catholic, yet Molloy answered that there were about a dozen Protestant medical male students and that he believed that some of the women students were also Protestants, among them the daughter of the late provost of TCD.[52] However, it is difficult to ascertain exact numbers of women from different religions at the Catholic University without the source of student registers, which often provided this information.

The QCC student registers give the most complete record of students' religious persuasions. For the first fifteen years in which women attended the QCC medical school, no Catholic women enrolled. After 1905, however, the majority of women taking medical courses at QCC were Catholic and from 1912 onwards there was a huge increase in Catholic women medical students. This increase may have occurred as a result of the Queen's Colleges' increased acceptability among Catholics from the early twentieth century and lessening of the Catholic hierarchy's hostility towards what they had previously called the 'godless' Colleges.[53]

Records for the other Queen's Colleges are incomplete, with the QCB registers listing students' religious persuasions in the cases of only some students. The QCG student registers do not list the religious persuasions of its students after 1904, although it is still possible to estimate students' religions from the 'officer at residence' to which the student had been assigned. Thirty of the thirty-five women who attended QCG for medical education between 1902 and 1922 listed Father Hynes as their officer at residence, so we could assume that these women were Catholic. Of the other five women, we know for certain that two were Anglican, and these were the first two women medical students at QCG; the third woman medical student at QCG was also possibly Anglican or Presbyterian; and the remaining two women matriculated later. The pattern of religious persuasions is essentially the same as that of QCC, with Anglican women being the first to enrol as medical students at QCG but Catholic women becoming the majority from 1914 onwards. At QCB, out of the thirty-eight medical women students for whom there was a record of religious persuasion, only two were Catholic; twelve were Church of Ireland and twenty-four were Presbyterians. This result is unsurprising.

Tables 3.2 and 3.3 demonstrate changes in religious denominations of female medical students over time. In the first two decades of their admission to medical schools, Church of Ireland women were in the majority. However, from 1903 to 1913 it is clear that there was an increase in women of all religions undertaking medical education, and by the period 1913–22 the numbers of Catholic women medical students had surpassed the numbers of Protestant women medical students.

Table 3.2 Religions of women medical students at Irish institutions over time

	Catholic	Church of Ireland	Presby-terian	Method-ist	Other Christ-ian	Jewish	Unknown/not given
1883–92	1	5	1	0	0	0	19
1893–1902	1	13	4	3	2	0	28
1903–12	22	11	5	5	4	0	33
1913–22	180	63	72	17	3	3	264
Total	*204*	*92*	*82*	*25*	*9*	*3*	*344*

Source: Student matriculation records, 1911 census.

Table 3.3 Numbers of Catholic and Protestant women medical students at Irish institutions over time

	Catholic	Protestant[a]
1883–92	1	6
1893–1902	1	22
1903–12	22	25
1913–22	180	155
Total	*204*	*208*

[a] Broadly incorporating Church of Ireland, Presbyterian, Methodist, Baptist, Brethren, Church of England, Congregationalist and Episcopal students.
Source: Student matriculation records, 1911 census.

In 1901, the Catholic share of the total Irish population was 74.2 per cent while the proportions of Church of Ireland and Presbyterian were 13.0 per cent and 9.9 per cent respectively, with figures remaining largely the same in 1911.[54] Thus, it is evident that Protestant women were more heavily represented as medical students than we might expect from their share of the general population.

For Amy Nash, from Dublin and of Church of Ireland background, the Royal College of Surgeons in Ireland was a cheaper alternative to TCD, and the Catholic University was a less likely option. Likewise, for Presbyterian Sarah Calwell, who was from Antrim, QCB would have been the obvious university to attend. For Harriet MacFaddin, it is unclear why she attended

QCG considering that she came from a Church of Ireland background and was from Kilkenny, when TCD may have been a more likely choice. It may have been because QCG was a less expensive option.

As well as religious factors, students' choice of university depended on how much time and money they, or more likely their parents, wished to spend on their education. Attending the College of Physicians or the College of Surgeons was a cheaper option for students; however, the qualification was not thought to be as venerable as the university degree. Some students may have chosen this option because it was cheaper but still meant that they could practise. TCD was the most expensive option but its degrees were thought to hold a certain prestige over those from the newer Queen's Colleges and the Catholic University. The *Irish Medical Student's Guide* in 1877 estimated that the total cost of a medical degree from TCD would be just over £198. (This was £49 12s for lectures, £33 12s for hospital fees, £32 for the cost of the degree, and £83 for a degree in arts, which was a requirement for TCD.) For a student at one of the Queen's Colleges, the guide estimated that the cost of education would be approximately £67, while the cost for the Royal College of Surgeons would be about £140.[55] In 1888, Mary Marshall, writing on 'Medicine as a profession for women' in *Woman's World* magazine, commented that the question of expense was an all-important one for the parents of any woman contemplating the study of medicine. She estimated that the actual cost of a complete medical education for a woman in the United Kingdom was just under £200, with this sum including all school, hospital and examination fees. She thought that students would require a further £50 for books, instruments and private teaching.[56]

By 1892, the Catholic University's *Guide for Medical Students* gave the following costs for a medical education at other institutions in Ireland, including the cost of lectures, hospital training, special courses and examinations (i.e. all professional expenses with the exceptions of books, instruments and private coaching or 'grindings'):[57]

Royal University, £146[58]
Conjoint Colleges of Physicians and Surgeons £162[59]
Conjoint College of Surgeons and Apothecaries Hall, £148

The guide stated that books would cost about £7–£12, instruments about £2 and grinding from £0 to £25, although it was recommended by Keetley's 1878 guide that 'an intelligent and industrious student requires little grinding in a school where the teaching is properly organised'.[60] The *Lancet* reported in 1897 that rent in Dublin was almost the same as in London (£1 per week), while in Cork rent was usually not higher than 15s a week and in the Irish provincial towns it was on average 5–6s a week.[61] The cost of living in Dublin depended on the individual, with Keetley's guide stating that most students could live comfortably on £4–£6 a month with everything included.[62] This would mean that four years of medical education through the RUI would cost a student approximately £434 in total. Keetley predicted that the total costs for four years of medical education including living costs for a student in London would be approximately £700, although he did point out that an education could be attained for much less.[63]

Considering that the largest number of women medical students were aged eighteen when they began their medical education, it is likely that they relied on the support of their parents in order to pay for their university careers. Therefore, it is unsurprising, as we shall see later, that they tended to come from affluent backgrounds. In some cases, students recorded their fathers as 'deceased', or gave the former occupation of their deceased father. The death of a father may have had serious repercussions for their children at university. Harriet MacFaddin was forced to leave university not long after beginning her medical studies. *QCG* magazine reported:

> Finally we regret the loss of the first lady who had the courage to rejoice the dissecting room with the sound of the divine feminine voice, and although we have another in her place, yet we think her loss will be felt, not alone in the medical school, but also in the various musical entertainments with which the ladies of the College raise us from things mundane to catch a glimpse of heaven. We also wish to express our sympathy with her in the sad bereavement she experienced during the summer in the loss of her father.[64]

However, there are several cases of women medical students who appear to have been supported by their widow mothers. Lucy Joly, for example, who matriculated at TCD in 1919, the middle daughter of three, was put through university by her mother, a widow who was living off dividends and interest.[65]

I was able to trace the occupations of the fathers of 542 of the 759 women medical students comprising the study cohort. As one might expect, a quick scan of the occupational categories listed in Table 3.4 and the more detailed breakdown given in Table 3.5 reveals a variety of occupations, the majority of which were respectable middle-class careers. This suggests that Irish medical schools were attracting 'ladies' rather than women from lower social classes. The largest proportion of women medical students (almost 30 per cent) came from commercial and industrial backgrounds, with another 18 per cent coming from agricultural backgrounds. Commercial and industrial occupations included careers such as merchants, grocers, shopkeepers, drapers and managers, while 'agriculture' could signify anything from a crofter to a substantial landowner.[66] Unsurprisingly, sixty-one women, like Amy Nash, came from medical backgrounds (11 per cent). Some of these women came from

Table 3.4 Occupational categories of fathers of women matriculating in medicine at all Irish institutions, 1885–1922

Occupation	Number	Percentage of all those traceable
Unknown/not given	198	
Deceased	19	
Commercial and industrial	158	29.15
Agriculture	97	17.90
Medicine	61	11.25
Religious life	48	8.85
Education	44	8.12
New professions	29	5.35
Local/central government	22	4.05
Armed forces	20	3.69
Land-related	18	3.32
Skilled working class	18	3.32
Law	18	3.32
Other	9	1.66
Total	*759*	

Source: Matriculation records for QCC, QCG, QCB, NUI; 1911 census records.

families where one or more of the siblings were also studying medicine. Alice Chance, for example, who matriculated at UCD in 1912, was the daughter of a doctor, Arthur Chance, and the fourth of seven children. Her brother Arthur, older by two years, was also a medical student.[67] Almost 9 per cent of the women medical students, such as Harriet MacFaddin, came from religious backgrounds with fathers working as clergymen. Margaret Heath Russell, the daughter of a missionary, matriculated at QCB in 1914, and followed in her father's footsteps in her own career as a medical missionary in India. Sarah Calwell was less typical of the cohort: her father's occupation was 'builder'. For Calwell's family, perhaps, a medical career for their daughter and Sarah's brother would have been a considerable step forward in social status and presumably sacrifices would have had to have been made to pay for the children's university education.

These statistics are similar to those relating to medical students at the Universities of Glasgow and Edinburgh in the late nineteenth century. Anne Crowther and Marguerite Dupree discovered that 25 per cent of students there (both male and female) came from commercial and industrial backgrounds, 17 per cent of students came from agricultural backgrounds, while 10 per cent

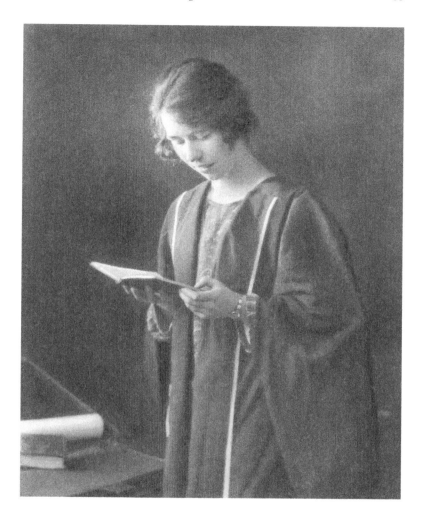

Plate I Rosaleen Hoskin, the daughter of a customs officer from Sandymount, matriculated at the Royal College of Surgeons in 1917, and graduated LRCPI & LM, LRCSI & LM in 1923, diploma in public health in 1924.

Table 3.5 Detailed occupations of fathers of women matriculating in medicine at Irish institutions, 1885–1922

Father's occupation	Number of students	% total traceable
Commercial and industrial	*158*	*29.15%*
Merchant	70	
Draper	14	
Grocer	11	
Shopkeeper	11	
Manufacturer	4	
Bank manager	4	
Manager	8	
Agent	8	
Commercial traveller	5	
Victualler	4	
Publican	3	
Seedsman	2	
Stationmaster	2	
Cashier bacon factory	1	
Caterer	1	
Cattle/horse dealer	2	
Coal importer	1	
Carriage proprietor	1	
Hotel proprietor	1	
Master of union	1	
Member of Dublin stock exchange	1	
Wholesale druggist	1	
Wholesale confectioner	1	
Director of companies	1	
Agriculture	*97*	*17.90%*
Farmer	97	
Medicine	*61*	*11.25%*
Doctor	46	
Chemist	5	
Dentist	3	
Pharmacist	3	
Vet	3	
Indian Medical Service	1	
Religious life	*48*	*8.85%*
Presbyterian clergyman	17	
Church of Ireland clergyman	13	
Undefined clergyman	11	
Wesleyan clergyman	2	
Methodist clergyman	2	
Missionary	1	
General secretary to mission house	1	
Chaplain at orphan house	1	
Education	*44*	*8.12%*
Teacher	31	
Inspector of national schools	5	
Headmaster	3	
Professor of mathematics	2	
Art master	1	
University president	1	
Secretary, Education Board	1	

New professions	29	*5.35%*
Engineer	10	
Clerk	8	
Secretary	4	
Accountant	2	
Journalist	2	
Architect	1	
Telegraphist	1	
Assurance company	1	
Local/central government	22	*4.05%*
Customs and excise officer	9	
Civil servant	6	
Member of Parliament	2	
Inland Revenue officer	1	
Overseer at general post office	1	
Consulate to Belgium	1	
National Health Insurance Commissioner	1	
Councillor	1	
Armed forces	20	*3.69%*
Royal Irish Constabulary	12	
Major, Royal Irish Fusiliers	2	
Army captain	2	
Armoured Marine Division	1	
Commander Royal Navy	1	
Royal Marines	1	
Pensioned officer	1	
Land-related	18	*3.32%*
Rate collector	4	
Gentleman	4	
Auctioneer	3	
Landowner	3	
Surveyor	3	
Land Commission inspector	1	
Skilled working class	18	*3.32%*
Builder/contractor	9	
Carriage builder	2	
Blacksmith	1	
Designer	1	
Felt maker	1	
Fish curer	1	
Hairdresser	1	
Hatter	1	
Jeweller	1	
Law	18	*3.32%*
Solicitor	14	
Barrister	3	
Justice of the peace	1	
Other	9	*1.66%*
Retired	1	
Bandmaster	1	
Doctor of music	1	
Musician	1	
Harbour officer	1	
Porter	1	
Shipowner	1	
Shipworker	1	
Warehouseman	1	

Source: Student matriculation albums, 1911 census records.

came from medical backgrounds.[68] Evidently, Irish women medical students
in the period, like their female counterparts in Scotland,[69] came from respectable backgrounds. Their matriculation into Irish medical schools and later
success in medical careers proved that it was possible to retain one's feminine
delicacy, or remain a lady, while pursuing a medical education and career.

Patterns of matriculation

IN 1904, when Calwell, MacFaddin and Nash matriculated, there were only
seven women medical students matriculating, in comparison with 271 men.
As Figures 3.1 and 3.2 demonstrate, the numbers of women matriculating in
medicine at Irish institutions were initially low, with only forty-one women
matriculating in the ten-year period between 1885 and 1895. After 1888, it
became uncommon for women to train at any of the smaller medical schools,
such as Carmichael College, which were by this stage largely extinct. These
low numbers are typical of numbers attending university in Ireland more
generally. In 1901, out of a population of 4.5 million, just 3,259 people were
attending university, of whom only ninety-one were women.[70] Indeed, in
1901, there were just two women matriculating in medicine, Anne Beamish

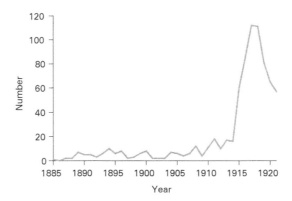

Figure 3.1 Numbers of women medical students matriculating in medicine
at all Irish institutions, 1885–1922.

Source: Matriculation records of QCB, QCC, QCG; *Medical Students' Register*, 1884–1922.

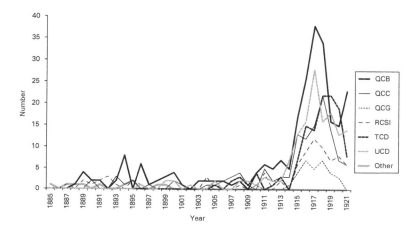

Figure 3.2 Numbers of women matriculating in medicine at individual
Irish institutions, 1885–1922.

Source: Matriculation records of QCB, QCC, QCG; *Medical Students' Register*, 1884–1922.

Reynolds at QCC and Maria Rowan at QCB. From 1895 to 1905, there were
forty-six women matriculating in medicine and numbers steadily increased
from the mid-1900s, with 104 matriculating between 1905 and 1915. This
was in line with patterns at Irish institutions more generally, which saw a
steady growth in women students occurring in this period, with increased
acceptance of women attending university. As is particularly evident from
Figures 3.1 and 3.2, the numbers of women medical students rose significantly
during the First World War. An article in the *Daily Graphic* in September
1914 stated that there were more places available for women in medical
schools as a result of the huge numbers of medical men who had gone off to
war.[71] The *Queen*, in February 1915, commented on the fact that the war had
given 'a most remarkable impetus to the demand, on the part of women for
fuller opportunities of gaining medical and surgical experience'.[72] At QCB, for
example, in 1912, one in twenty medical students were female, while by 1918
one in four were female. During the years of the war, 384 women matriculated
in medicine in Ireland. In 1914, just sixteen women had done so, but in 1915
numbers increased to sixty, and they rose again to eighty-five in 1916. In 1917
there were 112 women matriculating in medicine and in 1918 there were 111.

Table 3.6 Numbers of medical students, male and female, matriculating at Irish institutions, 1897–1906[a]

	CU		QCB		QCC		QCG		RCSI		TCD	
	Female	Male	Female	Male	Female	Male	Female	Male	Female	Male	Female	Male
1897	0	45	1	48	1	21	0	8	0	38	0	47
1898	0	55	2	36	0	37	0	10	0	35	0	56
1899	2	48	3	47	0	38	0	13	0	50	0	57
1900	2	70	4	42	2	30	0	10	0	43	0	48
1901	0	70	1	39	1	42	1	11	0	40	0	62
1902	1	71	0	35	0	45	0	12	0	25	0	45
1903	0	61	2	56	0	35	0	6	0	27	0	41
1904	0	65	2	56	1	46	1	10	3	38	0	56
1905	2	66	2	53	1	44	0	13	0	39	1	65
1906	0	71	2	37	2	33	0	7	0	46	0	42
Total	7	622	19	449	8	371	2	100	3	381	1	519
% females	1.1%		4.2%		2.11%		1.96%		0.78%		0.19%	

[a] Table compiled using Molloy's table in addition to my own statistics relating to women medical students. G. Molloy, *Progress of the Catholic University Medical School: Extract from the Evidence of the Right Rev. Monsignor Molloy, D.D. D.Sc., Given Before the Royal Commission on University Education in Ireland, 1901* (Dublin: Humphrey and Armour Printers, 1907), appendix A. Molloy's appendix A was compiled from the official *Medical Students' Register* published annually under the direction of the General Medical Council, which showed the number of medical students in each of the Irish medical schools during the years 1897–1906 inclusive.

However, with the return of men from the war after 1918, the numbers of women matriculating in medicine dropped to eighty-one in 1919 and sixty-five in 1920, with fifty-seven women matriculating in the 1921/22 term.[73] Unfortunately, no comprehensive set of figures survives for male medical students in Ireland. However, Molloy compiled statistics relating to numbers of medical students at Irish institutions between 1897 and 1906 which were published in 1907. Table 3.6 demonstrates the stark contrast between numbers of men and women medical students matriculating at Irish institutions in this period. This table is a compilation of statistics collected by Molloy in relation to numbers of students matriculating at Irish universities and my own statistics relating to numbers of women students. I attained these figures for male students by subtracting my numbers for female students matriculating from Molloy's totals for all medical students matriculating. Molloy gathered his statistics as part of his report on the progress of the Catholic University medical school which was given before the Royal Commission on Irish University Education in 1901. He extended these figures up to 1906 in the published edition of the report.[74] In this period, there were forty women matriculating in medicine in total and 2,442 men, indicating that women medical students comprised just 1.6 per cent of the overall number of medical students.

QCB had the highest number of women medical students of the universities in this period, with women representing 4.2 per cent of their medical student body. TCD had the lowest (under 0.2 per cent) but this is owing to the limited date range of the study, as TCD did not open its doors to women medical students until 1904. Despite having a greater intake of students, the Catholic University had a lower percentage of female students than QCB. However, this is likely to have been a result of the higher number of Protestant women taking up medical education in the twenty-year period from 1883 to 1903. In the next section, I will examine how many of the women medical students in the cohort made it through to graduation.

Graduation

WRITING IN HIS MEMOIRS in 1956, Bethel Solomons, an Irish doctor who trained at TCD in the early 1900s, commented:

Today the number of students wishing to enter the schools of Great Britain and Ireland is in excess of the number of vacancies. When I was a student, the schools were glad to get pupils, and in my year we started with fifty-eight and several dropped out. Probably fifty qualified. I think the student of today has to work harder than his brother of the past.[75]

Out of the 759 women who matriculated in medicine at Irish institutions between 1885 and 1922, 452 were successful in graduating with medical degrees, a success rate of 60 per cent. Unfortunately, we do not possess statistics on the drop-out rates for female students and medical students in general. For Irish students at the University of Glasgow between 1859 and 1900, approximately 35 per cent failed to make it to graduation.[76] The drop-out rate for medical students generally at the University of Glasgow in this period was 27 per cent.[77]

Two of the three women medical students we have been following, Sarah Calwell and Amy Nash, succeeded in qualifying, while Harriet MacFaddin did not. Calwell took eight years to graduate with a medical degree from QCB in 1912, while Nash was more typical, taking six years to graduate with her medical licence from the Royal College of Surgeons in 1910. We learnt earlier that MacFaddin was forced to leave university after the death of her father.[78] In their study of medical students at the University of Glasgow and the University of Edinburgh in the nineteenth century, Crowther and Dupree attributed the high drop-out rate among students to several factors. Often, ill-health and poverty prevented students from completing their studies.[79] Some students may have struggled with having to pay the yearly university fees, hospital fees and other necessary expenses. Medical students in particular would have faced risk of disease and illness through their practical experience working in hospitals and entering the homes of the poor. Failure at examinations may also have been a reason why some women did not graduate. Some students may have decided that a career in medicine was simply not for them: Matilda Caldwell Dagg, the first female medical student at QCG, failed to graduate; however, by 1911, at the age of twenty-nine, she was working as a teacher in Cork.[80] It is possible that women medical students may have had lower levels of support from their family for their chosen career than their male counterparts, meaning that they may have been less likely to graduate.

The time taken from matriculation to graduation varied. The average time for a female student to qualify was six years, although the greatest number of students (38 per cent) took five years to graduate with a medical qualification. Occasionally, there were instances of women students who took far longer to qualify, with fifteen students taking between ten and fourteen years. These students were often referred to as 'chronics'. In his account of his life as a medical student and doctor, Thomas Garry painted a grim picture of the chronic medical student:

> There were always innumerable 'chronics' leading a hopelessly precarious existence. At the beginning of each session, they lay in wait for new students who were generally unsophisticated and had plenty of money. Like all addicts whether of drink or drugs, they took immense delight in dragging others down to their own level.[81]

Bethel Solomons defined a chronic student as one who took as much as twelve years to qualify but emphasised that they 'often proved in the end to be good practical doctors', though Isaac Ashe, writing in 1868, claimed that these students often ended up working as unqualified assistants.[82] Kathleen Rose Byrne was one such student. She matriculated initially at TCD in the 1918/19 term but did not graduate with her degree until 1932, although we do not know why it took her and the other women in this category so long to qualify. She was listed in the *Medical Directory* at an address in Dublin from 1937 to 1947, so is likely to have worked as a general practitioner.

The types of qualifications that women medical graduates in the period succeeded in gaining are indicated in Figure 3.3. Evidently, the majority of students graduated with the MB BCh BAO degree, which was, as we saw earlier, generally viewed as being a superior qualification, albeit more expensive than the option of attaining the conjoint medical licence from the College of Surgeons and the College of Physicians. In a small number of cases, women medical students matriculated initially through Irish institutions but then went on to achieve their degrees elsewhere in the United Kingdom, or a licence from the Glasgow or Edinburgh Colleges of Physicians and Surgeons. It is unclear why women would have gone to Glasgow or Edinburgh to

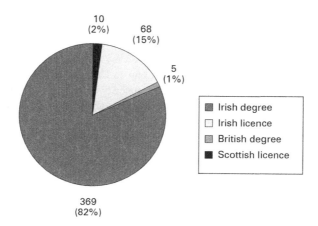

Figure 3.3 Qualifications of women medical graduates who matriculated at all Irish institutions, 1885–1922.

Source: *Medical Directory, Medical Register,* university calendars.

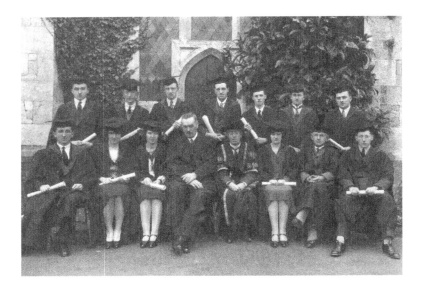

Plate II Medicine graduation day at University College Cork, 8 February 1927.

attain their licences but, according to Garry, who trained at QCG and at Dublin hospitals in the 1880s, this was a common practice and 'the periodic departure of students from Dublin to Edinburgh was always observed as a great event'.[83] It is clear that the majority of women medical students viewed a degree in medicine as being an important asset, and followed the advice of the student guides outlined earlier, which claimed that the achievement of a medical degree would allow students greater potential in their careers.

Conclusion

BY 1908, the numbers of women medical students were beginning to rise at Irish universities, leading the student magazine *QCC* to exclaim:

> The lady-medicals!!! No more – vide Cummins, Mockler, etc. In spite of all, we could not do without them. Picture the library, a wilderness without their interruptions, infer–eternal rustlings, bustlings, flirtings, and maddeningly irritating giggles.[84]

Although the numbers of women medical students matriculating at Irish institutions were small in the first three decades of their existence, numbers increased during the years of the First World War before falling in the years following it. This chapter has examined the social, geographical and religious backgrounds of these women medical students matriculating at Irish institutions from the 1880s to 1920s as well as discussing the possible reasons why a woman might have decided to take up medical education and the factors that might have affected her choice of university. Religious factors would have played some role in a woman's choice of university. Notably, the majority of early women undertaking medical education came from Protestant backgrounds. However, by the 1900s, following the opening of the Catholic University to women medical students in 1898, Catholic women students also began to take up medicine and there was an increase of Catholic women attending the Queen's Colleges also.

It is evident, however, that economic factors were most pertinent in both a student's decision to take up medical education and the type of qualification chosen. Students generally attended their local university, as this would have enabled them to save money through living at home. Additionally, the data have shown that the majority of women medical students in the period came from well-to-do backgrounds. Medicine would have been viewed as a respectable career for women of these backgrounds but their parents would also have had the finances to pay for their daughters' education. Of the 759 women who matriculated in medicine, 60 per cent succeeded in qualifying, with the majority (83 per cent) qualifying with the superior qualification of medical degree as opposed to licence (17 per cent). The following chapter will look at the experiences of these women while undergoing their medical training.

Notes

1 'The medical profession for women', *Freeman's Journal*, 18 August 1898, p. 4.
2 *Ibid.*
3 'Students in "Ye Citie of ye Tribes"', *QCG: A Record of College Life in the City of the Tribes*, 3:1 (1904), p. 25.
4 'Apologies', *Quarryman*, 1:2 (1914), p. 20.
5 Eibhlin Breathnach, 'Charting new waters: women's experience in higher education, 1879–1908', in Mary Cullen (ed.), *Girls Don't Do Honours: Irish Women in Education in the 19th and 20th Centuries* (Dublin: Women's Education Bureau, 1987), p. 58.
6 *Ibid.*, p. 60.
7 Matriculation refers here specifically to students enrolling in medicine in their first year of study and who appear in the matriculation albums/student registers of Irish universities.
8 One writer in the *UCG* student magazine in 1914 commented of the first-year medical students that year: 'And we hear too, that excessive mental exertion isn't apt to bring on any attacks of chronic meningitis amongst them. But you can't blame them really.'

That's all the ladies' fault. There are five of them, each taking out some of the lectures. It makes us sad to think of it. When we were young and promising jibs, there were no ladies in class with us. Otherwise we'd be First Medicals yet, we're afraid.' *UCG: A College Annual*, 1:2 (1914), p. 67.

9   'Medical notes', *UCG* (1919–20), p. 57. 'Chronics' are discussed later in the chapter.

10 Typed memoirs of Emily Winifred Dickson, private collection of Niall Martin, Edinburgh.

11 Florence Stewart papers, Public Record Office of Northern Ireland (D3612/3/1).

12 Maria Luddy, *Women and Philanthropy in Nineteenth-Century Ireland* (Cambridge: Cambridge University Press, 1995).

13 'Dublin university Fuh-Kien mission', *Irish Times*, 14 November 1914, p. 10; 'National Baby Week for Ireland', *BMJ*, 12 May 1917, p. 783.

14 'Anna Maria Dengel', in Leone McGregor Hellstedt (ed.), *Women Physicians of the World: Autobiographies of Medical Pioneers* (Washington, DC, and London: Medical Women's International Federation, Hemisphere Publishing Corporation, 1978), p. 92.

15 *Ibid.*, p. 93.

16 Sidney Elizabeth Croskery, *Whilst I Remember* (Belfast: Blackstaff Press, 1983), p. 13.

17 These two women are not in the cohort as they did not matriculate at Irish institutions.

18 Anne Digby, *The Evolution of British General Practice, 1850–1948* (Oxford: Oxford University Press, 1999), p. 163.

19 Matriculation records for QCC, QCB, QCG, respectively held at University College Cork Archives, Queen's University Belfast Archives, National University of Ireland, Galway (Registrar's Office).

20 Isaac Ashe, *Medical Education and Medical Interests*, Carmichael Prize Essay (Dublin: Fannin, 1868), p. 25.

21 *Ibid.*

22 *Guide for Medical Students, More Especially for Those About to Commence Their Medical Studies, by the Registrar of the Catholic University Medical School* (Dublin: Browne and Nolan, 1892), p. 6.

23 *Ibid.*

24 Anne Crowther and Marguerite Dupree, *Medical Lives in the Age of Surgical Revolution* (Cambridge: Cambridge University Press, 2007), p. 16.

25 1911 census record for Erskine family, Drumnadrough, Antrim, National Library Archives of Ireland, Dublin.

26 1911 census record for Moore Family, Ballyhelim, Bushmills, Antrim.

27 *Guide for Medical Students*, p. 5.

28 Ethel Lamport, 'Medicine as a profession for women', in *Education and Professions*, The Women's Library, vol. 1 (London: Chapman and Hall, 1903), p. 261.

29 *Ibid.*

30 *Guide for Medical Students*, p. 8.

31 Elizabeth Garrett Anderson, 'A special chapter for ladies who propose to study medicine', in Charles Bell Keetley, *The Student's Guide to the Medical Profession* (London: Macmillan, 1878), p. 43.

32 *Ibid.*, p. 44.

33 Keetley, *The Student's Guide to the Medical Profession*, p. 8.

34 Lamport, 'Medicine as a profession', pp. 262–3.

35 *Ibid.*, p. 262.

36 Ella Ovenden, 'Medicine', in Myrrha Bradshaw (ed.), *Open Doors for Irishwomen: A Guide to the Professions Open to Educated Women in Ireland* (Dublin: Irish Central Bureau for the Employment of Women, 1907), p. 35.

37 Lamport, 'Medicine as a profession', p. 261.

38 Digby, *The Evolution of British General Practice*, p. 153.

39 Edith J. Morley, 'The medical profession', in *Women Workers in Seven Professions: A Survey of Their Economic Conditions and Prospects* (London: Routledge, 1914), p. 138.

40 *Ibid.*
41 *Guide for Medical Students*, p. 9.
42 *Irish Medical Student's Guide* (Dublin: Dublin Medical Press, 1877), pp. 28–9.
43 *Ibid.*, p. 29.
44 *Ibid.*
45 Typed memoirs of Emily Winifred Dickson.
46 *Guide for Medical Students*, p. 10.
47 Keetley, *The Student's Guide to the Medical Profession*, p. 17.
48 1911 census record for Calwell family, 36 Old Park Road, Clifton, Antrim.
49 1911 census record for Nash family, 8 Rathdown Terrace, Circular Road, Dublin.
50 1911 census record for Burke family, 14 Palmyra Park, Galway.
51 In the nineteenth century, 65 per cent of all students were Presbyterian, 17 per cent
    Anglican, 6 per cent Catholic and 13 per cent classed as 'others'. From: Peter Froggatt,
    'The distinctiveness of Belfast medicine and its medical school', *Ulster Medical Journal*,
    54:2 (October 1985), pp. 89–108, on p. 97, taken from T. W. Moody and J. C. Beckett,
    Queen's Belfast 1849–1945: The History of a University (London: Faber and Faber,
    1959), vol. 2, appendix 2.
52 Gerald Molloy, *Progress of the Catholic University Medical School: Extract from
    the Evidence of the Right Rev. Monsignor Molloy, D.D. D.Sc., Given Before the Royal
    Commission on University Education in Ireland, 1901* (Dublin: Humphrey and Armour
    Printers, 1907), p. 24.
53 Matriculation albums for students at QCC.
54 Sean Connolly, *Religion and Society in Nineteenth-Century Ireland* (Dundalk: Econ-
    omic and Social History Society of Ireland, 1985), p. 3.
55 *Irish Medical Student's Guide*, p. 63.
56 Mary A. Marshall, 'Medicine as profession for women', *Woman's World*, January 1888,
    p. 108.
57 *Guide for Medical Students*, p. 6.
58 Breakdown of costs: first year, £16 6s; second year, £33 12s; third year, £30 9s; fourth
    year, £48 6s; examination fees, £17.
59 Breakdown of costs: first year, £35 14s; second year, £39 18s; third year, £39 18s; fourth
    year, £44 2s; fee for preliminary examination, £2 2s.
60 Keetley, *The Student's Guide to the Medical Profession*, p. 6.
61 'The cost of medical education', *Lancet*, 150:3860 (21 August 1897), pp. 437–8.
62 Keetley, *The Student's Guide to the Medical Profession*, p. 7.
63 *Ibid.*, p. 14.
64 'Medicine', *QCG*, 3:1 (1904), p. 16.
65 1911 census record for Joly family, Raglan Road, Pembroke West, Dublin.
66 Crowther and Dupree, *Medical Lives in the Age of Surgical Revolution*, p. 27.
67 1911 census record for Chance family, 90 Merrion Square, Trinity Ward, Dublin.
68 Crowther and Dupree, *Medical Lives in the Age of Surgical Revolution*, p. 28.
69 *Ibid.*, p. 43.
70 Susan M. Parkes, 'Higher education, 1793–1908', in W. E. Vaughan (ed.), *A New
    History of Ireland. Vol. 6: Ireland Under the Union II 1870–1921* (Oxford: Clarendon
    Press, 1996), pp. 539–70, on p. 540.
71 *Daily Graphic*, 23 September 1914. (From scrapbook relating to the Royal Free Hospital
    and the medical education of women, Royal Free Hospital Archive, London.)
72 *Queen*, 27 February 1915. (From scrapbook relating to the Royal Free Hospital and the
    medical education of women.)
73 Numbers calculated from university matriculation records and the *Medical Students'
    Register*.
74 G. Molloy, *Progress of the Catholic University Medical School: Extract from the Evidence
    of the Right Rev. Monsignor Molloy, D.D. D.Sc., Given Before the Royal Commission on*

University Education in Ireland, 1901 (Dublin: Humphrey and Armour Printers, 1907), appendix A.

75 Bethel Solomons, *One Doctor in His Time* (London: Christopher Johnson, 1956), p. 34.

76 Laura Kelly, 'Irish medical students at the University of Glasgow, 1859–1900' (MLitt thesis, University of Glasgow, 2007), p. 56.

77 Crowther and Dupree, *Medical Lives in the Age of Surgical Revolution*, p. 47.

78 'Medicine', *QCG*, 3:1 (1904), p. 16.

79 Crowther and Dupree, *Medical Lives in the Age of Surgical Revolution*, p. 47.

80 1911 census record for Matilda Caldwell Dagg.

81 Thomas Garry, *African Doctor* (London: John Gifford, 1939), p. 15.

82 Solomons, *One Doctor in His Time*, p. 34, and Ashe, *Medical Education and Medical Interests*, p. 28.

83 Garry, *African Doctor*, p. 16.

84 'Cherchez la femme', *QCC*, 5:1 (1908), p. 19.

4

Women's experiences of Irish medical education

... Though all the world's a stage and we are acting,
Yet still I think your part is not dissecting,
To me the art of making apple tarts
Would suit you better than those 'horrid parts'.
In times to come when queens at home you are,
There'll be more rapture in the light guitar.
Your knowledge – of the frog should only be
How they are cooked in France – or making tea!
And as for learning Chemistry and that
'Twould be a nicer thing to trim a hat.
I know your aims in medicine are true
But tell me is there any *need* of you?[1]

THIS POEM, entitled 'Ode to the lady medicals' and published in 1902, in *St Stephen's*, the student magazine of the Catholic University, questions the relatively recent undertaking of medical education by women. Although admittedly tongue-in-cheek, it highlights some of the prevalent attitudes towards the admission of women to medicine, a subject that had faced fierce criticism from some. Certainly, this poem strongly suggests that a woman's place should be in the home, learning how to cook frogs rather than how to dissect them, and that women should concern themselves with more feminine activities, such as hat-trimming. Moreover, it ends on the question of whether there was actually any need for women doctors, highlighting fears about the overcrowded medical marketplace. Thus, arts degrees were often proclaimed as being a more suitable alternative for lady students.[2]

We know little about the experiences of medical students of that time.[3] Even less work has been done on the educational experiences of women doctors in the first half of the twentieth century.[4] But how is it possible to find out what it was like to be a student in Ireland in the late nineteenth and early twentieth centuries? Barbara Brookes has utilised the unique source of Agnes Bennett's letters in order to gain an insight into the lives of women medical graduates of the University of Edinburgh, while Andrew Warwick has studied the mathematics curriculum of the University of Cambridge in the late nineteenth and early twentieth centuries in order to understand student experience there.[5] In this chapter, I will draw on medical student guides and university handbooks and calendars, which give us some idea of what students studied. The minute books of university medical societies go some way to revealing the extra-curricular activities of medical students. Additionally, the minute books of the Royal Victoria Hospital in Belfast give an insight into issues relating to the clinical experience of lady medicals. Of course, there are limitations in using official matter. University guides and minute books do not provide a complete record of student experience but rather tend to give us information on what students studied rather than their educational experiences. I therefore also draw on the memoirs of lady doctors and on student magazines for a better understanding of what student life was like.

Student magazines are valuable for gauging insight into attitudes towards lady medicals. Written by students for students, they give us an engaging view of their day-to-day life and it is surprising that few historians of science or medicine have used this resource.[6] Most Irish university magazines appeared at the turn of the century, such as *QCB*, the magazine of Queen's College Belfast. As a result, the magazines give the sharpest insight into the early twentieth century. Queen's College Galway and Queen's College Cork also had their own magazines, *QCG* and *QCC*.[7] The Catholic University, which later became University College Dublin, had its own magazine, *St Stephen's*, which later became the *National Student*. The magazine of Trinity College Dublin was *TCD: A College Miscellany*, while the *RCSI Student Quarterly* was the student publication of the Royal College of Surgeons in Ireland. It is difficult to determine what readership, apart from the students, these magazines had, but there is evidence that some, such as the *National Student*, had a readership outside the student population. For instance, the Irish writer and suffragist Francis Sheehy Skeffington often used it for the propagation of his political ideas.[8] And, although the editorial board was composed of students and most of the contributors were students, occasionally pieces by lecturers were published. Medical students were often contributors to these magazines, giving comment on subjects from medical education to university life and even amusing incidents that happened in a lecture one morning. Humour was an important element in the magazines, creating, as Janet Browne puts it, 'a common matrix: the social cement, as it were, of the undergraduate world'.[9]

Similarly, the memoirs of women doctors, although a rare source, are very useful because they are first-hand reports of their experiences. However, because they are personal accounts, they do not always give us a deep insight into women's experience more generally and they may also be biased or limited in terms of the information given about their education. I will draw on the unpublished memoirs of Emily Winifred Dickson (RCSI, 1891) and Florence Stewart (QUB, 1933) and the published memoirs of Anna Dengel (QCC, 1919) and Octavia Wilberforce (LSMW, 1920). Dickson and Stewart's memoirs were written presumably as accounts for their families, while Dengel's experiences were published in a collection of autobiographies of women doctors from around the world, and Wilberforce's autobiography was published for the general public.

I will also draw upon the minute books of the Belfast Medical Students' Association, which give an insight into the debates which took place in the university on matters relating to medical education and the medical profession. Sources relating to student societies are also under-utilised by historians but give an insight into the extra-curricular activities of students and thus deepen our knowledge of student experience.

In this chapter, I will suggest that, in contrast to Britain, Irish medical education from the 1880s to the 1920s was surprisingly egalitarian in nature, with women and men treated equally in terms of hospital experience, lectures, which they attended together, and prizes and scholarships, which were open to women on the same terms as to men. I will highlight important differences between Irish and British medical education with regard to the admission of women to hospital wards for clinical experience. However, despite Ireland's seemingly favourable attitude towards women medical students, there was one important exception: the dissecting room. Irish university authorities constructed separate dissecting rooms for male and female students, in addition to creating separate 'ladies' rooms' (i.e. common rooms for women). Not only did these physically separate spaces help to establish the identity of lady medicals students as a separate community but they also served a paternalistic function, providing them with protection from the men students who may have threatened to sully their 'sweet influence', 'good conduct and feminine modesty'.[10] Yet, as will be shown, this segregation went beyond the physical structure of the dissecting room and was not always promoted only by the university authorities. In some cases, women medical students separated themselves from the men as a distinct social group.

I will first examine students' experiences of medical education and attitudes to women medical students, in particular focusing on the topic of clinical education because this is where women students, in contrast to their counterparts in Britain, found themselves readily accepted. I will then discuss how Irish universities and hospitals showed themselves to be forward-thinking and egalitarian with regard to the medical education of women, with men and women being co-educated for most lectures. The one exception, which I will discuss in depth in the subsequent section of the chapter, was the dissecting room. The chapter will lastly examine how women also socially segregated themselves from the male students through their living arrangements and social activities. I will suggest that although Irish medical education from the 1880s to 1920s was more egalitarian than medical education elsewhere in the United Kingdom and women appear to have been strongly supported and incorporated, there still existed a distinct sense of separateness between the men and women students.

Studying medicine: attitudes and experiences

A SHORT STORY published in the *Quarryman* in March 1917, entitled 'How Lill got her M.D.', tells the tale of one woman student who, having succeeded in gaining an arts degree, also wanted to achieve a medical degree, solely, it seems, so that she could wear the 'becoming' scarlet graduation gown.[11] Lill crosses the quadrangle of the College and goes straight to the president of the university, threatening to expose him in the *Quarryman* and 'bribe the maid to put nettles in [his] Morphean couch' until the nervous president finally gives in and awards her the MD degree.[12] This story not only presents a view of women students as being more interested in fashion than academic pursuit but is indicative of the somewhat chauvinistic attitudes prevalent in the student magazines of the time. Arguably, it also shows cunning, determination and a scheming mind. In this section, I will examine attitudes to women medical students in the student press before looking at what it was like to study medicine in Ireland in the period.

Although the student press tended to mock women medical students, they were often seen as having a civilising effect on the men and were referred to affectionately. Male medical students were allegedly notorious for rowdy behaviour.[13] Thomas Neville Bonner argues that male medical students were characterised as being drunken, immature and irreverent, an image which persisted well into the second half of the nineteenth century and even into the early twentieth century.[14] As well as having a civilising effect on the male students, lady medicals were also said to be a distraction. In 1904, one writer in *TCD: A College Miscellany* stated that the presence of the female student in the physiological laboratory produced a 'laevo-rotatory action upon the eyes of mere man'.[15] However, university staff were also said to be affected. An article in the 1919–20 *UCG* annual claimed that the lady medicals of that year were very distracting to a certain impressionable young professor. The writer claimed: 'it is said that the closing of his eye in focusing a microscopic object for a certain Medica is a masterpiece of "Cupid Ophthalmology"'.[16] Lady students in general were thought to bring disadvantages. An article in *QCG* in 1904 commented that 'the continual rustling of skirts, the rattling of jewellery and the general "titivating" that a lady student thinks it her bounden duty to keep up during a lecture are – well, rather disconcerting'.[17] A comment in *QCB* drew attention to a female medical student who 'talks so frequently and affectionately to Male Medicals during lectures'.[18]

At the same time, women students were thought to have a positive effect on Irish medical institutions. A writer for *QCC* questioned where the medical school's peaceful charm would be 'without the same sweet faces that haunt our sanctum, not once, but twice, thrice and more times than we can count a day?'[19] More common, however, were pieces which poked fun at the women students. The author of a piece in *QCB* stated that he could not look at the lady medical 'without a pang at seeing so much sweet womanhood going astray ... if nature had intended woman to be a doctor she would have created her a man'.[20] Moreover, he added that he would refuse to let a woman operate on him, not because he feared her knife would slip through nervousness, but because he was afraid her 'infernal curiosity would tempt her to push the knife a little too far, just to see how [he] could stand it'.[21] Articles such as this, which use humour to convey the idea that medical education would potentially result in a loss of womanliness, also reinforce the male/female divide by drawing attention to other important arguments against women in medicine which proliferated at the time.

Often, the pursuit of a medical education was seen as a waste of time and money by the families of women medical students, and family support or lack of it could colour student experience. Parents may have been unwilling or unable to pay for the medical education of a daughter who could otherwise look after the home. It was believed by many that a career in medicine made a woman less suitable for marriage, as we learnt in Chapter 1. One commentator in 1886 stated that the family of a prospective woman doctor, 'not wishing to lose her pleasant companionship, plausibly object on the ground that as she will most likely marry soon, the cost of her medical education will be so much money wasted'.[22] Indeed, this was the case for Olive Pedlow, who trained at Queen's College Belfast in the early 1920s. Her father persuaded her to do an arts degree because he thought that she would 'waste' a medical degree on marriage. Pedlow obtained a first-class honours degree in French and German in 1917 and won enough prizes during her years as an arts student to enable her to pay for her first two years of medical study, at which point her father gave in.[23] Perhaps, Pedlow's determination to acquire a medical

Table 4.1 Proposed timetable for medical students in their second year at Queen's College Belfast, March 1901

	9–10	10–11	11–12	12–1	1–2	2–3	3–4	4–5
Monday	Hospital	Hospital	Practical chemistry	Anatomy		Physiology	Practical anatomy	Materia medica
Tuesday	Hospital	Hospital	Junior physiology	Anatomy		Physiology	Anatomy	Materia medica
Wednesday	Anatomy	Practical chemistry	Senior physiology	RUI men can continue practical chemistry or dissect		Practical histology after Xmas, practical anatomy before Xmas	Practical histology after Xmas, practical anatomy before Xmas	Materia medica
Thursday	Hospital	Hospital	Junior physiology	Anatomy		Practical histology after Xmas, practical anatomy before Xmas	Practical histology after Xmas, practical anatomy before Xmas	Materia medica
Friday	Anatomy	Practical chemistry	As on Wednesday	As on Wednesday		As on Wednesday	As on Wednesday	
Saturday	Hospital	Hospital						

Source: Minute book of the medical faculty of Queen's College Belfast, 1891–1907, Queen's University Belfast Archives (QUB/D/2/3/1).

Table 4.2 Proposed timetable for medical students in their third year at Queen's College Belfast, March 1901

	9–10	10–11	11–12	12–1	1–2	2–3	3–4	4–5
Monday	Hospital	Hospital	Hospital	Anatomy		Physiology	Practical anatomy	Surgery
Tuesday	Hospital	Hospital	Hospital	Anatomy		Practical physiology after Xmas, practical anatomy before	Practical physiology after Xmas, practical anatomy before	Surgery
Wednesday		Practical anatomy	Senior physiology	Anatomy		Practical anatomy	Practical anatomy	Surgery
Thursday	Hospital	Hospital		Anatomy		Practical physiology after Xmas, practical anatomy before	Practical physiology after Xmas, practical anatomy before	Surgery
Friday		Practical anatomy	Senior physiology	Anatomy		Practical anatomy	Practical anatomy	
Saturday	Hospital	Hospital						

Source: Minute book of the medical faculty of Queen's College Belfast, 1891–1907, Queen's University Belfast Archives (QUB/D/2/3/1).

education was her attempt to break out of the private sphere of marriage and instead enter the male-dominated public sphere of work. She nonetheless went on to marry and to combine a successful career with raising a family. In some cases, family commitments may partly explain the high drop-out rate for women medical students.

Medical students of both genders often struggled under the double burden of passing examinations and paying yearly fees. Anna Dengel, who graduated from Queen's College Cork in 1919, commented of her time at university:

> These were hard years for me. I was poor and had to do all sorts of work to pay the tuition, but kind people and my own determination saw me through to graduation with honours. It was 1919 by then. I needed a fee of five pounds in order to sit for the final examination. The sum was lent to me by Professor Mary Ryan[24] whose brother later became Bishop of Trinidad. This was the only debt I incurred, and I repaid it with part of my first salary.[25]

Like Dengel, Brigid Lyons Thornton, who trained at Galway, found that her time at university was a 'struggle and a constant financial worry'.[26] In addition to the yearly fees that students had to pay for their course of medical instruction, there were the added costs of travel home to see their families, and fees to the hospitals where they undertook their practical experience. Students also had the option of obtaining private instruction or 'grinding'.[27] This was conducted by private teachers, who were often connected with schools of medicine, for instance as a hospital physician or surgeon, and thus in a position to afford special advantages with regard to the clinical instruction of their pupils.[28]

The medical programme at the Queen's Colleges was intense, with second- and third-year students working from nine to five, Monday to Friday, as well as two hours gaining hospital experience on Saturday mornings as part of the requirement to gain nine months' hospital attendance each year. Surviving timetables are reproduced as Tables 4.1 and 4.2. These indicate the juxtaposition of hospital experience with other subjects and demonstrate the range of subjects taught at Queen's College Belfast in 1901 and the great emphasis on practical and clinical (hospital) work within the syllabus. This chapter will focus on these practical and clinical elements. The clinical work is demonstrative of an area where women medical students found themselves particularly supported, while the practical (the example here being anatomy) was an area of study in which separation was enforced.

Students intending to take the MB BCh BAO examination were required to show proof that they had clinical experience in a variety of areas.[29] In the first half of the nineteenth century, Irish medical students gained hospital experience from their first year of medical study. However, by the late 1880s, this hospital training had been postponed until their second year so that they might be provided with a stronger rudimentary education, which would benefit their later clinical experience.[30] Although by the late nineteenth century the place of the Dublin school of medicine in European medicine had declined, there were still thought to be good opportunities for clinical experience. One doctor, Sir William Bowman, at a meeting of the British Medical Association in Dublin in 1867, pronounced:

> The eminent spirit of Dublin as a clinical school of medicine and surgery has been perhaps less appreciated than it deserves by the world at large owing to its geographical position, somewhat aloof and insulated from the ordinary tracks of travel. The system of teaching is eminently honest, scientific, and practical, laboriously and richly turning to the best use of science and instruction great opportunities, the teachers exhibiting themselves to students as students themselves in the great field of nature.[31]

Stephen Jacyna has claimed that it was clinical experience on the wards that shaped medical students' attitudes and 'established their predominant patterns of practice'.[32] Opportunities existed for students to gain clinical experience at a range of institutions. For instance, Emily Winifred Dickson, who graduated in 1891, went to Sir Patrick Dun's Hospital, the Rotunda Lying-In Hospital, the National Eye and Ear Infirmary, Donnybrook Dispensary and the Richmond Lunatic Asylum, all of which were located in Dublin.[33] Yet, medical students were required to arrange this hospital experience themselves and had to pay a fee to the hospital concerned. Hospital instruction was incorporated into university timetables but students were also required to spend their summer holidays working in a hospital in order to fulfil all of the requirements for clinical experience. In fact, this was an important part of Irish medical education from the early nineteenth century and the stipulations of the bachelor of medicine degree of the Royal University of Ireland and later the National University of Ireland reflect this.

Medical scholarships, exhibitions and prizes were open to women on the same terms as to men from the beginning of women's admission to Irish institutions and women were sometimes successful in attaining these.[34] In contrast, at some universities in Britain, women did not have the opportunity to compete for prizes and scholarships on equal terms with men.[35] Irish women appear to have been successful in their academic achievements. In 1887, Eleanora Fleury came first in the list of the examinations in medicine at the Royal University and was commended in the *Dublin Medical Press*.[36] In 1901, Eva Jellett, a student at the Catholic University medical school at Cecilia Street, was successful in winning two medals for histology and physiology and, in 1905, Ella Ovenden won the Royal University's Travelling Medical

Scholarship.[37] In 1902, *QCG* reported on the arrival of Christina Caldwell Dagg, the first woman medical student at Queen's College Galway, and her brilliant success in the scholarship examinations.[38] Similarly, the success of Harriet MacFaddin was praised in a 1905 issue.[39] In addition, a 1904 issue of *St Stephen's* praised Ovenden for taking the blue ribbon in the bachelor of medicine examination.[40]

Examinations for the MB BCh BAO degree took place in Dublin at the Royal University of Ireland. One medical student at Queen's College Belfast described the train journey to Dublin to take the examination as nerve-racking and the examination hall itself as a 'sweating room'.[41] It was commented that lady medicals passed their examinations as easily as their male counterparts because they spent twice as long on a case in the wards as men did.[42] Humphrey Rolleston, an eminent English physician and president of the Royal College of Physicians in London from 1922 to 1926, commented that women were on average better students than men because they worked harder and 'take more pains – being more whole mindedly concentrated on the subject in hand'.[43] The reputation of women medical students as knowledgeable and hard-working is further evident in one humorous poem, 'To a surgeon's girl', which appeared in the *RCSI Student Quarterly*. The subject of the poem is a female medical student who, while in conversation with a smitten classmate, constantly refers to his romantic state in medical terms. For example, when the pair kiss for the first time, she states, 'You force me to confess / I fear your respiration is fifty-four or less'.[44]

In spite of the long hours and heavy workload involved, women were successful in their pursuit of medical education. In the president's report for Queen's College Belfast for the 1889–90 session, one year after the first female medical students were admitted to that institution, Dr Hamilton wrote:

> It has been a matter of great satisfaction to me ... that these young ladies have applied themselves to their work with the most laudable assiduity and success, and that their admission to the medical classes was attended with good results in every way.[45]

As the next section will demonstrate, the admission of women to medical classes does not appear to have caused complications for Irish universities. Rather, it seems that women students occupied a 'shared sphere' with the men, in all elements of medical education except anatomy.

Shared spheres?

IN 1896, Clara Williams, a student at the Royal College of Surgeons in Dublin, wrote to the magazine of the London School of Medicine for Women and Royal Free Hospital about what it was like to be a female medical student in Dublin.[46] The account was very positive. In Williams' view, the system of mixed classes in the Irish capital worked extremely well. In her words:

> nothing in the slightest degree unpleasant has ever occurred, and the professors are unanimous in stating that far from regretting the admission of women to their classes, they consider it has improved the tone of the College considerably. The students are all friendly, there is a healthy spirit of emulation aroused in working together for the various prizes, and an absence of jealousy which augurs well for the future of medical women in Ireland, and reflects favourably on the men as well; we all help each other, and I, for my own part, owe a great deal of my success to the assistance of a few of the senior men students.[47]

In the same year, the *Dublin Medical Press* had implied that the segregation of men and women for medical classes might lead to women missing out on the code of ethics of the profession and viewing their male classmates as competitors rather than colleagues in future professional life.[48] This view seems to have been shared by Irish universities, where, for the most part, women and men medical students were educated together. Percy Kirkpatrick, writing in 1912, commented that women and men were educated together for all lectures with the exception of anatomy and that 'in spite of the many prophecies to the contrary, the plan has worked well'.[49] In 1922, the *Irish Times* reported that at Trinity College Dublin and the Royal College of Surgeons, men and women were trained together without the slightest awkwardness.[50] Similarly, Colonel Sir William Taylor, then president of the Royal College of Surgeons, commented that he found no difficulty in giving clinical classes to men and women together at the Meath Hospital in the 1920s.[51]

This was in contrast to Britain, where women were initially educated at single-sex medical schools such as the London School of Medicine for Women (founded in 1874) and the Edinburgh School of Medicine for Women (founded in 1886), which were largely responsible for the medical education of British women until the opening up of other medical schools in Britain from the 1890s. At the University of Birmingham, following the admission of women medical students to the Birmingham medical school in 1900, female assistants were employed to teach women in separate classes for medicine, anatomy, surgery, midwifery and gynaecology. Moreover, a female assistant was requested to assist the chair of forensic medicine, 'as some issues, such as rape, were deemed too sensitive to discuss before a mixed group of young men and women'.[52] According to Carol Dyhouse, the existence of separate classes for women medical students suggests 'that a provincial medical education was very much characterised by a distinction of sex'.[53] Likewise, in America, the co-education of men and women had often been a problem for opponents of women in higher education. Late nineteenth-century women American physicians failed to share this concern.[54]

The co-education of women and men students did sometimes prove problematic in Ireland. Florence Stewart, who trained at Queen's College Belfast in the 1920s, commented that male and female medical students attended lectures together and that the lady medicals tended to sit together at the front of the lecture theatre. The only time that they were asked to leave was when 'sex problems' were being discussed.[55] Fundamentally, however, the system of mixed classes in Dublin, in Clara Williams' words, had been:

> productive of nothing but good, and they are helping in a large measure to destroy the prejudice against women studying medicine. The present generation of medical men having been educated with women, regard them exactly as their other fellow-students, and respect them according to their merits and capabilities, which is all any of us desire.[56]

The favourable attitudes towards women medical students in the lecture theatre extended into clinical experience too, with Williams stating that nearly all of the general hospitals and all of the special ones in Dublin were open to women and that they received precisely the same instruction there as the men. There do not appear to have been major issues with the introduction of women medical students to the wards of Irish hospitals. Moreover, women were entitled to hold the posts of clinical clerks and surgical dressers in the same way that men could.[57] In fact, it seems that Irish hospitals possessed an egalitarianism lacking in their British counterparts. At the teaching hospitals associated with the University of Birmingham, for example, separate ward classes were established for women students from 1905.[58] Meanwhile, in other parts of Britain, many hospitals would not accept women medical students on their wards and in some cases women doctors, such as Elizabeth Garrett Anderson, founded their own hospitals.[59] These hospitals, largely established in the late nineteenth and early twentieth centuries, served three purposes: they allowed for women's mission to care for women and children; they promoted professional success for women doctors; and they were important for the training of young professional women.[60]

It has been argued that Dublin's St Ultan's Hospital, established in 1919, served the same functions.[61] However, it appears that the main women doctors involved in its foundation, such as Kathleen Lynn, Katharine Maguire and Ella Webb (née Ovenden), were concerned primarily with improving the health and sanitary conditions of the city's poor, as was evident from their earlier involvement in organisations such as the Women's National Health Association, rather than the promotion of the professional interests of women doctors. Likewise, considering that Irish hospitals were open to women medical students, there was not a need for an additional hospital to serve this latter function.

Irish voluntary hospitals had a history of allowing women onto their wards for clinical experience and lectures and women medical students appear to have been readily accepted. Notably, the staff of the Royal Victoria Hospital in Belfast who received an application in 1889 from a female student to be admitted to practise on the hospital wards commented that they saw 'no reason why the application should be refused'.[62] Additionally, the medical staff minutes state that there 'should be no restrictions or objections made to their admission'.[63] Similarly, when, in 1903, a lady student asked about the possibility of becoming a resident medical pupil at the same institution, the staff requested that the board 'entertain the application and to take out such measures' as may facilitate the arrangement.[64] Margaret Ó'hÓgartaigh has highlighted one hospital that appears not to have been so welcoming to women students: the Adelaide in Dublin, to which Kathleen Lynn was refused admission in 1898. This was on account of the fact that there was no accommodation available for female students who wished to work as resident pupils. However, Lynn was successful in gaining a residency at the Royal Victoria Eye and Ear Hospital in Dublin.[65]

With regard to clinical education, it seems that women medical students occupied the same sphere as their male counterparts. The only time that objections were raised was in 1892, when the board of governors of Cork Infirmary refused to admit women medical students to their wards on the grounds that mixed classes had not been a success in Dublin. The Cork students appealed to their counterparts in Dublin for assistance and a letter of support was organised by Emily Winifred Dickson, dated October 1892 and signed by twenty-two lecturers from Dublin's medical schools and teaching hospitals. It read: 'Having been asked to express our opinion on the subject of the hospital education of women medical students, we, the undersigned, having had some years experience wish to state that we have had no difficulties arise in teaching men and women together'.[66] The Infirmary then opened its classes to women. Letters such as this one indicate that leading members of the Irish medical profession did not find problems with the introduction of women students to their wards.

Why were Irish hospitals more welcoming of women students than their British counterparts? It is possible that financial factors played their part. The Royal Victoria Hospital in Belfast was struggling as a result of the costs of building an extension to cater for increased demand, and its running and maintenance depended on donations.[67] Several of the best-known Irish hospitals were voluntary ones, founded by philanthropic bodies. They were run by a committee of local subscribers, with additional funds coming from grants from grand juries or municipal corporations. The most important of these hospitals included St Vincent's, the Mater Misericordiae, the Adelaide Hospital, the Rotunda Lying-In Hospital, Dr Steevens' Hospital, the Coombe Lying-In Hospital and the Royal Victoria Eye and Ear Hospital, which were all located in Dublin.[68] Their institutional histories provide evidence that they were under significant financial pressure in the late nineteenth century. At the Royal Victoria Eye and Ear Hospital there were constant appeals for financial support. In the last quarter of 1876, funds became so depleted that only the most urgent cases were admitted to the hospital, and pleas for expansion continued into the twentieth century.[69] The dire state of the voluntary hospital system in Ireland resulted in the Dublin Hospitals Commission report of 1887, which recommended the amalgamation of certain voluntary hospitals as well as the provision of state grants to others that were in particular need.[70] Accordingly, therefore, the admission of women students to the wards of Irish hospitals made sound financial sense, as it increased income from teaching fees.

At the Rotunda, teaching fees played an important part in the financing of the hospital including, in particular, the master's salary, although Robert Harrison, in his study of education at that institution, does not specify what fraction of the hospital income these fees constituted. In 1896, fees were 20 guineas for six months, which included lodging at the hospital.[71] At the Royal Victoria Hospital in Belfast, fees from students gaining their clinical experience at the hospital produced considerable income.[72] Similarly, at the Meath Hospital, Dublin, such fees from medical students were significant. According to Peter Gatenby, the medical board minutes in 1905 noted that the total fees collected for the summer session amounted to £163 6s 11d, with this amount being divided up between the seven members of the board.[73]

Clearly, the income received from women students contributed significantly to the finances of the hospitals. Moreover, given that many of the British teaching hospitals were closed to women, Irish hospitals and their teaching staffs would have benefited financially from British women, like Octavia Wilberforce, a student at the London School of Medicine for Women, who came to Ireland in order to gain their clinical experience.

The Rotunda Lying-In Hospital in Dublin is a prime example of institutions which supplemented their income in this way. It had a reputation for being the best lying-in hospital in the United Kingdom and many medical students from universities all over the country gained their midwifery experience there.[74] In addition, the hospital attracted American, English and Scottish medical students wishing to study obstetrics, as it offered one advantage over the hospitals of Vienna, Prague and Dresden, in that the English language was spoken in it.[75] Wilberforce went to the Rotunda Hospital in July and August 1918 in order to gain practical midwifery experience. While there, she remarked on the pervading atmosphere of equality between the sexes:

> The best part of this place is the way men and women work together, and the younger men, Simpson, Gilmour and English make one feel just as capable as the men students.... Here in Dublin, men and women students have worked together at Trinity College for years. At Arthur Ball's hospital,[76] I was so pleased to see the perfect naturalness and equality of men and women. They forget half the time that there's any difference between the men and women students, and that's what you need in Medicine. Equality and absence of sex.[77]

Clearly, Wilberforce, as someone who had experienced educational segregation at the London School of Medicine for Women, found the Irish system to be refreshing, at least with regard to hospital experience. Florence Stewart also commented on the friendly attitude towards women medical students at the Rotunda. In 1932, when she gained her clinical experience there, the master of the hospital and his wife took all of the medical students who were free out for a picnic on Easter Sunday to the Sugar Loaf, where they all played football together.[78]

In contrast, the London Hospital Medical College, the Westminster Medical School and St Mary's Medical School, which were all affiliated to the University of London, as well as St George's Hospital and University College Hospital Medical School began admitting women to their wards only during the First World War, but most of these hospitals closed their doors to women after the war and did not re-admit them until the 1940s.[79] Notably, St Thomas' Hospital and Guy's Hospital in London did not admit women medical students to their wards until 1947. At the medical school in Birmingham, the medical faculty created separated ward classes for women medical students from 1905.[80] In comparison, it appears that Irish hospitals did not take issue with women's admission to their wards or classes. However, as the next section will demonstrate, there were some exceptions to women's complete incorporation into medical education.

Educational segregation

So far, I have demonstrated that women and men medical students in Ireland were for the most part educated together, and successfully so. In this section, I will discuss the one instance where this was not the case. Although women and men walked the wards and attended medical lectures

together, dissections were seen as an exception to the rule and the co-
education of men and women in this setting was thought to be inappropriate.
The problem with anatomy dissections was complex. On the one hand, there
were those who viewed the practice as unsuitable for women students under
any conditions. In the United States, it was thought to have a hardening
effect on women students.[81] Opponents of the medical education of women,
such as Harvard's Professor Ware, believed that dissection would guarantee
the 'defilement of women's moral constitution'. Anatomy dissections had
the potential to 'desex' the female dissector.[82] On the other hand, advocates
of women's medical education argued that the practice had the potential to
'fortify the character and moral sensibilities of the physician in training'.[83]
However, Irish institutions appear to have taken issue specifically with the
idea of men and women dissecting together and the sexualised nature of
anatomy dissections.

Irish university authorities attempted to remedy the controversy sur-
rounding anatomy dissections by building separate dissecting rooms for men
and women. The construction of separate dissecting rooms was not unique
to Irish medical schools, which could be seen to be following international
trends.[84] In May 1897, the council of the medical faculty of the Catholic
University met to discuss the subject of women medical students and came to
the decision that the medical faculty should be authorised to make any special
arrangements relating to them as they saw fit and to report back the following
year about their decisions.[85] The council agreed that male and female medical
students ought to attend lectures together; but not courses of anatomy dissection. The council set up a special dissecting room with a waiting room
attached for women students in the summer of 1897 so that they could carry
out their dissections away from the male students.[86] The council reported
that 'the results have proved most satisfactory and encouraging, and the
Faculty are satisfied that the step taken in this decision is one which will add
considerably in the future, to the success and usefulness of the School'.[87]
Women demonstrators were appointed to teach the women students in
their dissection room. As we will see in the next chapter, this was an area
of employment in the academic field for newly qualified women graduates.
For example, Lily Baker (TCD, 1906) worked as an anatomy demonstrator
at Trinity College Dublin, Ina Marion Clarke (RCSI, 1909) at the Royal
College of Surgeons in Ireland, Alice Chance (UCD, 1917) at the University
of Oxford and Amy Connellan McCallum (QCB, 1918) at Queen's College
Belfast. Evidently, not only did college councils feel that it was inappropriate
for men and women to conduct dissections together but they also believed
that women students should be educated by female demonstrators. This was
a common practice in British universities.

Separation of students for anatomy dissections took place in all of the Irish medical schools. The new buildings of the Royal College of Surgeons, renovated in 1892, included a ladies' dissecting room.[88] Trinity College Dublin had a separate dissecting room for women medical students which remained in existence until 1937.[89] The dissecting room had cost the university £1,500 to build.[90] At Queen's College Galway, in 1916, *UCG* magazine reported that women medical students had been 'moved to the museum', although it is unclear whether this was for anatomy dissections.[91]

At Queen's College Cork, part of the dissecting room was initially screened off so that men and women would be able to carry out their dissections separately from one another. In addition, women were not permitted to undertake dissections unless there were at least two women medical students taking anatomy.[92] There were at least two women students matriculating every year from 1906, so this rule would not have applied. And, in 1907, a separate dissecting room was constructed for the 'fascinating scalpel-wielders' and 'fair dissectors' so that they could conduct their dissections in complete isolation from their male counterparts.[93] Clearly, the College council felt that it was an improper thing for women and men medical students to look at the body together.

One of the women students at Queen's College Cork, Janie Reynolds, wrote to the College council to complain: 'in being limited to one "subject" and in not being allowed to see the dissections of the other students, women are severely handicapped and prevented from forming an earlier and more intimate acquaintance with the subject of Anatomy'.[94] Reynolds also pointed out the fact that she and the other women medical students were used to attending lectures with the men, and she wondered why anatomy dissections were an exception to the rule.

What was it about women's contact with corpses in an academic setting that universities appear to have found difficult? The topic of anatomy had been problematic in the 1860s when women were forbidden from attending some meetings of the Ethnological Society in London on the grounds that certain subjects were deemed unsuitable for women, such as, ironically, the 'indelicate' topic of childbirth.[95] Likewise, we may gain an insight into Victorian attitudes of feminine 'delicacy' through examining the case of English anatomy museums.[96] At some anatomy museums in England, such as Kahn's museum in the 1850s, women were permitted to attend the display on certain days, a practice that the *Lancet* objected to at the time because it was believed to undermine one of the most common arguments against women studying medicine: that they would find anatomy distressing.[97] Revealingly, women were not allowed to view any models 'that could offend the most prudish taste' and only nurses and midwives were entitled to view the syphilitic models.[98] However, considering that women and men were allowed to attend all lectures at Irish institutions together, including anatomy, and they were also allowed to walk the wards together with no restrictions on the living bodies they could see, it seems that it was not the subject of anatomy itself that was deemed unsuitable but, rather, the specific issue of dissecting dead corpses and, in particular, dissecting dead corpses in the company of men, which was problematic. What were the reasons for this?

Historians have drawn attention to the highly sexualised nature of anatomy dissections in general.[99] Alison Bashford has argued that there was significant cultural investment in a gendered and sexualised understanding of dissection, whereby the masculine scientist/dissector penetrated and came to 'know' the feminised corpse in a process clouded by desire. The female dissector, or woman medical student, not only disrupted this desire when she entered the dissecting room but also inverted the sexualised and gendered dynamics that took place there.[100] At one university, it seems that it was the issue of women dissecting the male body that was problematic. Tellingly, at Trinity College, when the segregation of women and men for anatomy dissections came to an end in 1937, women medical students were then allowed only to 'poke around with the female anatomy'.[101]

However, the key issue seems to have been that university authorities were not favourable to the idea of men and women dissecting together. Revealingly, Queen Victoria, who disapproved of women in the professions, had a particular dislike of the 'awful idea of allowing young girls and young men to enter the dissecting room together, where the young girls would have to study things that could not be named before them'.[102] Similar opinions were repeated in the medical press. The *British Medical Journal* commented in 1870 that it was 'an indelicate thing for young ladies to mix with other students in the dissecting-room and lecture theatre'.[103] At the University of Edinburgh, it was the issue of women and men dissecting together which gave rise to the famous riot in protest against women medical students in the university in 1870.[104] Through separating men and women students for anatomy dissections, it is possible that college authorities wished to protect their budding young male doctors and indeed staff from the 'distracting influence' of female medical students. At the same time, one male medical student claimed that the 'refining influences' exercised by the women in the dissecting room upon their male brethren was 'of greatest practical importance'.[105] A further interpretation could be that Irish university authorities felt that, in the case of a female student becoming distressed by the dissection process, she would find support among the other women and would not have to face the embarrassment of revealing her weakness before the male students.

The sight of corpses and the dissection of them may also have been seen as a corrupting influence on lady medicals if they were working alongside the male students. At Trinity College Dublin there was a joke that 'the dissection "parts" for the ladies [were] decorated in pink ribbon as to render them prettier and more attractive'.[106] Furthermore, the dissecting room may have been viewed as a place where sexual thoughts were liable to develop. By separating the women from the men, university authorities might have felt that they were protecting the 'delicate' female students from the threat of male advances, or perhaps even male humour and seedy discussion that may have been particularly prevalent in such a context.[107] A poem entitled 'For the dissecting room', published in *QCB* in 1907, is indicative of this black humour. The writer composes a list of irritating characters in the College, from the 'pestilential footballer' to 'the sorry cranks whose aim in life is running QCB' whom he would like to use as dissecting room cadavers.[108] One student in 1900 claimed that it was 'a well established rule that a man's dissecting ability is generally inversely proportional to the elaborate nature of his toilet'.[109] Another student, writing in 1917, claimed that 'the dissecting-room is to the student a club, a smoke room, a common research room – one in all'.[110]

Clearly, the separation of female medical students from their male counterparts for anatomy dissections was a complex issue and not unique to Irish universities. Fundamentally, it seems that objections to women medical students conducting dissections were raised on two main points: first, that anatomy dissection was an indelicate practice for women; and second, that if in such situations women and men were together, the influence of the male students might corrupt the women. It is also possible that women may have been separated so that they could be protected from awkward situations and provide support for each other. As the next section will demonstrate, this separation was not limited to the dissecting room. Women medical students created their own social network within the university, sometimes assisted by the university authorities.

Social segregation

AS WELL AS BEING segregated from the men for certain educational purposes, women and men students were sometimes socially separated by university authorities through the construction of women's common rooms, often called 'ladies' rooms'. These provided a place for women students to meet and chat between classes. At the Catholic University medical school on Cecilia Street, a room was built specifically for the women students. Accounts of this room were extremely positive and it appears to have served not only as a haven and place for the women to socialise, but also as a separate sphere to keep the women medical students from mixing with the male medical students. One female writer commented in *St Stephen's* in 1902 that she and some of the other women students had 'a most pleasant experience at Cecilia Street recently'.[111] They were invited for tea at the ladies' room of the medical school, where they 'dissected nothing more gruesome than plum cake, nor concocted any more baleful potion than distilled essence of the tea-vegetable, tempered with H_2O and lacteal fluid'.[112]

Twelve years later, a letter to the *National Student* mentioned the 'extraordinary tenderness shown by the College authorities for the lady students'.[113] The male writer asserted that the ladies' room of the medical school had just been fitted out in a lavish manner, with 'cheerful green and white wall-paper, comfortable furniture, a carpet, curtains to the window, and ... a plentiful supply of magazines'.[114] There was, however, no such provision for the male students and the writer asked 'why should a dozen women students have every comfort while a couple of hundred men have to put up with the hall, the street, or the neighbouring taverns?'[115] Clearly, some of the male medical students felt that the lady medicals were being treated with undue favour by the university authorities and begrudged them this.

This theme of social separation was not unique to Irish universities. Women medical students at American universities socially separated themselves from the men through their integration into sororities.[116] At Johns Hopkins University, in the early twentieth century, women medical students created their own 'fraternity', discussing journal articles together, meeting for tea and organising social activities among themselves.[117] At Irish universities, special reading rooms for female students allowed for this social separation. At Trinity College, a special reading room was constructed within the anatomy department (which also had a separate entrance for women students) for lady medicals.[118] The Royal Victoria Hospital in Belfast had a special sitting room for female students in the early twentieth century.[119] And, at the Royal College of Surgeons, from 1892 there existed a 'suite of apartments' specifically for women medical students.[120] There were also 'ladies' rooms' for female students at Queen's College Belfast.[121] We may wonder why the authorities of some Irish universities constructed these special ladies' rooms. It is true that male medical students, in particular those in their first year, were infamous for their boisterous behaviour, and it may be that the authorities felt that separation from their boorish male counterparts was necessary if the women's delicate natures were not to be corrupted. At the same time, there is a sense that the universities wanted to nurture the women medical students, to make them feel welcome, and so provided them with a sanctum to which they could retreat between classes. This private space afforded the women students a sphere where they could congregate and identify themselves as a separate group, a space which served both to separate and to protect them from the male students. The fact that lady medicals were few in number sometimes worked to their advantage. Mary McGivern, who matriculated at University College Dublin in 1918, was one of few women medical students in her class. According to her daughter:

> She seemed to be very happy there and because there were very few women, they got a lot of attention from the males. So it was quite social, and she enjoyed that social aspect of it all. But she was a student, and she did study and, you know, she made it in the time that she was supposed to make it ... and listening to her, whenever I would question her, it just seemed more like she was having a good time than studying.[122]

By the 1930s and 1940s, the situation had changed. Writing about her experiences as a medical student at Trinity College Dublin in the 1940s, Joyce Delaney commented that in her class there were ten men to every female medical student but, to her disappointment, their priorities were drinking and horses rather than paying attention to the opposite sex.[123] By this point, perhaps the female medical student was no longer seen as a unique anomaly.

Women medical students were also socially segregated with regard to their living arrangements. Undoubtedly, for first-year women, it would have added greatly to their comfort to live together and to prepare their meals in common.[124] By sharing accommodation, these young women could provide each other with the support and encouragement that were of vital importance for students whose first year at university would also have been their first year away from home. This pattern was not unique to Ireland: at Johns Hopkins University, women medical students from the very beginning of their admission tended to live together.[125] At Queen's College Galway, first-year female students commonly lived at the same address.[126] This pattern perhaps suggests that friendships between first-year lady medicals were formed early on, and the same pattern exists for male medical students. In addition, some students, for example, Anne Kelly and Winifred O'Hanlon, who began their studies at Queen's College Galway in the 1917/18 term, had both attended the same secondary school, suggesting that school-friends commonly lived together. Two rooms at 10 Dominick Street in Galway were rented out to first-year women medical students every year between 1915 and 1918, suggesting that perhaps some landlords and landladies were known for renting rooms to women medical students.

Dublin hospitals also provided separate accommodation for women students gaining their clinical experience. At the Coombe Lying-In Hospital, women students were boarded in a house twelve minutes' walk away.[127]

Similarly, at the Rotunda Hospital, men students were boarded in the hospital itself, while women students resided in two boarding-houses in the local area, at Granby Row and Gardiner's Place.[128] At the Royal Victoria Hospital in Belfast, women resident pupils slept in the same quarters as the nurses, while, interestingly, the men slept in the same quarters as the sisters.[129]

Like their male counterparts, some women medical students lived in digs while at university, a cheap form of accommodation including meals, costing about fifteen shillings a week in 1907.[130] For female medical students in particular, accommodation in digs would perhaps have been seen as a more favourable option than renting a room in a house. The arrangement provided women students with a place to stay that was probably more similar to their family home and would have perhaps reduced their families' worries about their living conditions. Brigid Lyons Thornton, who began her first year of medical studies at Queen's College Galway in 1915, resided in the house of Maud Kyne on Francis Street, which, as her biographer has described, 'turned out to be warm, hospitable and chatty'.[131] Digs were often a subject of satire in student magazines. In the May 1907 issue of *QCB*, one article claimed that the student in digs was a distinct class of individual – 'the ordinary common or garden student, who pays his bills weekly, who stubbornly fights every inch of his road to a dinner which he can eat and contests several items on his bill'.[132] The food provided by the landladies of digs was in ill-repute and the author commented: 'From the first day that a student becomes a lodger he begins to look upon the world with different eyes. He begins to firmly believe that hens lay only stale eggs; that a cow, when living, yields only adulterated chalk, and that when dead, the carcase is entirely composed of steak.'[133]

At Queen's College Belfast, some women students lived at Riddel Hall, a residence specially established for them.[134] Florence Stewart commented that she felt she owed a big debt of gratitude to Riddel Hall because her father 'would not have allowed me to go to Queen's unless I had been able to reside there'.[135] Similarly, Clara Williams commented that parents often did not like their daughters to go to study medicine in Dublin because there was no residence specifically for women. However, this problem was remedied by the establishment of a committee of women doctors, among them Emily Winifred Dickson, to advise women students on their work and also to help them find suitable lodgings.[136]

The women medical students' sense of being a separate community was also clearly evident from their representation on the student council at Queen's College Belfast, where there was a position for 'lady medical' from 1901 (Plate III).[137] Lady medicals also formed a group for fundraising efforts. At Queen's College Belfast in 1907, the chairman of the student council complained that male medical students were making no effort to engage

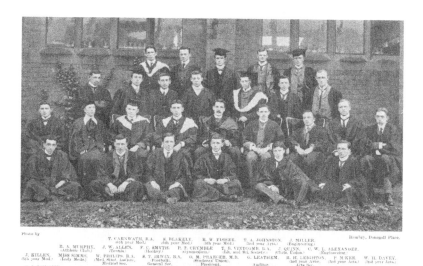

Plate III　Student representative council at Queen's University Belfast, 1900–01, in which Evelyn Simms (second from the left in the second row from the front) is the representative 'Lady Meds'.

in charity fundraising efforts, unlike the female medical students, who had displayed zeal by organising a stall.[138] Similarly, in 1915, the women banded together in order to put on a concert to fundraise for wounded soldiers and sailors.[139] They also came together in social settings such as at the meetings of the Belfast Medical Students' Association, in which they appeared to have played an important role. Between 1899 and 1925, with the exception of four years, there was at least one female medical student on the committee of the Association.[140] The Association held debates and talks on matters relating to the interests of medical students of Belfast and women medical students often participated in these, especially when they themselves were the subjects of the debate.

In February 1900, there was a debate on the topic 'Should ladies practise medicine?'[141] A student called Graham Campbell, arguing the affirmative, 'flitted like a gladsome bee from Homer to Tennyson, then via Ruskin to Euripides and a lady medical at Athens', while a Mr W. Phillips spoke against the motion, arguing that the profession was bound up in what he called a 'frock hat'.[142] The debate was won by Phillips, in spite of an apparently strong case made by many of the women medical students when the debate was opened up to the floor.[143] In March 1905, at another meeting of the Belfast Medical Students' Association, a student called A. V. McMaster spoke on 'Women as medical men' and expressed a favourable attitude towards lady medicals.[144] Following that paper, one speaker from the floor, a Mr W. McCready, spoke against women doctors, in response to which one of the female medical students called him 'Grandfather'.[145] According to the Association's minutes, a considerable discussion ensued, in which prominent contributions came from Maria Rowan, a fourth-year medical student, and Jemima Blair White, in her fifth year, 'the latter being so irrepressible as to necessitate her being called to order by the chairman'.[146] Evidently, women medical students felt the need to defend their attendance at Irish medical schools and some felt particularly strongly about their place in the medical profession. A similar debate, on the topic of 'Will the advent of women to the medical profession be beneficial or otherwise to the community?', was held by the Biological and Debating Society of the Royal College of Surgeons in 1917.[147] Through attending meetings of such associations, and arguing for their right to be members of the medical profession, women medical students asserted their claim to be part of the public sphere but also affirmed their separate identity.

As this section has demonstrated, not only were women medical students physically segregated from the men through the construction of ladies' rooms, but they also self-consciously separated themselves through their living arrangements and socially at societies like the Belfast Medical Students' Association. This reinforces the point that women students occupied a separate sphere from the men, one which was both physically constructed by the universities and self-consciously constructed by the students themselves.

Conclusion

Mary had a little book,
And in the bone-room daily
She flaunted it before our gaze
And read its pages gaily.

Mary came to Queen's, alas!
(We're sorry this to say)
One morning in a hurry,
Without her little Gray.

But nevermore we saw her,
No longer was she free,
And Mary did not come to Queen's –
She'd joined the W.A.A.C.'s, you see.

We missed her in the bone-room,
That loved her presence gay;
We missed her really just because
We missed her little Gray.[148]

HISTORIANS OF MEDICAL WOMEN have drawn attention to the sense of separateness that British and American women tended to feel, both with regard to their university education but also later in their professional lives.[149] Certainly, with regard to Irish medical education, there existed a sense of separatism between the men and women students which may be seen in poems such as the one above, which pokes fun at the lady medical. Yet, as this chapter shows, Irish universities possessed a surprisingly inclusive attitude to women medical students. Similarly, albeit for financial reasons, Irish hospitals appear to have welcomed women to their wards.

Nevertheless, it is clear that, in the context of Irish universities, women medical students came to occupy a world which was very much separate from that of the men. This was constructed literally through special dissecting rooms so that the women might practise anatomy without the difficulties that might arise from the proximity of the men, as well as through the creation of special ladies' rooms. By providing ladies' rooms and dissecting rooms in order to protect the women students, the university authorities demonstrated their fears about women mixing with men and this could be viewed as paternalistic action. Spiritually, women students had always been seen as a separate and unique group; however, lady medicals came to be seen as a particularly distinctive cohort. At the same time, women medical students themselves reinforced this sense of distinction through their self-identification as a cohort, at social events and lectures, in their representation on student councils or through their living arrangements. In a sense, we may view their banding together in this way as an attempt to reconcile the distinctions constructed by university authorities between them and the male students. Through their self-enforced social segregation, women accepted that they were different from the men, and thus distanced themselves from the stereotype of the rowdy male medical student.

Notes

1 'Girl graduates chat', *St Stephen's*, 1:5 (1902), p. 93.

2   For instance, one writer for *UCG* claimed: 'It is a great pity that more of the gentler sex do not enter the portals of the magic studio of "The First of Arts, without whose light, all others would fade into the night". Do they not hear the cries of the sick little children as St. Patrick heard the children of the Gael?' 'Medical notes', *UCG: A College Annual* (1919–20), p. 57.

3   Keir Waddington, 'Mayhem and medical students: image, conduct and control in the Victorian and Edwardian London teaching hospital', *Social History of Medicine*, 15:1 (2002), pp. 45–64, on p. 45.

4   Carol Dyhouse, 'Driving ambitions: women in pursuit of a medical education, 1890– 1939', *Women's History Review*, 7:3 (1998), pp. 321–43, on p. 322.

5   See: Barbara Brookes, 'A corresponding community: Dr Agnes Bennett and her friends from the Edinburgh Medical College for Women of the 1890s', and Andrew Warwick, *Masters of Theory: Cambridge and the Rise of Mathematical Physics* (Chicago, IL: University of Chicago Press, 2003).

6   Janet Browne, 'Squibs and snobs: science in humorous British undergraduate magazines around 1830', *History of Science*, 30 (June 1992), pp. 165–97, on p. 167.

7   These were respectively succeeded by *UCG: A College Annual* and the *Quarryman*.

8   Francis Sheehy Skeffington, 'The position of women', *St Stephen's*, 1:12 (1903), pp. 252–3.

9   Browne, 'Squibs and snobs', p. 193.

10 'Medicine', *QCG*, 5:2 (1907), p. 50; and 'My impressions of the lady students by X.Y.Z.', *UCG: A College Annual*, 1:1 (1913), p. 33.

11 'How Lill got her M.D.', *Quarryman*, 4:5 (1917), p. 101.

12 *Ibid.*

13 Thomas Neville Bonner in *Becoming a Physician: Medical Education in Britain, France, Germany and the United States, 1750–1945* (Oxford: Oxford University Press, 1996), p. 215, and M. Jeanne Peterson, *The Medical Profession in Mid-Victorian London* (Berkley, CA: University of California Press, 1978), p. 40.

14 Bonner, *Becoming a Physician*, p. 215.

15 'News from the schools: medical school', *TCD: A College Miscellany*, 10:179 (1904), p. 166.

16 'Medical notes', *UCG: A College Annual* (1919–20), p. 57.

17 'Students in "Ye Citie of ye Tribes"', *QCG*, 3:1 (1904), p. 25.

18 'Things we would like to know', *QCB*, 11:1 (1919), p. 28.

19 'Cherchez la femme', *QCC*, 5:1 (December 1908), p. 19.

20 'Winsome women at Q.C.B. (with apologies to no-one)', *QCB*, 6:3 (1905), p. 7.

21 *Ibid.*

22 Robert Wilson, *Aesculapia Vitrix* (London: Chapman and Hall, 1886), p. 28.

23 Details in personal letter from Joyce Darling, daughter of Olive Pedlow.

24 Mary Ryan was the first female professor to be appointed to an Irish university. She was made Professor of Romance Languages at Queen's College Cork in 1910.

25 Leone McGregor Hellstedt (ed.), *Women Physicians of the World: Autobiographies of Medical Pioneers* (Washington, DC, and London: Medical Women's International Federation, Hemisphere Publishing Corporation, 1978), p. 93.

26 John Cowell, *A Noontide Blazing. Brigid Lyons Thornton: Rebel, Soldier, Doctor* (Dublin: Currach Press, 2005), p. 44.

27 *Irish Medical Student's Guide* (Dublin: Dublin Medical Press, 1877), p. 33.

28 *Ibid.*

29 Nelson Hardy, *The State of the Medical Profession in Great Britain and Ireland in 1900* (Dublin: Fannin, 1902), p. 61.

30 Henry Bewley, 'Medical education: a criticism and a scheme', *Dublin Journal of Medical Science*, 129 (1910), pp. 81–97, on p. 82.

31 See E. D. Mapother, 'The medical profession and its work', *Dublin Journal of Medical Science*, 82 (1886), pp. 177–206, on pp. 193–4.

32 L. S. Jacyna, 'The laboratory and the clinic: the impact of pathology on surgical diagnosis in the Glasgow Western Infirmary, 1875–1910', *Bulletin of the History of Medicine*, 62:3 (1988), pp. 384–406, on p. 405.

33 MB BCH BAO RUI degree certificate for Emily Winifred Dickson, 1893, National University of Ireland Archives, Dublin.

34 Royal Commission on University Education in Ireland, *Final Report of the Commissioners* (London: HM Stationery Office, 1903), p. 8.

35 For example, at the University of Glasgow women were unable to apply for bursaries when they were first admitted to the medical school. And in later years women were still restricted with regard to the bursaries they could apply for. See Wendy Alexander, *First Ladies of Medicine: The Origins, Education, and Destination of Early Women Medical Graduates of Glasgow University* (Glasgow: Wellcome Unit for the History of Medicine, 1988), p. 19.

36 'Medical honours to ladies', *DMP*, 8 June 1887, p. 552.

37 'Girl graduates chat', *St Stephen's*, 2:1 (1901), p. 50, and an untitled article, *St Stephen's*, 2:8 (1905), p. 182.

38 'Medicine', *QCG*, 1:1 (November 1902), p. 6.

39 'Medicine', *QCG*, 4:1 (November 1905), p. 23.

40 'From the ladies' colleges', *St Stephen's*, 2:5 (1904), p. 111.

41 'Medical Students' Association', *QCB*, 1:3 (1900), p. 11.

42 'Winsome women at Q.C.B.', p. 7.

43 Humphrey Rolleston, 'An address on the problem of success for medical women', *BMJ*, 6 October 1923, pp. 591–4, on p. 592.

44 'To a surgeon's girl', *RCSI Student Quarterly*, 1:1 (1917), p. 13.

45 Quoted in Richard H. Hunter, 'A history of the Ulster Medical Society', *Ulster Medical Journal*, 5:3 (1936), pp. 178–95, on p. 168.

46 Clara L. Williams, 'A short account of the school of medicine for men and women, RCSI', *Magazine of the London School of Medicine for Women and Royal Free Hospital*, no. 3 (January 1896), pp. 91–132, on p. 104.

47 *Ibid.*, p. 105.

48 'Medical advertising by ladies', *DMP*, 1 April 1896, p. 358.

49 T. Percy C. Kirkpatrick, *History of the Medical Teaching in Trinity College Dublin and the School of Physic in Ireland* (Dublin: Hanna and Neale, 1912), p. 330.

50 'Women medicals', *Irish Times*, 3 March 1922, p. 4.

51 'Women medical students: barred by London hospital: attitude of Irish schools', *Irish Times*, 3 March 1922, p. 6.

52 Jonathan Reinarz, *Health Care in Birmingham: The Birmingham Teaching Hospitals 1779–1939* (Woodbridge: Boydell Press, 2009), p. 161.

53 Carol Dyhouse, *No Distinction of Sex? Women in British Universities, 1870–1939* (London: UCL Press, 1995), p. 238, cited in Reinarz, *Health Care in Birmingham*, p. 163.

54 Carroll Smith-Rosenberg and Charles Rosenberg, 'The female animal: medical and biological views of woman and her role in nineteenth-century America', *Journal of American History*, 60:2 (1973), pp. 332–56, on p. 342.

55 Florence Stewart papers, Public Record Office of Northern Ireland (D3612/3/1).

56 Williams, 'A short account', p. 109.

57 *Ibid.*, p. 106.

58 Reinarz, *Health Care in Birmingham*, p. 163.

59 Anne Crowther and Marguerite Dupree, *Medical Lives in the Age of Surgical Revolution* (Cambridge: Cambridge University Press, 2007), p. 157.

60 Mary Ann Elston, '"Run by women (mainly) for women": medical women's hospitals in Britain, 1866–1948', in Laurence Conrad and Anne Hardy (eds), *Women and Modern Medicine*, Clio Medica Series (Amsterdam: Rodopi, 2001), pp. 73–108, on p. 77.

61   Margaret Ó hÓgartaigh, *Kathleen Lynn: Irishwoman, Patriot, Doctor* (Dublin: Irish Academic Press, 2006), p. 68.

62   Staff report dated 10 September 1889, Medical staff reports, 1881–99, Royal Victoria Hospital, Belfast.

63   Medical staff minutes, 1875–1905, 10 September 1889, p. 205, Royal Victoria Hospital, Belfast.

64   Staff report dated 15 April 1903, Medical staff reports, 1899–1936, Royal Victoria Hospital, Belfast.

65   Ó hÓgartaigh, *Kathleen Lynn*, p. 11.

66   Letter dated October 1892, signed by twenty-two lecturers from the Dublin teaching hospitals, the King and Queen's College of Physicians and the Royal College of Surgeons, private collection of Niall Martin, Edinburgh.

67   Richard Clarke, *The Royal Victoria Hospital Belfast: A History, 1797–1997* (Belfast: Blackstaff Press, 1997), p. 65.

68   Mary E. Daly, 'An atmosphere of sturdy independence: the state and the Dublin hospitals in the 1930s', in Greta Jones and Elizabeth Malcolm (eds), *Medicine, Disease and the State in Ireland, 1650–1914* (Cork: Cork University Press, 1999), pp. 234–52, on pp. 235–6.

69   Gearoid Crookes, *Dublin's Eye and Ear: The Making of a Monument* (Dublin: Town House, 1993), pp. 34–5.

70   'Dublin Hospitals Commission report', *Irish Times*, 23 April 1887, p. 5. These Dublin voluntary hospitals later faced financial crisis in the 1930s, which resulted in the establishment of the Irish Hospitals' Sweepstake by the Irish Free State. See Marie Coleman, 'A terrible danger to the morals of the country: the Irish hospitals' sweepstake in Great Britain', *Proceedings of the Royal Irish Academy*, 105:5 (2005), pp. 197–220.

71   Robert F. Harrison, 'Medical education at the Rotunda Hospital 1745–1995', in Alan Browne (ed.), *Masters, Midwives and Ladies-in-Waiting: The Rotunda Hospital, 1745–1995* (Dublin: A. and A. Farmar, 1995), p. 72.

72   Clarke, *The Royal Victoria Hospital Belfast*, p. 21.

73   P. Gatenby, *Dublin's Meath Hospital: 1753–1996* (Dublin: Town House, 1996), p. 73.

74   Walter Rivington, *The Medical Profession of the United Kingdom, Being the Essay to Which Was Awarded the First Carmichael Prize by the Council of the Royal College of Surgeons in Ireland, 1887* (Dublin: Fannin, 1888), p. 658.

75   H. Hun, *A Guide to American Medical Students in Europe* (New York: William Wood, 1883), p. 146.

76   Arthur Ball, a graduate of Trinity College Dublin, was house-surgeon to Sir Patrick Dun's Hospital and was later appointed Regius Professor of Surgery at Trinity College Dublin. See 'Obituary: Sir Arthur Ball, Bt., M.D., M.Ch.', *BMJ*, 5 January 1946, p. 33.

77   Pat Jalland (ed.), *Octavia Wilberforce: The Autobiography of a Pioneer Woman Doctor* (London: Cassell, 1994), p. 101.

78   Florence Stewart papers.

79   Medical Women's Federation Archives, Wellcome Library (SA/MWF/C.10). The archive consists of letters dated from 1951 from universities and hospitals around Britain (in response to a request from the secretary of the Federation) giving details of the dates of the first women to be admitted for medical study.

80   Reinarz, *Health Care in Birmingham*, p. 163.

81   John Harley Warner and Lawrence J. Rizzolo, 'Anatomical instruction and training for professionalism from the 19th to the 21st centuries', *Clinical Anatomy*, 19:5 (2006), pp. 403–14, on p. 404.

82   Michael Sappol, *A Traffic of Dead Bodies: Anatomy and Embodied Social Identity in Nineteenth-Century America* (Princeton, MA: Princeton University Press, 2001), pp. 88–9.

83   Warner and Rizzolo, 'Anatomical instruction', p. 405.

84 At the University of Oxford, there was a separate dissecting room for women medical students between 1917 and 1937, where women were instructed in anatomy by a female Irish instructor, Dr Alice Chance. See A. M. Cooke, *My First 75 Years of Medicine* (London: Royal College of Physicians, 1994), p. 7. At the University of Manchester, one small room was allocated to lady medical students which served as a dissecting room, cloakroom and a place for lady medicals to take their lunch. See Dyhouse, *No Distinction of Sex?*, p. 34. In South Africa, at the Capetown Medical School, there was a separate dissecting room for women students, although women and men medical students attended the same lectures and demonstrations. See 'University of Capetown new medical school', *BMJ*, 3 November 1928, p. 813. And at the University of Ontario, men and women medical students were also separated for dissections. See C. M. Godfrey, 'The origins of medical education of women in Ontario', *Medical History*, 17:1 (1973), pp. 89–94, on p. 90.

85 'Meeting: Friday May 28th 1897', Catholic University School of Medicine, Governing body minute book, vol. 1, 1892–1911, University College Dublin Archives (CU/14).

86 'Annual report of the faculty: May 20th 1898', *ibid.*

87 *Ibid.*

88 'The new schools of the Royal College of Surgeons in Ireland', *Irish Times*, 29 January 1892, p. 3.

89 'Ireland: from our special correspondent', *Lancet*, 6 February 1937, p. 343.

90 'Trinity College and women graduates: address by the provost', *Irish Times*, 20 December 1905, p. 8.

91 'Medical notes', *UCG: A College Annual*, 1:4 (1916), p. 33.

92 Letter (undated but c.1895–1905) from Janie Reynolds to the members of council, Queen's College Cork Archives (UC/Council/19/51).

93 'Editorial', *QCC*, 4:1 (1907), p. 15.

94 Letter from Janie Reynolds.

95 Evelleen Richards, 'Huxley and woman's place in science: the "woman question" and the control of Victorian anthropology', in James R. Moore (ed.), *History, Humanity and Evolution: Essays for John C. Greene* (Cambridge: Cambridge University Press, 1989), pp. 253–85, on p. 275.

96 See A. W. Bates, '"Indecent and demoralising representations": public anatomy museums in mid-Victorian England', *Medical History* 52:1 (2008), pp. 1–22, and A. W. Bates, 'Dr Kahn's museum: obscene anatomy in Victorian London', *Journal of the Royal Society of Medicine*, 99:12 (2006), pp. 618–24.

97 Bates, 'Indecent and demoralising representations', p. 11.

98 Bates, 'Dr Kahn's museum', p. 620.

99 Waddington, 'Mayhem and medical students', p. 53, and Alison Bashford, *Purity and Pollution: Gender, Embodiment and Victorian Medicine* (London: Macmillan, 1998), p. 114.

100 Bashford, *Purity and Pollution*, p. 114.

101 'An Irishwoman's diary', *Irish Times*, 21 July 1992, p. 9.

102 A. M. Cooke, 'Queen Victoria's medical household', *Medical History*, 26:3 (1982), pp. 307–20, on p. 308.

103 'Lady surgeons', *BMJ*, 2 April 1870, p. 338.

104 Bashford, *Purity and Pollution*, p. 112. The Edinburgh male medical students protested on the grounds that women dissecting alongside men signified a 'systematic infringement of the laws of decency'.

105 Untitled article, *QCB*, 18:2 (1917), p. 15.

106 'News from the schools: medical school', *TCD: A College Miscellany*, 10:179 (1904), p. 166.

107 Daragh Smith, *Dissecting Room Ballads from the Dublin Schools of Medicine Fifty Years Ago* (Dublin: Black Cat Press, 1984).

108 'For the dissecting room', *QCB*, 8:6 (1907), p. 11.
109 'The medical school', *QCB*, 2:1 (1900), p. 9.
110 Untitled article, *QCB*, 18:2 (1917), p. 15.
111 'Girl graduates chat', *St Stephen's*, 1:5 (1902), p. 93.
112 *Ibid.*
113 'Letters to the editor: a long-felt want', *National Student*, 4:4 (1914), p. 102.
114 *Ibid.*
115 *Ibid.*
116 Helen Lefkowitz Horowitz, *Campus Life: Undergraduate Cultures from the End of the Eighteenth-Century to the Present* (New York: Alfred A. Knopf, 1987), p. 17.
117 Regina Markell Morantz-Sanchez, *Sympathy and Science: Women Physicians in American Medicine* (Chapel Hill, NC: University of North Carolina Press, 1985), p. 123.
118 'Consultation with the sphinx', *Irish Times*, 25 April 1914, p. 20.
119 Information from Professor Richard Clarke, archivist of the Royal Victoria Hospital, Belfast.
120 'The new schools of the Royal College of Surgeons in Ireland', *Irish Times*, 29 January 1892, p. 3.
121 'Five years at Queen's: a retrospect', *QCB*, 12:8 (1911), p. 14.
122 Oral history interview with Mary Mullaney.
123 Joyce Delaney, *No Starch in My Coat: An Irish Doctor's Progress* (London: P. Davies, 1971), p. 15.
124 Elizabeth Garrett Anderson, 'A special chapter for ladies who propose to study medicine', in C. B. Keetley, *The Student's Guide to the Medical Profession* (London: Macmillan, 1878), p. 45.
125 Morantz-Sanchez, *Sympathy and Science*, p. 124.
126 Matriculation albums for students at QCG, 1902–22, National University of Ireland, Galway (Registrar's Office).
127 Julia Pringle, 'Coombe Lying-In Hospital and Guinness Dispensary', *Women Students' Medical Magazine*, 1:1 (1902), p. 42.
128 C. Muriel Scott, 'Rotunda Hospital', *Women Students' Medical Magazine*, 1:1 (1902), p. 44.
129 Monthly staff meeting, 7 May 1912, Medical staff minutes, 1905–37, p. 153, Royal Victoria Hospital, Belfast.
130 'The student in digs', *QCB*, 8:7 (1907), p. 15.
131 Cowell, *A Noontide Blazing*, p. 43.
132 'The student in digs', p. 15.
133 *Ibid.*, p. 16.
134 Gillian McClelland, *Pioneering Women: Riddel Hall and Queen's University Belfast* (Belfast: Ulster Historical Foundation, 2005).
135 Florence Stewart papers.
136 Williams, 'A short account', p. 107.
137 Photograph of student representative council in which Evelyn Simms is the representative 'lady medic', supplement to *QCB*, 2:8 (1901).
138 'Fete news: medical students' stall', *QCB*, 7:4 (1907), p. 14.
139 'Editorial', *QCB*, 16:3 (1915), p. 3.
140 Belfast Medical Students Association, Minute book (internal committee meetings), 1899–1925, Queen's University Belfast Archive.
141 'Medical Students' Association', *QCB*, 1:3 (1900), p. 11.
142 *Ibid.*
143 *Ibid.*
144 'Medical Students' Association', *QCB*, 6:6 (1905), pp. 13–14.
145 *Ibid .*

146 Belfast Medical Students' Association, Minutes, 1898–1907 (9 March 1905), Queen's University Belfast Archive.

147 *RCSI Students' Quarterly*, 1:4 (1917), p. 76.

148 'Nursery rhymes for young medicals', *QCB*, 19:3 (1918), p. 18.

149 See, for example, Virginia G. Drachman, 'The limits of progress: the professional lives of women doctors, 1881–1926', *Bulletin of the History of Medicine*, 60:1 (1986), pp. 58–72.

5

Careers and opportunities

I N 1879, Stewart Woodhouse, then physician to the Richmond, Whitworth
and Hardwicke Hospitals in Dublin, wrote in his advice to medical
graduates:

> Never, perhaps, more than at the present time has it been so necessary for medical
> students to balance the relative advantages and drawbacks of the careers open to
> them when they will be fairly launched in life, and to choose one which will best
> accord with their circumstances and their tastes.[1]

Woodhouse's words rang true into the twentieth century. Following their
course of medical study, in which women students at Irish institutions from
the 1880s to 1920s found themselves to be readily accepted and treated
fairly, while maintaining a sense of distinction from their male brethren,
new women graduates had to set about finding a career. This was a difficult
task and for women doctors it may have been particularly so, as a result of
increased competition for posts or the possibility of prejudice from patients
as well as medical professionals.

Guides written for medical students in the period advised them of their
career options and how to go about attaining a career in the sector of their
choosing. In the view of Michael Foster Reaney, an Irish doctor writing in
1904, opportunities for women graduates were 'naturally limited'. He claimed
that 'women can never really rival men in medical work in the sense that they
have done in office and city life. Their spheres of activity are strictly limited
and must remain rightly so.'[2] Among careers open to women, he listed appointments such as junior resident officerships in the special hospitals and
occasionally in the Poor Law infirmaries and staff appointments at hospitals
for women and children, as well as at larger post offices. Sentiments such as
these concerning women doctors' supposed limited employment prospects

were not uncommon in the early years of the twentieth century. However, Reaney also commented that 'the arrival of the medical woman is to be welcomed, and wherever her lot may be cast, she should be certain of the courteous support of her male colleagues'.[3]

Other commentators, such as Ella Ovenden (later Webb, CU, 1904), were more optimistic. Writing three years after Reaney, she claimed that opportunities for women doctors were improving every year as the woman doctor began to take 'a more established place in the community' but the only way her position could be secured was if she could show 'that she has taken up medicine, not as a fad, but as a serious scientific or philanthropic undertaking'.[4] Another doctor, Howard Marsh, writing in 1914, claimed that there was a need for women doctors in the realms of public health, in hospitals for women and children, in women's wards of the general hospitals, in the missions and also in general practice.[5]

As we learnt in Chapter 1, supporters of the admission of women to the medical profession in the late nineteenth century and early twentieth century had claimed that women were eminently suited to work in women's and children's health, and that there was a special role for female doctors within the missionary field. In the early 1900s, it was indeed believed that women doctors were generally employed within the sectors of women and children.[6] I will demonstrate that Irish women medical graduates were in fact less likely to attain posts in these sectors than they were in other areas of medical employment. Rather, it was more common for Irish female medical graduates to secure posts in general practice, hospital appointments in general hospitals

Table 5.1 Numbers of traceable and untraceable women among the 452 female medical graduates who matriculated 1885–1922 five to thirty-five years after graduation[a]

	5 years	10 years	15 years	25 years	35 years
Traceable graduates	429 (95.0%)	359 (79.4%)	317 (70.1%)	276 (61.1%)	243 (53.8%)
Untraceable graduates	23 (5.0%)	93 (20.6%)	135 (29.9%)	176 (38.9%)	209 (46.2%)
Total	*452*	*452*	*452*	*452*	*452*

[a] The period in fact spans 1891, five years after the year of graduation of the first female graduate of the Royal College of Surgeons, Mary Emily Dowson, to 1969, thirty-five years after graduation of the last of the women graduates who matriculated in 1922, Mary Rose McQuillan (LRCP LRCS Edin, 1934, matriculated at QCB).
Source: *Medical Directory*.

Table 5.2 Careers of the 452 women medical graduates who matriculated 1885–1922 five to thirty-five years after graduation, c.1891–1969

	5 years	10 years	15 years	25 years	35 years
Traceable graduates	429	359	317	276	243
	(95.0%)	(79.4%)	(70.1%)	(61.1%)	(53.8%)
Untraceable graduates	23	93	135	176	209
	(5.0%)	(20.6%)	(29.9%)	(38.9%)	(46.2%)
General practice	*300*	*223*	*157*	*128*	*108*
	(70.0%[a])	*(65.0%)*	*(50.0%)*	*(46.4%)*	*(44.4%)*
Address but no post	299	219	151	125	106
(presumed GP)					
GP (listed as GP)	1	4	6	3	2
Hospital appointments	*70*	*61*	*48*	*44*	*31*
	(16.3%)	*(17.0%)*	*(15.1%)*	*(15.9%)*	*(12.8%)*
General hospital	42	38	29	33	20
Asylum	11	10	11	5	7
Children's/maternity	17	13	8	6	4
Public health	*22*	*40*	*70*	*57*	*52*
	(5.1%)	*(11.1%)*	*(22.1%)*	*(20.7%)*	*(21.4%)*
Assistant medical officer	5	5	14	15	13
Schools medical officer	8	12	19	14	9
Dispensary	6	13	18	14	10
Medical officer of health	2	4	10	8	12
Aurist	0	0	1	0	0
Child welfare centre	1	5	5	3	6
Medical examiner	0	0	0	1	0
Vaccinations	0	1	0	0	0
Ministry of Health	0	0	1	1	1
Registrar	0	0	1	0	0
Tuberculosis officer	0	0	1	1	1
Missions/	*14*	*15*	*20*	*15*	*13*
humanitarian work	*(3.3%)*	*(4.2%)*	*(6.3%)*	*(5.4%)*	*(5.3%)*
Specialists	*7*	*4*	*6*	*12*	*9*
	(1.6%)	*(1.1%)*	*(1.9%)*	*(4.3%)*	*(3.7%)*
Gynaecologist	2	0	0	0	0
Anaesthetist	4	2	3	4	3
Pathologist	1	1	2	2	1
Radiologist	0	1	0	2	2
Dermatologist	0	0	1	2	1
Psychiatrist	0	0	0	2	2
University appointment	*6*	*3*	*2*	*2*	*3*
	(1.4%)	*(0.8%)*	*(0.6%)*	*(0.7%)*	*(1.2%)*
War-related work	3	1	0	0	0
Convent	0	0	1	0	0
Company doctor	5	7	4	4	2
Research	2	4	3	2	1
Deceased	0	0	4	8	12
Not practising/retired	0	1	2	4	12
Total	*429*	*359*	*317*	*276*	*243*

[a] These are percentages of the traceable graduates only.
Source: *Medical Directory.*

and asylums and, later on, within the public health service. It should also be acknowledged that making a medical living often involved collecting a number of part-time posts. Thus, for example, a doctor listed as working for an insurance company may also have been working in general practice and other branches of medicine.[7] In this chapter, I will discuss these careers and their popularity with Irish women doctors. I will start with postgraduate opportunities before moving on to investigate their careers in general practice, hospital work, public health, specialist and academic work and overseas (missionary) employment.

Table 5.1 gives details of the numbers of graduates whom it was possible to trace while Table 5.2 lists their careers. Five years after graduation, 95 per cent of graduates were listed in the *Medical Directory*. However, as years goes on, it is clear that some graduates drop off from the *Medical Directory* and are untraceable. There are three main reasons why graduates were untraceable: some may have married and thus were no longer listed under their maiden names in the *Medical Directory*; some may have stopped practising or chosen a different career; and others may have died and thus no longer have been listed. When discussing the careers of women doctors, I will refer to percentages of women working in the different fields as percentages of the traceable cohort. This means that this method is most accurate for graduates five years after graduation; however, one can still make a fairly accurate generalisations about women doctors' careers in the later years.

Postgraduate study

B Y THE END of the nineteenth century, British and Irish universities had begun to offer postgraduate courses to medical graduates.[8] In Britain, unlike Ireland, many of these postgraduate courses, which often were run through hospitals, were not open to women. According to Louisa Garrett Anderson, the British suffragette, female doctor and daughter of the first woman to gain a medical qualification in Britain, writing in 1913:

> To obtain good postgraduate work women are forced to go to Berlin or Vienna or America. It is withheld from them in England. On qualification a man, if ambitious and able, finds the medical world open to him. A woman's difficulties begin after she qualifies. She has no postgraduate opportunities in London.[9]

In the late nineteenth century, prior to the advent of postgraduate courses at Irish universities, women students tended to go abroad for study. Emily Winifred Dickson (RCSI, 1891) won a travelling studentship which enabled her to undertake postgraduate study in Vienna and Berlin.[10]

Postgraduate work was seen as essential for women who wished to get ahead in the medical profession. Miss Cummins, a student at Queen's College Cork, in a university prize-winning paper, remarked that in order to be 'really successful in this profession in England or Ireland, a woman has to be superior to or better qualified than her male rivals. How is she to do this? Obviously by taking up and specialising in some particular branch of her profession. This means for the woman additional expense, and specialist training in addition to that required for the ordinary practitioner.'[11] In order to work in the sphere of public health, for example, it was necessary to have a diploma in public health.[12] At least 21 per cent of the women graduates went on to obtain postgraduate qualifications such as diplomas in public health and MD degrees.

Postgraduate study involved the specialised study of a particular area of medicine, for example state medicine or tropical medicine.[13] In Ireland, there were opportunities for postgraduate study in Belfast, Cork and Dublin from the early twentieth century and courses were open to both men and women. Queen's College Belfast offered postgraduate courses in clinical pathology and bacteriology for MD degrees in state medicine and diplomas in public health. Research grants were available to students who wished to pursue these courses. At Cork, there was a course for the diploma in public health. In Dublin, postgraduate instruction could be obtained at Trinity College and the Royal College of Surgeons in conjunction with the major hospitals there. Instruction was given in the following subjects: medicine, surgery, gynaecology, diseases of eye, diseases of the throat, nose and ear, diseases of the skin, pathology, anatomy, physiology, X-ray work and cystoscopy. The courses in pathology, anatomy and physiology were designed to have a special bearing on clinical problems. The composite fee for the entire course in 1914 was £5 5s.[14]

Postgraduate qualifications would have enabled women doctors to make the claim that they were qualified to specialise in certain areas. The majority of women doctors, however, were most likely to work in the realm of general practice, within which there appear to have been genuine opportunities.

General practice

MICHAEL FOSTER REANEY, writing in 1904, commented on 'the whole position of the female sex in the social economy of the world':

> passive, as opposed to the active male, [which] makes it extremely undesirable that a woman should engage in ordinary general practice, or should include men among her patients. To the writer's mind this fact is unalterable and as such is seemingly recognised by the majority of lady practitioners.[15]

Table 5.3 Numbers of women graduates who matriculated 1885–1922 who were likely to have been working as general practitioners five to thirty-five years after graduation, c.1891–1969

	5 years	10 years	15 years	25 years	35 years
General practice total	300 (70.0%[a])	223 (65.0%)	157 (50.0%)	128 (46.4%)	108 (44.4%)
Address but no post (presumed GP)	299	219	151	125	106
GP (listed as GP)	1	4	6	3	2

[a] These are percentages of the traceable graduates only.
Source: *Medical Directory.*

Reaney suggests here that general practice was an undesirable sphere of the medical profession for women doctors to concern themselves with, because women would have to treat male patients. However, his statement that 'the majority of lady practitioners' recognised this fact is untrue, considering that general practice represents the most common career choice for the early generations of Irish women doctors, especially among those from the post-war cohort. Irene Finn has argued that for most women doctors, private practice was the only viable career option.[16] It is difficult to determine exactly how many of the cohort practised as general practitioners. General practitioners are notoriously difficult to trace through the *Medical Directory*.[17] In many cases, doctors list their addresses in the *Medical Directory* but no posts. In a few cases, it is possible to determine women who were working as general practitioners as they list the name of the practice they were working in. Otherwise, if we assume that most of those doctors who listed their address but no post in the *Medical Directory* were working as general practitioners, then 70 per cent of the total traceable cohort worked as general practitioners five years after qualification (Table 5.3). Women who remained in Ireland were more likely to work as general practitioners than their counterparts who migrated to England, as will be discussed below. For women who wished to remain in Ireland after graduation, it is evident that there was a niche for them in general practice.

In the late nineteenth and early twentieth centuries, newly qualified doctors most commonly entered into general practice by becoming assistants to established practitioners and working their way up to achieving a partnership in the practice.[18] Assistantships were often intense: Anna Dengel (QCC,

1919) worked as an assistant to two general practitioners in Claycross, near Nottingham, while she waited for her visa which would allow her to go to India to work as a missionary. The position paid £500 per year and Dengel was expected to take all the night calls and a turn at the surgery each day.[19] Women doctors were advised to be content to wait for their practice to build up, which was an expensive task, as the waiting had to be done in a house on a reputable street, which meant high rent.[20] By the 1920s, more women may have sought careers in general practice because the prospect of promotion for them in other branches of medicine was low. One British woman doctor in 1924 commented that young women medical graduates should consider a career in general practice over public health, a branch of the profession she called 'overcrowded and often disappointing'.[21] Another writer in the same year commented that genuine opportunities existed for women medical graduates in the realms of general practice, both in the crowded quarters of big cities and in small country towns. Women starting out in general practice were advised to try to save enough money to keep themselves for one year while they built up their place in the community in which they had chosen to work.[22]

Another option was to purchase an established practice from a retiring general practitioner but partnerships were seen as being a safer option for new graduates.[23] Some women set up joint practices with their husbands or sisters or other women doctors. Georgina Collier (LRCP LRCS Edin, 1897), for example, who studied at QCB in the 1890s, worked in a general practice in Wimbledon, London, alongside her husband Joseph Harvey for her entire career.[24] By the 1930s, medical women in general practice partnerships together were a well established phenomenon.[25] Mary Florence Broderick (later Magner, UCD, 1922) and her sister Henrietta (RCSI, 1925) had a general practice together in south-west London, while Henrietta also worked as assistant chest physician for the Dartford area. Similarly, sisters Margaret (QCC, 1918) and Kate Enright (year and place of graduation unknown) had their own practice at Waterloo Terrace, Cork,[26] and the Baker sisters, Madeline (CU, 1907) and Lily (TCD, 1907), whom we will meet again in Chapter 7, ran a general practice together in Dublin after they graduated.

Some women doctors were able to build up practices consisting mainly of women patients. Margaret Smith Bell (KQCPI/RCSI, 1894) built up a large practice of chiefly women patients in Manchester while also acting as a member of the Midwives Supervisory Committee and working as a medical officer at both the Ancoats Day Industrial School and 'The Grove' retreat in Fallowfield.[27] Her older sister, Elizabeth (Eliza) Gould Bell (QCB, 1893), who practised in Belfast, also built up a practice largely of female patients.[28] In addition to her general practice work, Eliza also took an active part in the suffrage movement and acted as honorary physician to the Women's Maternity Home, Belfast, and the Babies' Home at The Grove, Belfast, in addition to being involved in the babies clubs welfare scheme.[29] Cecilia Williamson (RCSI, 1909) went to Ipswich in 1913, where she worked as an assistant to a female doctor with an established practice. After a short time, she took full charge of the practice and became well known for her maternity work.[30]

Patients were not always receptive to women doctors, however: Margaret McEnroy (QCG, 1926) recalled one elderly female patient of hers in the late 1920s commenting, 'Ah girleen, would you ever get me a real doctor?'[31]

Certain addresses were occupied by successions of female general practitioners, for example 18 Upper Merrion Street, Dublin. From 1895 to 1899, the address was the practice of Emily Winifred Dickson. Five years later, it was occupied by Lizzie Beatty, a graduate of Queen's College Belfast who went on to work as a medical missionary. And from 1908 to 1912, it was the address of the practice of sisters Lily and Madeline Baker. It is highly likely that this address had a reputation for being the practice of women doctors.[32]

General practice enabled women doctors to combine family life and professional commitments, although it might also be combined with part-time positions such as work as medical inspectors of schools or as factory surgeons. Women general practitioners could also supplement their income through giving 'grinds' to medical students, lecturing under bodies such as the Technical Board and through literary work.[33] In the next sections, I will examine some of the other career options which could sometimes be held alone or in concurrence with running a general practice.

Hospital appointments

ALTHOUGH GENERAL PRACTICE was the most common career path for Irish women medical graduates, nevertheless over 16 per cent of women were successful in achieving hospital posts within five years of graduation (Table 5.4). Ella Ovenden, writing in 1907, claimed that the numbers of hospital appointments open to women were few and that they were not very highly paid. Thus, in her view, a newly qualified woman doctor 'ought to be content to take an unpaid post for the purpose of gaining new experience'. Once the new graduate had gained experience, there were more opportunities open to her, such as posts in some of the infirmaries and asylums, worth from £40 to £100 or more a year but Ovenden acknowledged that there was a great deal of competition for these and that 'personal interest' was needed to obtain them.[34]

Certain Irish hospitals appear to have been renowned for their employment of women doctors, such as the Richmond Hospital in Dublin, an asylum,

Table 5.4 Numbers of women medical graduates who matriculated 1885–1922 working in hospital appointments five to thirty-five years after graduation, c.1891–1969

	5 years	10 years	15 years	25 years	35 years
Hospital appointments (total)	70 (16.3%[a])	61 (17.0%)	48 (15.1%)	44 (15.9%)	31 (12.8%)
General hospital	42	38	29	33	20
Asylum	11	10	11	5	7
Children's/ maternity	17	13	8	6	4

[a] These are percentages of the traceable graduates only.
Source: *Medical Directory*.

which employed women medical attendants to take charge of its female wards from the 1890s.[35] Emily Winifred Dickson, for example, worked as assistant master at the Coombe Lying-In Hospital from 1895 to 1898 and then spent three to four years as a gynaecologist at the Richmond.[36] The appointment of women doctors to these Irish hospitals received great attention in the Irish press, suggesting that the lady doctor was seen as something of a novelty. For example, in 1903, the appointment of three women doctors to the residential staff of the Richmond Hospital led *St Stephen's* magazine to declare: 'We hear that an epidemic – not of small pox, so don't be alarmed – but of Lady Medicals, has broken out in a certain hospital in town'.[37]

One English female medical graduate, Muriel Iles, claimed in 1901 that the men doctors of Dublin hospitals treated their female counterparts chivalrously, as a result of the system of mixed classes in Irish medical schools as discussed in Chapter 4:

> On coming to Dublin, one of the first things that strikes you as a medical woman is the extreme kindliness of the men doctors. This is probably largely due to the system of mixed medical education in vogue here. The men and women (or boys and girls) are accustomed to meet one another on equal terms at college and hospital, and are consequently not afraid of each other afterwards.[38]

Evidently, in Iles' view, as someone who had experienced the English system of segregation for medical education, Irish hospitals were a positive place to work, in which women were treated well by the men doctors.

Hospital appointments represented the second largest career grouping for women medical graduates. Notably, women medical graduates were most likely to obtain hospital appointments in general hospitals, rather than in asylums or children's/maternity hospitals (Table 5.4), thus indicating that there were genuine opportunities for them outside their expected spheres of employment. This differed from the situation for women medical graduates in England, as Mary Ann Elston's work has suggested. She has shown that a sample of English women doctors holding hospital 'house posts' in 1899 and 1907 were most likely to be in women-run hospitals than in other types of institutions.[39] These women-run hospitals had close connections with the female medical schools such as the London School of Medicine for Women and the Edinburgh School of Medicine for Women. In contrast, women medical graduates in Ireland were more likely to work in posts in general

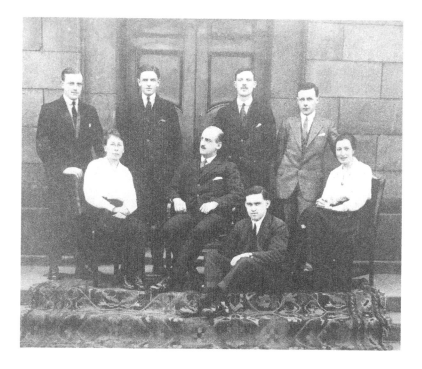

Plate IV Resident staff of Sir Patrick Dun's Hospital, November 1918–May 1919. Photograph includes Eileen Dowse (TCD, 1920) on the left and Enid Baile (RCSI, 1922) on the right.

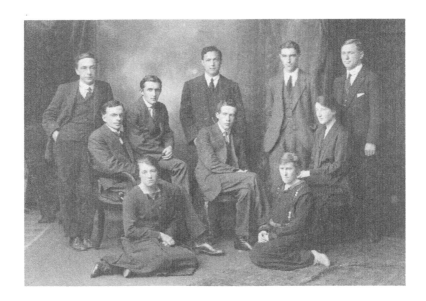

Plate V Residential medical staff of Adelaide Hospital, 1921. Photograph shows Charlotte Annie Stuart (TCD, 1922) and Dorothy Herbert Benson (RCSI, 1922) seated at the front and Enid Baile (RCSI, 1922) in the second row, to the right.

hospitals rather than in women-run institutions or hospitals for women and children. It is possible that this was due to the system of co-education in Irish medical institutions and the liberalism of the Irish medical profession.

The most common hospital appointments available to newly qualified doctors were as house surgeons and house physicians. House surgeons were members of the surgical staff, while house physicians were members of the general medical staff of a hospital. These appointments served as 'a buffer between an education with a large theoretical content and the everyday requirements of the profession'.[40] Alfreda Baker (QCB, 1921), for example, secured the post of house surgeon at the Royal Victoria Hospital in Belfast after graduation. This first post provided her with a step on to the medical career ladder and by 1931 she held the more senior position of resident house surgeon at the Hounslow Hospital in Middlesex, England. By 1936, she was assistant consultant surgeon at the same hospital and from 1946 she worked as a consultant surgeon at the Elizabeth Garrett Anderson Hospital in London.[41] Early graduates tended to prefer the post of house physician to that of house surgeon, as it was believed that this would prepare them better for a career in general practice. However, because complaints such as skin diseases, venereal diseases and urinary and bone and joint disorders also lay within the domain of surgery, newly qualified doctors were advised to take up a house surgeon position if it was offered.[42]

One writer for the *Women Students Medical Magazine* (a periodical published in Edinburgh from 1902 to 1904 by a group of women medical students) wrote in 1903 of her experiences working as a house surgeon for an Irish ophthalmic hospital. She commented that house surgeons tended to patients in the hospital as well as out-patient cases, which might number sixty daily.[43] Her salary was £30 a year and she found the experience positive, as it offered the opportunity to study the work of more senior surgeons while gaining further experience in the field.[44] As in the case of Alfreda Baker, an initial post as a house surgeon allowed the young doctor to gain valuable experience which would further her medical career.

Another hospital appointment that graduates could seek was that of resident medical officer. These appointments differed from house surgeon and physician posts in that the resident medical officer was provided with lodging and boarding while working at the hospital in question and these positions also had the added advantage of introducing the doctor to a locality, making it much easier for them to practise there afterwards.[45] Miss Cummins, writing in 1914, commented that women had not yet won the same opportunity of medical work as men and that men were more likely than women to obtain resident appointments in most of the hospitals in Britain and Ireland.[46] Nevertheless, Isobel Addy Tate (QCB, 1899) and Mary Ellen Logan (QCB, 1902) gained resident hospital posts. Tate held a resident physician appointment at Hailet Sanatorium, Oxford, after graduation, before becoming a resident medical officer at Burnley Union Infirmary, while Logan worked as resident medical officer at the Infirmary in Belfast.

Some women took up appointments working in asylums and mental hospitals. Among them was Lucia Strangman Fitzgerald (RCSI, 1896), who secured a post as a medical officer in charge of the female wards of the District Lunatic Asylum in Cork, where she remained until the end of her career. Amelia Grogan (RCSI, 1895) was principal doctor in charge of the women's wing of the Mullingar Lunatic Asylum in 1900, before moving to England, where she worked as a medical officer at a women's hospital in Brighton.[47] Asylums offered new graduates a good salary and a comfortable position, and Charles Bell Keetley's 1878 medical student guide advised that persons 'of lively disposition with musical accomplishments and a taste for private theatricals' were often preferred as officers at these institutions.[48]

Public health

THE PUBLIC HEALTH SECTOR was an important area of employment for women graduates, especially those who moved to England. It was the third largest area of employment for the cohort, with 5 per cent of women graduates working in the field five years after graduation and 22 per cent working in the field fifteen years after graduation. This sector of medicine was claimed to be an appealing area of work for new graduates because it did not require the time and capital necessary to build up a private practice.[49] As Table 5.5 demonstrates, women doctors working in public health were commonly employed as schools medical officers, dispensary doctors, assistant medical officers of health and medical officers of health.

In Ireland, graduates commonly worked as Poor Law (dispensary) medical officers. The post of dispensary medical officer had been created in Ireland by legislation in 1851 which resulted in the country being divided into 723 dispensary districts, each with one or more medical officers.[50] The election of new Poor Law medical officers in Ireland was often corrupt in nature. According to the *Irish Medical Students' Guide*, politics and religious feeling often entered into the election of Poor Law medical officers and family interest also possessed great weight in the late nineteenth century.[51]

Table 5.5 Numbers of women medical graduates who matriculated 1885–1922 working in public health five to thirty-five years after graduation, c.1891–1969

	5 years	10 years	15 years	25 years	35 years
Public health total	22	40	70	57	52
	(5.1%[a])	(11.1%)	(22.1%)	(20.7%)	(21.4%)
Assistant medical officer	5	5	14	15	13
Schools medical officer	8	12	19	14	9
Dispensary	6	13	18	14	10
Medical officer of health	2	4	10	8	12
Aurist	0	0	1	0	0
Child welfare centre	1	5	5	3	6
Medical examiner	0	0	0	1	0
Vaccinations	0	1	0	0	0
Ministry of Health	0	0	1	1	1
Registrar	0	0	1	0	0
Tuberculosis officer	0	0	1	1	1

[a] These are percentages of the traceable graduates only.
Source: *Medical Directory*.

In many instances, an appointment was 'virtually made before the advertisement appears for a Medical Officer, in which case also candidates are put to unnecessary trouble and expense under false pretences'.[52] Poor Law appointments were often eagerly sought by new graduates because they provided a salary which a graduate could supplement with his or her private earnings, in addition to gaining practice in the field. The average salary for a Poor Law medical officer was £116 a year in 1907.[53] One doctor in Cashel, Tipperary, in 1903, estimated that dispensary officers attended on an average 1,000 cases a year, and that they received 4–6*d* for each town case and an average of about 20*d* for each country case.[54] The duties of Poor Law medical officers were twofold. They were expected to attend their dispensary on a given day or days during each week. In addition, Poor Law medical officers were issued with visiting tickets by members of the Poor Law committee or by the relieving officer for sick persons in need of relief. They were then expected to visit the sick person at any hour of the day or night as needed and to provide medical attendance as often as was necessary until the termination of the patient's case. Moreover, these doctors were expected to keep up with many registry books and returns, as well as making up the medicines for the poor in many districts.[55] Overall, Poor Law medical officers had a heavy workload. They were expected to undertake medical duties (attending the dispensary and visiting patients in their homes), sanitary duties (acting as the medical officer of health for the district), registration duties (to register births, marriages and deaths), vaccination duties and constabulary, certifying, factory, coastguard and lighthouse duties, as required. The remainder of his or her time, if there was any available, could be devoted to private practice.[56]

The Public Health Act 1872 dictated that all English authorities were to follow London's lead and appoint medical officers of health who would deal with issues of sanitation and public health.[57] The act also called for further professionalisation of these officers and universities began to offer diplomas in public health in order to deal with this demand.[58] In 1874, Irish dispensary doctors became medical officers of health for their districts, for which they received an extra salary, which by the 1900s averaged £19 per year.[59] Anne Hardy has argued that the foundation of the medical officer of health resulted in the creation of a new dimension to the medical profession's involvement in government and social reform.[60]

Despite the fact that the position of medical officer of health existed from the 1870s, public health came to be associated with women only from the early twentieth century. In 1911, for example, the *Dublin Medical Press* suggested that women should take a leading role in the public health movement, and organisations such as the Women's National Health Association, founded by Lady Aberdeen in 1908, supported such suggestions.[61] Certainly, in Britain, women doctors found a niche for themselves within the public health movement, working initially as assistant medical officers of health and, after 1907, as schools medical officers. Despite claims by the Irish medical profession that there was greater urgency for medical inspection of schoolchildren within the country considering the general death rate (which was higher than that in England or Scotland), it was not until 1919 that school health inspection and treatment services were introduced to Ireland, under the Public Health: Medical Treatment of Children Act.[62] Eleanor Lowry, who initially matriculated at Queen's College Belfast (LSMW, 1907), commented that work as a school officer offered many benefits for those interested in improving the social conditions of children, although, for some, medical inspection often had the potential to become mere routine.[63] By the 1920s, women doctors came to be employed as medical officers at child welfare centres, a role which, it was claimed, they were eminently suited to undertake.[64]

Prospects of promotion were slim for women doctors who worked in the public health sector, with some women doctors, such as Clara Scally (UCD, 1921), holding the position of assistant medical officer of health in Barnsley for almost her entire career with no promotion. It was claimed that women faced discrimination within the British public health service and that male doctors were more likely to achieve promotion than women. One woman doctor, Letitia Fairfield, wrote in 1924:

> the worst drawback of the Public Health Service at the present time is however, the poor prospect of promotion. The women are worse off [than the men], as even in large services where many women are employed, promotion is usually reserved for the men and no effort is made to organise the work so that women can be heads of departments. A woman will often find herself after ten years of meritorious service precisely where she started as regards salary, less efficient professionally owing to the monotonous nature of her duties and with no prospect for the future except that of seeing junior men step over her head. Perhaps a score of important Government or semi-public appointments are now held by medical women, but this is not enough to mitigate the stagnation among rank and file.[65]

Certainly, in Ireland, in spite of the favourable attitudes towards women in medical education, it seems that there were fewer opportunities in public health work than in other spheres of medical employment, although it is difficult to determine whether this was due to discrimination against women doctors or simply a result of a lack of posts.

Specialist and academic career options

A s TABLE 5.6 SHOWS, not all women worked in general practice, hospitals or the public health sector. A small proportion of women worked as specialists. Five years after graduation, just 1.6 per cent of the cohort were working as gynaecologists, anaesthetists or pathologists, and this proportion remained stable for the cohort ten and fifteen years after graduation. However, by twenty-five years after graduation, the proportion increased to over 4 per cent, with women graduates working as anaesthetists, pathologists, radiologists, dermatologists and psychiatrists. This is unsurprising as, by this point in their careers, women doctors would have worked their way up to these positions and undergone the necessary training required. What is interesting here is the lack of women working as specialists within the realms of women's health – as gynaecologists – giving further proof that women did not necessarily enter into the careers that were expected of them.

Table 5.6 Alternative careers of women medical graduates who matriculated 1885–1922 working five to thirty-five years after graduation, c.1891–1969

	5 years	10 years	15 years	25 years	35 years
Missions/ humanitarian work	14 (3.3%[a])	15 (4.2%)	20 (6.3%)	15 (5.4%)	13 (5.3%)
Specialists	7 (1.6%)	4 (1.1%)	6 (1.9%)	12 (4.3%)	9 (3.7%)
Gynaecologist	2	0	0	0	0
Anaesthetist	4	2	3	4	3
Pathologist	1	1	2	2	1
Radiologist	0	1	0	2	2
Dermatologist	0	0	1	2	1
Psychiatrist	0	0	0	2	2
University appointment	6 (1.4%)	3 (0.8%)	2 (0.6%)	2 (0.7%)	3 (1.2%)
War-related work	3	1	0	0	0
Convent	0	0	1	0	0
Company doctor	5 (1.1%)	7 (1.5%)	4 (0.9%)	4 (0.9%)	2 (0.4%)
Research	2	4	3	2	1
Deceased	0	0	4	8	12
Not practising/retired	0	1	2	4	12

[a] These are percentages of the traceable graduates only.
Source: *Medical Directory*.

A small number of women graduates worked as company doctors. Henrietta Ball-Dodd (RCSI, 1922), for example, worked as a medical examiner to the Britannic and Co-operative Assurance Company from 1927 to 1937, while Sybil Stantion (later Magan, QCC, 1921), worked as a medical officer for the Post Office from 1931 until 1946. Similarly low numbers of women worked in the areas which will be discussed next: those of academic work and humanitarian work.

In the previous chapter, we learnt that anatomy demonstrators were often female as a result of the separation of women and men students for dissection classes. Occasionally, women medical graduates attained such posts at universities. Of the ninety-seven women who graduated before 1918, five worked as demonstrators in anatomy at Irish and English universities. One female medical graduate, Alice Carleton (née Chance, UCD, 1917), the daughter of Arthur Chance, former president of the Royal College of Surgeons in Ireland, achieved a post as an anatomy demonstrator at Oxford University straight after qualification and held this post for much of her career. She was initially employed to teach anatomy to the women medical students but, after the end of the First World War, she was lecturing to both men and women.[66] She was apparently both admired and feared by her students.[67] Carleton published widely in the field of dermatology and after her retirement from Oxford she worked as a visiting lecturer at the University of California and later as a visiting lecturer at Yale.[68] Eveline McDaniel (QCB, 1921) worked as professor of therapeutic pharmacology and material medica at University College Galway in the early 1930s. McDaniel was crucial in spear-heading the birth-control movement in Ireland and this seems to have been of more interest to her than a career in academia. She went to London in 1934 to train at the Marie Stopes' clinic before returning to Belfast to work as a schools medical officer and as the first doctor of the Marie Stopes' Mothers' Clinic in Belfast, from 1936 to 1940.[69]

Research was an area in which a few women worked. Ethel Luce (TCD, 1918) was the most prestigious researcher of the cohort. She attained a research fellowship in London before moving to America, where she achieved the position of Sterling senior fellow and professor of paediatrics at Yale University. Fifteen years after graduation, she worked as a research fellow in biology at the University of Rochester, while the remaining years of her career saw her working as assistant professor of zoology at the same university. Bacteriology in the early 1920s had been pronounced by one commentator as being 'the most romantic and most promising of all the branches of modern medicine' and it offered many opportunities for women graduates.[70] Teresa Jones (UCD, 1922) worked as a bacteriologist at St Ultan's Hospital.[71] Similarly, Anna O'Reilly (RCSI/RCPI, 1922) worked as an assistant to the professor of bacteriology at the Royal College of Surgeons in Ireland after graduation. It was, though, uncommon for women doctors to publish research in medical journals. Of the 452 women graduates in total, just 30 (6 per cent) published articles in medical journals.[72] The same number worked abroad in missionary and secular organisations which required women doctors.

Humanitarian medical work overseas

FROM THE 1920s, with growing fears that the medical marketplace was becoming overcrowded, women were increasingly being encouraged to go to India and other countries and work among the poor. According to Anne Digby, 'society's anxieties about female entrants to the medical profession were calmed to some extent by the perception that medical women would work in zenanas in India and hence not provide any competition at home'.[73] Indeed, those women doctors who moved overseas tended to go to places where there was a humanitarian need for them, such as India and Africa. It was often suggested that the best opening for a female physician was in India or Burma under the new government service for women in those countries, the aim of which was to provide adequate medical attention for native women.[74] However, strikingly, only 6 per cent of women medical graduates who matriculated between 1885 and 1922 worked abroad in humanitarian and missionary roles, despite claims that this would have been an important area of work for new graduates.

The Irish missionary movement grew significantly in the closing years of the nineteenth century.[75] Myrtle Hill has outlined the work of some Irish women doctors in Protestant missionary societies, among them Elizabeth Beatty (matriculated at QCB but qualified Edinburgh/Glasgow, 1899) and graduates from the Scottish medical schools such as Margaret McNeill and Isobel Mitchell.[76] In this section, I will discuss the lives of medical graduates who went abroad for humanitarian and missionary work. In Chapter 7, I will examine some members of the Irish Presbyterian Missionary Society in detail, but here I will also examine some Catholic women missionaries and Irish women who worked in secular organisations like the Dufferin Fund.

There had been cries for women doctors for India since 1882, when Frances Hoggan, one of the first licentiates of the King and Queen's College of Physicians of Ireland, published her paper 'Medical women for India', in which she argued that the medical needs of Indian women were not being met by the new civil wing of the Indian Medical Service, which had been established in 1880 in order to provide Western medical care to the Indian population.[77] In 1882, the Medical Women for India Fund for Bombay was established, while in 1885 the Dufferin Fund was established by Lady Dufferin, the wife of the then viceroy to India. The aim the Fund was to provide medical relief to Indian women in addition to establishing new hospitals and encouraging women, both British and Indian, to study medicine.[78] Both organisations recruited British women doctors to practise medicine in India in secular rather than missionary settings. The movement placed emphasis on social reform and philanthropy and defined itself as a 'self-consciously secular movement quite distinct from the medical missionary work which was already well underway in India'.[79] Edith Pechey, a contemporary of Sophia Jex-Blake, whom we met in Chapter 2, was one of the many women who played a role in the development of the Dufferin Fund.[80]

One Irish woman, Elizabeth Stephenson Walker (QCB, 1915), took an ap-pointment within the Indian Women's Medical Service. Walker had started her career as a medical attendant for the Royal Army Medical Corps, before moving to India and working for the Dufferin Fund. (She then disappears from the *Medical Directory*.) Women working in the Indian Women's Medical Service were not remunerated on the same scale as men working in the Indian Medical Service, although one commentator speculated that the career nevertheless provided a newly qualified female doctor with a good starting salary. Additionally, it allowed doctors to have a private practice in conjunction with their work, as well as entitling them to a pension on retirement. However, the same commentator argued that the majority of Irish women doctors did not wish to go so far afield and would prefer to work at home, in spite of the difficulties in securing a successful career as a general practitioner or employment in one of the general hospitals.[81] Working abroad was a compromise which provided some women with useful experience that might help them to secure a hospital appointment at home afterwards. However, the evidence seems to suggest that Irish women who went abroad as medical missionaries remained working in the missionary field for their entire careers, while those working in secular organisations such as the Dufferin Fund were likely to return home after a time. Moreover, it was more likely for Irish women doctors to work in missionary organisa-tions than in secular ones, as Table 5.7 shows.

Women doctors who wished to work as missionaries commonly aligned themselves with missionary societies, such as the Irish Presbyterian Missionary Society, the Zenana Medical Missions, the Methodist Missions, the Dublin University Missions and the Catholic Missionary Society, among others. Classmates at Queen's College Belfast Alexandrina Crawford Huston, Elizabeth Beatty and Emily Martha Crooks (all graduated in 1899, with Beatty taking the Scottish conjoint examinations) became members of the Irish Presbyterian Missionary Society. Huston was based in Bombay five years

Table 5.7 Numbers of women medical graduates who matriculated 1885–1922 engaged in missionary and secular humanitarian work five to thirty-five years after graduation, c.1899–1955[a]

	5 years	10 years	15 years	25 years	35 years
Total working in missions/ humanitarian field	14	15	20	15	13
Missions	10	13	14	12	11
Secular humanitarian work	4	2	6	3	2

[a] 1899 refers to five years after the graduation of the first of the women in the cohort who appears to have worked in the humanitarian field, while 1955 refers to the last recorded year when there was a member of the cohort engaged in humanitarian work.
Source: *Medical Directory*

after graduation, although there is no trace of her after this time. Beatty went to Kwangning, Manchuria, in China, in 1906, where she established her own hospital. She occasionally returned to Ireland in order to give lectures to Presbyterian societies and churches about her missionary work in China in order to fundraise for her hospital.[82] She remained in China for about eleven years.[83] For a small number of women doctors, missionary work was a lifelong commitment rather than simply about gaining valuable and varied medical experience. Crooks, for example, worked as a medical missionary in China, first at Newchwang and later in Kirin, Manchuria, where she was still based thirty-five years after graduation.

Anna Dengel (QCC, 1920) was the most famous missionary to graduate from an Irish medical school. Dengel had always wanted to become a missionary and with encouragement from Dr Agnes McLaren (KQCPI, 1877), an older doctor who worked in India, she trained at Queen's College Cork.[84] After her visa arrived, Dengel took up duty at St Catherine's Hospital in Rawalpindi, India, a hospital founded by McLaren.[85] She wrote of her experiences there:

The work was overwhelming. Besides the study of language, there was hospital work, the dispensary, and home visits. I quickly realised that this was a task for many and not for one. I could not have endured it longer than the four years I was there. No matter where I looked, I saw unrelieved, although preventable suffering. Malaria was common, epidemics were a constant threat, and government facilities were very limited. The marriage age was about fifteen, and the mortality of young mothers was very high, as midwifery was just being introduced. The awareness of the need for cleanliness was still rare. The hospital, although small, was not always full because the women, especially the Moslem women, could not easily come to stay. We had many obstetric cases, very often complicated ones. The few sisters present in the hospital were, owing to Church laws, prevented from assisting in midwifery, which in view of the haphazard care of women in childbirth, presented a serious gap in a women's hospital. This attitude, as well as our inability to help mothers in their hour of need under the prevailing conditions in India, touched me deeply and spurred me on to find a solution.[86]

Dengel, a Catholic, noted that most of the missionary work undertaken in India was carried out by Protestant missionary societies. This suggests that there may have been confessional rivalries between Catholic and Protestant missionary societies which may have influenced some Irish women medical graduates' decision to work in the missionary field. Feeling dismayed about how much of a difference she was making in India, she decided that it was necessary to make the plight of Indian women known to the Western world. She went to Washington, DC, and in 1925 founded her own order of women medical missionaries called the Medical Mission Sisters and toured around America and England giving lectures about missionary work and fundraising.[87] The Medical Mission Sisters trained Indian nurses and medical personnel for work in India, while Dengel informed readers of the work of her order and the plight of Indian women through her periodical the *Medical Missionary*, which she edited from 1927 into the 1950s.[88] Because of the pressures of public relations, fundraising and the administration of the organisation, she did not return to medical practice. However, she returned many times during her life to India, and later Pakistan, to visit members of the Medical Mission Sisters and the hospitals founded under the auspices of the organisation.[89]

India, China and, later, African countries such as Kenya, Nigeria, South Africa and Uganda were common destinations for Irish women medical missionaries. Evelyn Connolly (UCD, 1919) worked at the Nsambya Mission Hospital, Kampala, Uganda, for at least thirty-five years.[90] Alongside Mother Kevin, the first superior general of the Franciscan Missionary Sisters for Africa, she established a Catholic nurses' training school at Nsambya.[91] Similarly, Margaret Mary Nolan (UCD, 1925) first worked in India at the Dufferin Fund Eden Hospital in Calcutta before migrating to Nigeria, where she worked as a gynaecologist at a mission hospital until the end of her career.

Conclusion

IT WAS CLAIMED in the late nineteenth century that there was a need for women doctors in the sphere of women and children's health and in the missionary field. Those arguing in favour of women in medicine in the period stressed this need, while members of the medical profession, who were concerned about future pressure on the already overcrowded medical marketplace, also encouraged women doctors to work in the missionary field. However, as this chapter has demonstrated, early women graduates from Irish medical institutions were more likely to work in other areas.

Overall, women graduates were most likely to work as general practitioners; however, hospital and public health work were also common areas of employment. Hospital appointments were more likely to be in general hospitals rather than in women and children's hospitals or wards, suggesting that women doctors entered into realms of medical practice which were not expected of them. It seems likely that the sense of inclusion in Irish medical education that women students experienced continued into their careers in Ireland and there was not the same sense of separatism that historians have argued existed for women doctors in Britain and the United States.

Notes

1 Stewart Woodhouse, 'To students', *Dublin Journal of Medical Science*, 68:4 (1879), p. 351.
2 Michael Foster Reaney, *The Medical Profession: The Carmichael Prize Essay for 1904* (Dublin: Browne and Nolan, 1905), p. 104.
3 *Ibid.*
4 Ella Ovenden, 'Medicine', in Myrrha Bradshaw (ed.), *Open Doors for Irishwomen: A Guide to the Professions Open to Educated Women in Ireland* (Dublin: Irish Central Bureau for the Employment of Women, 1907), p. 36.
5 Letter from Howard Marsh, 'Women doctors and the war', *Times* (London), 8 December 1914, p. 9.
6 Reaney, *The Medical Profession*, p. 103.
7 For more on this topic, see Anne Digby, *Making a Medical Living: Doctors and Patients in the English Market for Medicine, 1720–1911* (Cambridge: Cambridge University Press, 1994).
8 Anne Crowther and Marguerite Dupree, *Medical Lives in the Age of Surgical Revolution* (Cambridge: Cambridge University Press, 2007), p. 244.
9 Louisa Garrett Anderson, 'Why medical women are suffragists', *Votes for Women*, 6:273 (1913), p. 509.
10 Typed memoirs of Emily Winifred Dickson, private collection of Niall Martin, Edinburgh.
11 'Women in the learned professions (extracts from a paper given by Miss Cummins which received the gold medal from the Cork University Philosophical Society)', *Irish Citizen*, 28 July 1914, p. 66.
12 'For mothers and daughters: choosing a profession', *Catholic Bulletin and Book Review*, 12:2 (1922), p. 732.
13 'Postgraduate study', *Lancet*, 26 September 1914, p. 799.
14 *Ibid.*, p. 803.
15 Reaney, *The Medical Profession*, p. 103.
16 Irene Finn, 'Women in the medical profession in Ireland, 1876–1919', in Bernadette Whelan (ed.), *Women and Paid Work in Ireland, 1500–1930* (Dublin: Four Courts Press, 2000), pp. 102–19, on p. 112.

17 See Anne Crowther and Marguerite Dupree, 'The invisible general practitioner: the careers of Scottish medical students in the late nineteenth century', *Bulletin of the History of Medicine*, 70:3 (1996), pp. 387–413. Crowther and Dupree have outlined the difficulties involved with tracing general practitioners through the *Medical Directory*. They comment that the *Medical Directory* (published annually by the General Medical Council since 1845), with the exception of early editions, does not identify general practitioners, who are simply 'taken for granted' (p. 389).

18 *Irish Medical Student's Guide* (Dublin: Dublin Medical Press, 1877), p. 21.

19 'Anna Maria Dengel', in Leone McGregor Hellstedt (ed.), *Women Physicians of the World: Autobiographies of Medical Pioneers* (Washington, DC, and London: Medical Women's International Federation, Hemisphere Publishing Corporation, 1978), p. 93.

20 Ovenden, 'Medicine', p. 36.

21 Letitia Fairfield, 'Women and the public health service', *Magazine of the London School of Medicine for Women and Royal Free Hospital*, 19:87 (1924), p. 14.

22 Elizabeth Kemper Adams, *Women Professional Workers: A Study Made for the Women's Educational and Industrial Union* (New York: Macmillan, 1924), p. 69.

23 C. B. Keetley, *The Student's Guide to the Medical Profession* (London: Macmillan, 1878), pp. 33–4.

24 General Medical Council, *Medical Directory*, entries for Georgina Collier, later Harvey.

25 Anne Digby, *The Evolution of British General Practice, 1850–1948* (Oxford: Oxford University Press, 1999), p. 168.

26 'Social and personal', *Irish Times*, 26 June 1934, p. 6.

27 'Obituary: Margaret Smith Bell', *BMJ*, 8 September 1906 (from Kirkpatrick Archive, Royal College of Physicians, Dublin).

28 'Obituary: Dr Eliza Gould Bell', *Irish Times*, 10 July 1934, p. 8.

29 'Woman doctor's death', *Irish Press*, 12 July 1934 (from Kirkpatrick Archive, Royal College of Physicians, Dublin).

30 'Obituary: Cecilia F. Williamson', *BMJ*, 15 August 1964, p. 453.

31 Oral history interview with Brian McEnroy, nephew of Margaret.

32 Source: *Medical Directory*.

33 Ovenden, 'Medicine', p. 36.

34 *Ibid.*

35 'The Richmond lunatic asylum', *Freeman's Journal*, 8 December 1894, p. 4.

36 Typed memoirs of Emily Winifred Dickson.

37 Untitled article, *St Stephen's*, 1:13 (1903), p. 244.

38 Muriel Iles, 'Notes on two centres of post-graduate work', *Magazine of the London School of Medicine for Women and Royal Free Hospital*, no. 18 (1901), p. 730.

39 Mary Ann Elston, '"Run by women (mainly) for women": medical women's hospitals in Britain, 1866–1948', in Laurence Conrad and Anne Hardy (eds), *Women and Modern Medicine*, Clio Medica Series (Amsterdam: Rodopi, 2001), pp. 73–108, on p. 84.

40 Crowther and Dupree, *Medical Lives in the Age of Surgical Revolution*, p. 127.

41 *Medical Directory* entries for Alfreda Baker, from 1926 to 1956.

42 Keetley, *The Student's Guide to the Medical Profession*, p. 28.

43 'Medical posts held by women, no. 3: house surgeonship in an ophthalmic hospital, Ireland', *Women Students Medical Magazine*, 1:4 (1903), p. 111.

44 *Ibid.*

45 Keetley, *The Student's Guide to the Medical Profession*, p. 29.

46 'Women in the learned professions', p. 66.

47 'College news', *Alexandra College Magazine*, no. 16 (1900), p. 46.

48 Keetley, *The Student's Guide to the Medical Profession*, p. 30.

49 'For mothers and daughters: professions for girls', *Catholic Bulletin and Book Review*, 12:2 (1922), p. 732.

50 Ruth Barrington, *Health, Medicine and Politics in Ireland 1900–1970* (Dublin: Institute of Public Administration, 1987), pp. 7–8.
51 *Irish Medical Student's Guide*, p. 17.
52 *Ibid.*, p. 18.
53 Barrington, *Health, Medicine and Politics*, p. 9.
54 'Correspondence', *St Stephen's*, 1:10 (1903), p. 218.
55 *Irish Medical Student's Guide*, p. 17.
56 Reaney, *The Medical Profession*, p. 86.
57 Crowther and Dupree, *Medical Lives in the Age of Surgical Revolution*, p. 215.
58 Anne Hardy, 'Public health and the expert: the London medical officers of health, 1856–1900', in Roy MacLeod (ed.), *Government and Expertise: Specialists, Administrators and Professionals, 1860–1919* (Cambridge: Cambridge University Press, 2003), pp. 128–42, on p. 130.
59 Barrington, *Health, Medicine and Politics*, p. 9.
60 Hardy, 'Public health and the expert', p. 130.
61 'Women and public health', *DMP*, 20 September 1911, p. 311.
62 Sir William J. Thompson, 'Medical inspection of school children', *Dublin Journal of Medical Science*, 136:3 (1913), pp. 161–73, on p. 163, and Finola Kennedy, *Family, Economy and Government in Ireland* (Dublin: Economic and Social Research Institute, 1989), p. 133.
63 Eleanor Lowry, 'Some side paths in the medical inspection of school children', *Magazine of the London School of Medicine for Women and Royal Free Hospital*, 7:48 (1911), p. 362.
64 Lydia Henry, 'Medical women and public health work', *Medical Women's Federation Quarterly Newsletter*, February 1922, p. 18 (Wellcome Library, London, SA/MWF/B.2/1).
65 Fairfield, 'Women and the public health service', pp. 13–14.
66 'Obituary: Alice B. Carleton', *BMJ*, 12 January 1980, p. 124.
67 A. M. Cooke, *My First 75 Years of Medicine* (London: Royal College of Physicians, 1994), p. 7.
68 'Obituary: Dr Alice Chance', *Times*, 4 December 1979, p. 14.
69 *Medical Directory* entries for Eveline McDaniel, and Greta Jones, 'Marie Stopes in Ireland: the Mother's Clinic in Belfast, 1936–47', *Social History of Medicine*, 5:2 (1992), pp. 255–77.
70 'Introductory address by Viscount Burnham to open winter session of London School of Medicine for Women', *Magazine of the London School of Medicine for Women and Royal Free Hospital*, 17:83 (1922), p. 129.
71 *Medical Directory.*
72 *Medical Directory*, obituaries.
73 Digby, *The Evolution of British General Practice*, p. 162.
74 'Women in the learned professions', p. 66.
75 Edmund M. Hogan, *The Irish Missionary Movement: A Historical Survey 1830–1980* (Dublin: Gill and Macmillan, 1990), p. 7.
76 Myrtle Hill, 'Gender, culture and "the spiritual empire": the Irish Protestant female missionary experience', *Women's History Review*, 16:2 (2007), pp. 203–26, on pp. 209–10.
77 Anne Witz, '"Colonising women": female medical practice in colonial India, 1880–1890', in Laurence Conrad and Anne Hardy (eds), *Women and Modern Medicine*, Clio Medica Series (Amsterdam: Rodopi, 2001), pp. 23–52, on p. 27.
78 Geraldine Forbes, 'Medical careers and health care for Indian women: patterns of control', *Women's History Review*, 3:4 (1994), pp. 515–30, on p. 516.
79 Witz, 'Colonising women', p. 26.
80 Forbes, 'Medical careers and health care for Indian women', p. 518.

81 'Women in the learned professions', p. 66.
82 Classified advertisement 191, *Irish Times*, 25 November 1911, p. 6.
83 'Obituary: Dr. Elizabeth Beatty', *Irish Times*, 13 August 1924, p. 6.
84 Hellstedt, *Women Physicians of the World*, p. 93.
85 Ann Ball, *Faces of Holiness: Modern Saints in Photos and Words* (Huntington, IN: Our Sunday Visitor Publishing, 1998), p. 19.
86 Hellstedt, *Women Physicians of the World*, pp. 93–4.
87 D. Donnelly, 'Catholic medical missions', *Studies: An Irish Quarterly Review*, 19:76 (December 1930), pp. 661–70, on p. 665.
88 Angelyn Dries, 'Fire and flame: Anna Dengel and the medical mission to women and children', *Missology*, 27:4 (1999), pp. 495–502, on p. 498. With thanks to Ryan Johnson for alerting me to this source.
89 Information courtesy of Sr Jane Gates, Medical Mission Sisters.
90 *Medical Directory.*
91 Website: 'Mother Kevin: a prophetic woman', www.catholicireland.net/pages/index.php?nd=53&art=440, consulted 7 July 2009.

Trends in the careers of Irish women doctors: emigration, marriage and the First World War

IN THIS CHAPTER, I will examine the themes of emigration and marriage and how these affected the careers of Irish women medical graduates. Following this, I will investigate whether the First World War resulted in a change of opportunities for Irish women in medicine. Historiographically, the war is seen as a turning point in history, in that it inaugurated significant life and career changes for women.[1] Such views have been challenged by feminist historians, who have argued that, after the war, powerful groups such as trade unions, government ministries and doctors 'tried successfully to limit the alterations in gender relations created by the demand for women's labour and hence, that underlying structures remained the same'.[2] Gail Braybon has argued that the 1920s proved to be challenging years for many women workers, with some commenting that life was more difficult than it had been during the war.[3]

I will consider the women medical graduates in two distinctive cohorts – those who qualified prior to 1918 and those who qualified after 1918 – as a means of investigating the oft-cited impact of the war. As in the previous chapter, tables of data based on my database lie throughout the chapter. Ninety-seven women graduated with medical qualifications from Irish institutions prior to 1918, and the remaining 355 of the cohort qualified after 1918. The difference in the sizes of these two cohorts is very striking; however, it may not be entirely a result of the war but rather reflect trends in increased acceptance of women pursuing university education. The careers of the two cohorts are summarised in Tables 6.1 and 6.2.

Evidently, the first cohort graduated in a twenty-five-year period when the lady doctor was less common. By the post-war period, however, into the 1920s and 1930s, female doctors were more established in numbers and would have been less of an exception. I will focus on the changes in attitude

Table 6.1 Posts of the ninety-seven pre-1918 women medical graduates five to thirty-five years after graduation, c.1891–1953

	5 years	10 years	15 years	25 years	35 years
Traceable graduates	91	76	72	57	57
	(93.8%)	(78.4%)	(74.3%)	(58.8%)	(58.8%)
Untraceable graduates	6	21	25	40	40
	(6.2%)	(21.6%)	(25.7%)	(41.2%)	(41.2%)
General practice	*33*	*21*	*20*	*20*	*21*
	(36.3%ᵃ)	*(27.6%)*	*(27.8%)*	*(35.0%)*	*(36.8%)*
Address but no post	33	21	16	16	16
(presumed to be GPs)					
GP (listed as GPs)	0	0	4	4	5
Hospital appointments	*30*	*30*	*21*	*12*	*7*
	(33.0%)	*(39.5%)*	*(29.2%)*	*(21.1%)*	*(12.3%)*
General hospital	16	15	10	5	1
Asylum	6	4	4	3	3
Children's/maternity	8	11	7	4	3
Public health	*8*	*12*	*17*	*11*	*10*
	(8.8%)	*(15.8%)*	*(23.6%)*	*(19.3%)*	*(17.5%)*
Assistant medical officer	4	3	1	1	1
Schools medical officer	4	7	10	6	2
Dispensary	0	2	4	2	3
Medical officer of health	0	0	1	0	3
Aurist	0	0	1	0	0
Child welfare centre	0	0	0	1	1
Medical examiner	0	0	0	1	0
Missions	*6*	*5*	*5*	*4*	*4*
	(6.6%)	*(6.6%)*	*(6.9%)*	*(7.0%)*	*(7.0%)*
Specialists	*3*	*0*	*1*	*0*	*1*
	(3.3%)		*(1.4%)*		*(1.8%)*
Gynaecologist	2	0	0	0	0
Anaesthetist	1	0	1	0	1
University appointment	*5*	*2*	*2*	*1*	*2*
	(5.5%)	*(2.6%)*	*(2.8%)*	*(1.8%)*	*(3.6%)*
War-related work	3	1	0	0	0
Company doctor	2	2	0	0	0
Research	1	2	2	2	1
Women's Medical Service	0	1	1	0	0
for India					
Deceased	0	0	3	7	11
Not practising/retired	0	0	2	3	5
Total	*91*	*76*	*72*	*57*	*57*

ᵃ These are percentages of traceable graduates only.
Source: *Medical Directory.*

Table 6.2 Posts of the 355 post-1918 women medical graduates five to thirty-five years after graduation, c.1924–69

	5 years	10 years	15 years	25 years	35 years
Traceable graduates	338	283	245	219	186
	(95.2%)	(79.7%)	(69.0%)	(61.7%)	(52.4%)
Untraceable graduates	17	72	110	136	169
	(4.8%)	(20.3%)	(31.0%)	(38.3%)	(47.6%)
General practice	*267*	*202*	*139*	*111*	*92*
	(79.0%[a])	*(71.4%)*	*(56.7%)*	*(50.7%)*	*(49.5%)*
Address but no post (presumed to be GPs)	266	198	135	109	90
GP (listed as GPs)	1	4	4	2	2
Hospital appointments	*40*	*31*	*27*	*32*	*24*
	(11.8%)	*(11.0%)*	*(11.0%)*	*(14.6%)*	*(12.9%)*
General hospital	26	23	19	28	19
Asylum	5	6	7	2	4
Children's/maternity	9	2	1	2	1
Public health	*14*	*28*	*53*	*46*	*42*
	(4.1%)	*(9.9%)*	*(21.6%)*	*(21.0%)*	*(22.6%)*
Assistant medical officer	1	2	13	14	12
Schools medical officer	4	5	9	8	7
Dispensary	6	11	14	12	7
Medical officer of health	2	4	9	8	9
Child welfare centre	1	5	5	2	5
Medical examiner	0	0	0	0	0
Vaccinations	0	1	0	0	0
Ministry of Health	0	0	1	1	1
Registrar	0	0	1	0	0
Tuberculosis officer	0	0	1	1	1
Missions	*8*	*9*	*14*	*11*	*9*
	(2.4%)	*(3.2%)*	*(5.7%)*	*(5.0%)*	*(4.8%)*
Specialists	*4*	*4*	*5*	*12*	*8*
	(1.2%)	*(1.4%)*	*(2.0%)*	*(5.5%)*	*(4.3%)*
Anaesthetist	3	2	2	4	2
Pathologist	1	1	2	2	1
Radiologist	0	1	0	2	2
Dermatologist	0	0	1	2	1
Psychiatrist	0	0	0	2	2
University appointment	1	1	0	1	1
Convent	0	0	1	0	0
Company/factory doctor	3	5	4	4	2
Research	1	2	1	0	0
Deceased	0	0	1	1	1
Not practising/retired	0	1	0	1	7
Total	*338*	*283*	*245*	*219*	*186*

[a] These are percentages of traceable graduates only.
Source: *Medical Directory*.

as a result of the war and the involvement of Irish women doctors in it. I will then examine the effect of the war in the three main areas where Irish graduates worked: general practice, hospital appointments and public health.

Emigration

EMIGRATION TO ENGLAND was a common theme in the stories of many of these women doctors, with few women migrating to Scotland or Wales for work. Greta Jones has argued that throughout the late nineteenth and early twentieth centuries, there was a constant flow of doctors emigrating from Ireland.[4] She has claimed that Irish doctors who emigrated did not necessarily do so because they faced diminished opportunities. Rather, she opines that 'the anticipation of a good living in England, the excitement of the metropolis or larger town, and the opportunities provided by an empire' were the main factors which encouraged Irish medical graduates to migrate.[5] It was uncommon for Irish women doctors to migrate to traditional Irish emigrant destinations such as Australia, the United States and Canada, which suggests that there were ample opportunities for women medical graduates within the United Kingdom (Table 6.3).[6]

Table 6.3 Destinations of the 452 women medical graduates who matriculated 1885–1922, five to thirty-five years after graduation, c.1891–1969

Location	5 years	10 years	15 years	25 years	35 years
Africa	5	4	8	6	7
America	0	3	4	3	4
Australia	0	2	2	0	0
China	2	5	5	4	2
Egypt	0	1	1	0	1
England	78 (18.3%[a])	101 (28.0%)	128 (40.3%)	107 (38.8%)	89 (36.8%)
India	6	8	7	4	5
Ireland	332 (77.8%)	230 (64.0%)	153 (48.1%)	138 (50.0%)	116 (47.9%)
Italy	0	1	0	0	0
Pakistan	0	0	0	0	1
Persia	0	1	0	0	0
Scotland	3	2	1	1	2
Wales	1	3	5	5	3
Deceased	0	0	4	8	12
Unknown	25	91	134	176	210

[a] These are percentages of traceable graduates only.
Source: *Medical Directory*.

Table 6.4 Destinations of the ninety-seven pre-1918 women medical graduates five to thirty-five years after graduation, c.1891–1953

Location	5 years	10 years	15 years	25 years	35 years
Africa	1	1	1	1	1
America	0	1	1	1	1
Australia	0	0	1	0	0
China	2	2	3	2	2
England	30 (33.3%[a])	36 (47.4%)	35 (48.6%)	28 (48.3%)	22 (38.6%)
India	2	3	2	1	1
Ireland	53 (58.9%)	32 (42.1%)	26 (36.1%)	18 (31.0%)	19 (33.3%)
Scotland	2	1	0	0	0
Deceased	0	0	3	7	11
Unknown	7	21	25	39	40

[a] These are percentages of traceable graduates only.
Source: *Medical Directory*.

Of the ninety-seven women in the cohort who graduated in medicine prior to 1918, thirty-six were based in England ten years after graduation, while thirty-two remained in Ireland (Table 6.4). Small numbers migrated to places such as Africa, China, India, Scotland and America. We do not have any equivalent statistics relating to the careers of Irish male doctors in the early twentieth century but Bethel Solomons (TCD, 1907) claimed that of the doctors of his generation, only 15 per cent remained in Ireland, with many male doctors entering 'the Army, Navy, Indian and Colonial Medical Services, some went to Great Britain as assistants or partners; the remainder stayed in Ireland as general practitioners or specialists'.[7]

The other 355 women in the cohort graduated after the First World War (Table 6.5). For these women, opportunities were said to be more limited than they were for their predecessors. By the 1920s, there were growing fears concerning career openings in Ireland for newly qualified doctors. In 1921, an article appeared in the *Irish Times* concerning opportunities for women doctors. The writer stated:

> We wonder what all the women doctors are going to do. They are entering a profession which, for the time being at least, seems to be over-crowded. The end of the war brought back a large number of doctors from foreign parts and filled the medical schools with young men who recently have qualified for practice. In the near future the competition for work is likely to be very severe. Many women doctors have found good appointments in women's hospitals and with local authorities, but the number of such positions is not unlimited. The young male doctor

who fails to find his chance at home can try his luck in the Dominions and usually is prepared to face a certain amount of hardship before he 'settles down'. His woman competitor's opportunities seem to be fewer and more restricted.[8]

Even Irish women doctors appeared to be acknowledging the problem that was now facing women medical graduates. Mary Strangman (RCSI, 1896) remarked in 1925:

A considerable number of Irishwomen who qualified in the Irish schools in the past have not been able to find openings for practice in Ireland, and it is probable that in the near future there will not be a sufficient number of such openings to make it worth the while of any woman to take out an Irish degree.[9]

This statement suggests that Irish women doctors had little choice but to go abroad in order to gain a medical post but it also seems to indicate that Irish women might be more successful in attaining a post if they undertook their medical training in Britain.

As Table 6.5 demonstrates, women in the post-war cohort were more likely to remain in Ireland than their predecessors. It is likely that this was due to increased opportunities opening up for women in Ireland after 1918 in the field of general practice, while their counterparts who graduated before

Table 6.5 Destinations of the 355 post-1918 women medical graduates five to thirty-five years after graduation, c.1924–69

Location	5 years	10 years	15 years	25 years	35 years
Africa	4	3	7	5	6
America	0	2	3	2	3
Australia	0	2	1	0	0
China	0	3	2	2	0
Egypt	0	1	1	0	1
England	48 (14.2%[a])	65 (22.8%)	93 (37.8%)	79 (36.2%)	67 (36.2%)
India	4	5	5	3	4
Ireland	279 (82.8%)	198 (69.5%)	127 (51.6%)	120 (55%)	97 (52.4%)
Italy	0	1	0	0	0
Pakistan	0	0	0	0	1
Persia	0	1	0	0	0
Scotland	1	1	1	1	2
Wales	1	3	5	5	3
Deceased	0	0	1	1	1
Unknown	18	70	109	137	170

[a] These are percentages of traceable graduates only.
Source: *Medical Directory.*

Table 6.6 Comparison of the careers of pre-1918 women medical graduates in Ireland with those in England five to fifteen years after graduation, c.1891–1933

	5 years		10 years		15 years	
	Ireland	England	Ireland	England	Ireland	England
General practice	26	5	13	8	10	8
	(49.0%)	*(16.7%)*	*(40.6%)*	*(22.2%)*	*(38.5%)*	*(22.9%)*
Address but no post (presumed to be GPs)	26	5	13	8	10	6
GP (listed as GPs)	0	0	0	0	0	2
Hospital appointments	17	13	13	15	10	12
	(32.0%)	*(43.3%)*	*(40.6%)*	*(41.7%)*	*(38.5%)*	*(34.3%)*
General hospital	9	7	6	7	5	5
Asylum	4	2	3	1	3	1
Children's/maternity	4	4	4	7	2	6
Public health	2	6	3	9	4	12
	(3.8%)	*(20.0%)*	*(9.4%)*	*(25.0%)*	*(15.4%)*	*(34.3%)*
Assistant medical officer	1	3	0	3	0	1
Schools medical officer	1	3	1	6	2	7
Dispensary			2	0	2	2
Medical officer of health	0	0	0	0	0	1
Aurist	0	0	0	0	0	1
Child welfare centre	0	0	0	0	0	0
Medical examiner	0	0	0	0	0	0
Mission hospital	0	1	0	1	0	0
		(3.3%)		*(2.8%)*		
Specialists	2	0	0	0	0	1
	(3.8%)					*(2.9%)*
Gynaecologist	1	0	0	0	0	0
Anaesthetist	1	0	0	0	0	1
Other						
University appointment	3	2	0	2	0	2
	(5.6%)	(6.7%)		(5.6%)		(5.7%)
War-related work	3	0	1	0	0	0
	(5.6%)		(3.0%)			
Company doctor	0	2	1	1	0	0
		(6.7%)	(3.0%)	(2.8%)		
Research	0	1	1	0	1	0
		(3.3%)	(3.0%)		(3.8%)	
Deceased	0	0	0	0	0	0
Not practising/retired	0	0	0	0	1	0
					(3.8%)	
Total	53	30	32	36	26	35

Source: *Medical Directory.*

Table 6.7 Comparison of the careers of post-1918 women medical graduates in Ireland with those in England five to fifteen years after graduation, c.1924–49

	5 years		10 years		15 years	
	Ireland	England	Ireland	England	Ireland	England
General practice	*238*	*27*	*155*	*40*	*79*	*52*
	(85.3%ª)	*(56.3%)*	*(78.3%)*	*(61.5%)*	*(62.2%)*	*(56.0%)*
Address but no post (presumed to be GPs)	238	26	154	36	79	48
GP (listed as GPs)	0	1	1	4	0	4
Hospital appointments	*25*	*15*	*17*	*12*	*13*	*13*
	(8.9%)	*(31.3%)*	*(8.6%)*	*(18.5%)*	*(10.2%)*	*(14.0%)*
General hospital	16	10	11	10	8	10
Asylum	3	2	4	2	5	2
Children's/maternity	6	3	2	0	0	1
Public health	*9*	*5*	*17*	*10*	*29*	*23*
	(3.2%)	*(10.4%)*	*(8.6%)*	*(15.4%)*	*(22.8%)*	*(24.7%)*
Assistant medical officer	0	1	0	2	2	11
Schools medical officer	1	3	3	2	5	4
Dispensary	5	1	10	2	13	1
Medical officer of health	2	0	4	0	6	2
Child welfare centre	1	0	1	4	2	3
Medical examiner	0	0	0	0	0	0
Registrar	0	0	0	0	0	1
Ministry of Health	0	0	0	0	0	1
Tuberculosis officer	0	0	0	0	1	0
Specialists	*3*	*0*	*3*	*1*	*4*	*1*
	(1.0%)		*(1.5%)*	*(1.5%)*	*(3.1%)*	*(1.0%)*
Anaesthetist	2	0	2	0	2	0
Pathologist	1	0	1	0	1	0
Radiologist	0	0	0	1	0	0
Dermatologist	0	0	0	0	1	0
Other						
University appointment	1	0	1	0	0	0
	(0.3%)		(0.5%)			
Company doctor	2	1	3	2	2	2
	(0.7%)	(2.0%)	(1.5%)	(3.0%)	(1.6%)	(2.0%)
Research	1	0	2	0	0	1
	(0.3%)		(1.0%)			(1.0%)
Not practising/retired	0	0	1	0	0	0
			(0.5%)			
Convent	0	0	0	0	0	1
						(1.0%)
Total	*279*	*48*	*198*	*65*	*127*	*93*

ª These are percentages are of those working in the respective countries.
Source: *Medical Directory.*

Table 6.8 Comparison of the numbers of women medical graduates in Ireland and England working in general practice, hospital appointments and public health five to fifteen years after graduation, c.1891–1969

	5 years		10 years		15 years	
	Ireland	England	Ireland	England	Ireland	England
General practice	264	32	168	48	89	60
	(79.5%[a])	(41.0%)	(73.0%)	(47.5%)	(58.2%)	(46.9%)
Hospital appointments	42	28	30	27	23	25
	(12.7%)	(36.0%)	(13.0%)	(26.7%)	(15.0%)	(19.5%)
Public health	11	11	20	19	23	35
	(3.3%)	(14.0%)	(8.7%)	(18.8%)	(15.0%)	(27.3%)

[a] These are percentages of those working in the respective countries.
Source: *Medical Directory.*

1918 may have moved to England because it offered more opportunities for employment in the public health sector and hospitals (compare Tables 6.6 and 6.7). Alternatively, because of the large number of post-war graduates, opportunities for hospital and public health appointments may have been severely diminished as a result of increased competition. Thus, for the post-war cohort, general practice may have been a more obvious career choice.

Table 6.8 outlines the numbers of women graduates working in the three main areas of practice: general practice, hospital work and the public health sector. Evidently, women who remained in Ireland were more likely to work in general practice, while their counterparts in England had a greater likelihood of securing posts within hospitals or public health. However, there were not great discrepancies in the numbers of posts in these fields available in the two countries. Rather, it is possible that women who remained in Ireland were more likely to work in general practice because it was easier to set up a practice in one's home town in Ireland than in a new city in England.

Marriage and family

As DISCUSSED in Chapter 1, opponents of women in medicine often claimed that such a career was detrimental to a woman's family life. Additionally, it was often wondered how women doctors could possibly combine a career with marriage and family. Mary Putnam Jacobi, an early American woman doctor and supporter of women in medicine, responded to such claims by arguing in 1882 that medicine was in fact an ideal career choice for a woman who also wished to have a family. She stated:

> a healthy girl of eighteen, with an ultimate view to the study of medicine, enters upon a university course, and, at the age of twenty-two, begins medical study. She is ready for practice at twenty-seven, marries at the same time or a year later. Her children are born during the first years of marriage, thus also during the first years of practice, and before this has become exorbitant in its demands. The medical work grows gradually, in about the same proportion as imperative family cares grow lighter. The non-imperative duties – the sewing, cooking, dusting, even visiting – are susceptible of such varied modifications of arrangement as it would be trivial to discuss in these pages. So great is the division of labour in medical work that it is indeed rather the minority of physicians who can consider themselves fortunate in being 'overwhelmed' with practice.[10]

Such claims continued into the twentieth century. 'A Woman Professor' in a letter to the *Times* in 1922, for instance, claimed that medicine was a profession which a woman could carry on just as well if she married. Because there were no set hours, a woman doctor could 'work when she can do and look after the family in the intervals'.[11] The letter was torn apart by a writer for the *Times* who claimed:

> It [the medical profession] is the last occupation for a woman; a 'hybrid' may do better by getting some clerical post under the health or municipal departments but sound practice, never, as they are totally unfitted for it and cannot do it. The whole of this woman movement is an attempt to shirk a woman's responsibilities – house work and maternity – and may, perhaps be an attempt of Nature, not yet recognised, to approximate the female to the male type and thus obviously limit procreation – as the general effect is certainly not calculated to increase the attractiveness of the female, decidedly the reverse.[12]

Evidently, even by the 1920s, there were still some opponents of women in medicine who continued to argue that a career in the medical profession defeminised women and that women should concentrate on their responsibilities within the home and concerning their families.

Surprisingly, some women doctors were also against the idea that a woman could be a successful doctor while married. Octavia Wilberforce, an English woman doctor who did not go on to marry, claimed that:

> To be anything of a good doctor, if you want to live up to any kind of ideal (women doctors have higher ideals naturally than the common run of men) you'd be no use – or at least never in the higher class – if you were married (lower class doesn't satisfy my ideas); and you'd be never any use with a lot of close ties.[13]

It is difficult to determine the exact number of women doctors who married. When tracing women doctors in the *Medical Directory*, there is no definitive way of finding out women's marital status, unless they have changed their surname to that of their husband, in which case they may be listed as, for example, Murphy (née Kelly). Similarly, some women doctors list themselves as, for example, Dr Mary Kelly (Mrs Murphy). However, in many cases, women doctors changed their surnames upon marriage and were simply listed under their new surnames, thus meaning that a large number of women doctors from the cohort simply became untraceable. In some cases also, women doctors married but retained their maiden name for practice, so, similarly, there is no way of knowing whether they married, unless it is known through other biographical information such as an obituary.

What can be said is that at least eighty-four women in the cohort (18.6 per cent) married.[14] Table 6.9 outlines the areas in which these women worked. The proportions do not differ greatly from those for the overall cohort (see for example Table 5.2, p. 112). Evidently, as in the case of the overall cohort, general practice was the most common choice, with 69 per cent of the women graduates known to be married working in this field five years after they had graduated. Emily Winifred Dickson (RCSI, 1891), Jane D. Fulton (TCD, 1925) and Mary McGivern (UCD, 1925), whom we will meet in the following chapter, managed to balance successful careers as general practitioners with raising their families. However, it should be noted that a small number of women also succeeded in juggling hospital and public health appointments with marriage and family life. These women doctors proved wrong those who had argued against women in the medical profession on the grounds that a medical career and marriage were incompatible.

The *Freeman's Journal* commented in 1877 that women doctors tended to marry other doctors.[15] This is certainly true of the cohort, with several examples in the 'Biographical index' at the end of this book of women who married other doctors. Humphry Rolleston commented in 1923 that the number of women giving up a career in medicine before or after qualifying was much greater than in the case of men and that marriage seriously depleted the ranks of women doctors. Accordingly, marriage was sometimes viewed as a handicap to women doctors.[16] Joyce Delaney, who qualified in 1940, in her autobiography, told the story of Ann, a woman doctor who had worked at the same hospital as her in England in the 1940s and who, aged nearly thirty, decided to leave the medical profession in order to marry. In Ann's view:

> England's teeming with bright young registrars who are as good or better than I am. Oh, I could probably get a consultant's job in surgery eventually. But I'd have to join the rat-race, attach myself to a Professional Unit, say the right things to the right people and move around, and eventually, after ten years or so, what'll I get? A job in some crummy place that a man doesn't want to work in and I'll be nearly forty, and who wants to marry an ageing woman who happens to be natty with a

Table 6.9 Careers of the eighty-four women medical graduates known to be married, five to fifteen years after graduation

	5 years	10 years	15 years
General practice	*58 (69.0%ᵃ)*	*46 (54.8%)*	*43 (51.2%)*
Address but no post	58	46	41
(presumed to be GPs)			
GP (listed as GPs)	0	0	2
Not listed	*9 (10.7%)*	*12 (14.3%)*	*14 (16.7%)*
Hospital appointments	*8 (9.5%)*	*13 (15.5%)*	*5 (6.0%)*
General hospital	2	4	2
Asylum	3	4	2
Children's/maternity	3	5	1
Public health	*4 (4.8%)*	*8 (9.5%)*	*13 (15.5%)*
Assistant medical officer of health	0	0	2
Schools medical officer	2	2	2
Dispensary	0	3	4
Medical officer of health	1	0	3
Aurist	0	0	0
Child welfare centre	1	2	2
Medical examiner	0	0	0
Vaccinations	0	1	0
Missions/humanitarian work	*0*	*0*	*3 (3.6%)*
Specialists	*2 (2.4%)*	*2 (2.4%)*	*1 (1.2%)*
Gynaecologist	0	0	0
Anaesthetist	1	1	1
Pathologist	1	1	0
Other			
University appointment	1 (1.2%)	0	1 (1.2%)
Company doctor	2 (2.4%)	3 (3.6%)	2 (2.4%)
Research	0	0	0
Deceased	0	0	1 (1.2%)
Not practising/retired	0	0	1 (1.2%)

ᵃ These are percentages of the cohort known to be married.
Source: *Medical Directory.*

knife? And if I don't marry I end up with high blood pressure like Murdoch or a lonely personal life like Fitzie, or go to the States and make ten thousand dollars a year in Shitsville.[17]

Ann's words led Delaney to consider her position concerning marriage and she decided to apply for the Malayan Colonial Service because 'I'd always heard that the tropics were full of lonely, womenless men, one of whom, I thought, might settle for me'.[18] Unlike Ann, however, Delaney managed to combine a career as a general practitioner (upon her return to Ireland) with marriage and family life, and it was not uncommon for Irish women doctors to succeed in doing this.

Changes in attitudes

THE FIRST WORLD WAR is said to have represented a distinct watershed for women doctors in both Britain and Ireland. As in other spheres of work, women became recognised as a valuable contribution to the workforce. The effect of wartime work, as Deborah Thom has outlined, was to demonstrate that women were capable of undertaking a variety of tasks but it did not demonstrate that they were entitled to do them.[19] Advocates of women doctors claimed that qualified women had the right 'to take an active part in the national emergency as the professional equals of male doctors, both at home and abroad'.[20] Medical journals such as the *Lancet* claimed that these years represented an exceptional time for women to enter into medicine, as a result of the great shortage of doctors in consequence of the war.[21]

Suffragists seized the war as an opportunity to make demands for an increased role for women in the professions.[22] A distinct change in attitude became discernible, as women doctors were 'no longer looked at with suspicion' and came to be of crucial importance in managing hospitals at the front, as well as at home, during wartime.[23] Some suffrage magazines, such as *Votes for Women*, claimed that 'the success of women doctors has long ago put such arguments [against the admission of women] to rout; but the war has completed the rout'.[24] In addition, women came to be offered many appointments that had not been open to them before. In 1915, at a meeting to promote the London School of Medicine for Women, Dr Florence Willey pointed out that many medical women were working among the French and Belgian soldiers as well as filling gaps at home in hospitals.[25] The suffragette Millicent Fawcett claimed that 'the advocates of the principle of equal pay for equal work have an encouraging precedent in the successful stand which women doctors have made from the outset that they would not undersell the men in the profession'.[26]

From the first year of the war, a distinct change in attitude took place, with the increase in women medical students at universities being praised in Britain by some as a 'great benefit to the nation'.[27] By the time of the war, the rate of remuneration for women doctors was equal to that paid to men.[28] The role of women doctors in the war effort came to be praised and some newspapers asserted that the war had justified many of the claims made by women, as well as giving added impetus to the demand on the part of many women for fuller opportunities to gain clinical and surgical experience.[29] Wendy Alexander has commented that women's war services provided collective as well as individual benefits. In the first stages of the war, a few individuals proved by their actions that women were well capable of running large mixed general hospitals. This meant that, after the war, 'it was no longer possible for opponents of women doctors to claim with any legitimacy that they had been excluded on grounds of competency'.[30] The contribution of Scottish women doctors through the Scottish women's hospitals helped to convince many sceptics that women doctors were just as competent as their male counterparts.[31] In England, there existed a military hospital at Endell Street, London, staffed entirely by women doctors under the command of Louisa Garrett Anderson and the doors of the London teaching hospitals – Charing Cross, St Mary's, Paddington and St George's – were thrown open to women medical students as a war emergency.[32]

Despite the tensions between Britain and Ireland at the time, it was not only British women doctors who volunteered to help in the war effort. Some Irish women doctors also played important roles. Elizabeth (Eliza) Gould Bell (QCB, 1893) was in charge of the ward in a Malta hospital during the war.[33] Isobel Addy Tate (QCB, 1899) was stationed at a hospital in Serbia, before going to a hospital in Malta, where she contracted typhoid fever and died in January 1917.[34] Lily Baker (CU, 1903) replaced the honorary obstetrical surgeon at the Bristol Royal Infirmary when he left for military service, 'taking entire charge in his absence'. After his return, she volunteered for the war and held the rank of honorary major in the Royal Air Force Medical Service during the war. When peace was declared, she was sent overseas to act as gynaecologist to the Rhine Army of Occupation.[35] Elizabeth Stephenson Walker (QCB, 1915) worked as a medical attendant to the Royal Army Medical Corps during the war years, while Mary Josephine Farrell (UCD, 1916) worked as a medical referee for the Longford War Pensions Committee.[36] Elizabeth Budd (RCSI, 1916) was appointed medical director of the Women's Army Auxiliary Corps in 1917, a position she held until the corps was disbanded in September 1921.[37]

Some medical journals held a cynical view of women doctors' work during the war. The *Dublin Medical Press* commented on the 'snuffling sentimentality' that had been expended upon the work being done by medical women in the war. Without wishing to detract from the efficiency of the lady doctors who had helped in the war effort, the writer wondered 'why it is that these ladies, who consistently claim to be the equals of men, should be advertised as having done something superhuman when they have done no more than five or six times their number of men, at possibly much great sacrifice, have done and are doing, unsung and unnoticed, in the service of their country'.[38] Despite the praise given to women doctors for their work in the war effort, this article seems to be suggesting that they were not doing anything that the men were not and seems to be advocating a more balanced attitude towards women doctors.

It was argued that the First World War and the work of women doctors within the war effort resulted in a more positive attitude among some towards women in the medical profession. However, did the war result in increased opportunities for women doctors? In the next section, I will examine the effects of the war on three main areas of employment for Irish women medical graduates: hospital appointments, general practice and public health. I will argue that, rather than experiencing increased opportunities, the cohort who graduated after the war experienced severe difficulties in attaining employment, leading to a far greater number of women doctors seeking careers within the field of general practice.

The effect of the war on women's medical careers

IF WE EXAMINE Table 6.10, it is evident that, for the post-war generation of women medical graduates, there was less likelihood of attaining a hospital appointment. The numbers of hospital appointments appear to have remained similar but the growth in numbers of medical graduates meant that an individual's chance of securing a hospital appointment was one-third of what it had been prior to the war.

Whereas almost 40 per cent of the traceable pre-1918 graduates had been successful in attaining hospital appointments ten years after graduation, only 11 per cent of their successors were able to achieve the same. However, those who did attain hospital appointments were more likely to be working in general hospitals and, additionally, the actual numbers of women working in hospital occupations are higher in the post-war cohort. It seemed that the medical marketplace had become overcrowded as a result of male doctors

Table 6.10 Numbers of pre-1918 and post-1918 women medical graduates working in hospital appointments five to fifteen years after graduation, c.1891–1949

		5 years	10 years	15 years
Pre-1918	Total	30 (33.0%)	30 (39.5%)	21 (29.2%)
	General hospital	16	15	10
	Asylum	6	4	4
	Children's/maternity	8	11	7
Post-1918	Total	40 (11.8%)	31 (11.0%)	27 (11.0%)
	General hospital	26	23	19
	Asylum	5	6	7
	Children's/maternity	9	2	1

Source: *Medical Directory.*

Table 6.11 Comparison of the numbers of women medical graduates with hospital appointments in England and Ireland, pre-1918 and post-1918 cohorts, five to fifteen years after graduation, c.1891–1949

		5 years		10 years		15 years	
		Ireland	England	Ireland	England	Ireland	England
Pre-1918	Total hospital appointments	17 (32.0%[a])	13 (43.3%)	13 (40.6%)	15 (41.7%)	10 (38.5%)	12 (34.3%)
	General hospital	9	7	6	7	5	5
	Asylum	4	2	3	1	3	1
	Children's/maternity	4	4	4	7	2	6
Post-1918	Total hospital appointments	25 (8.9%)	15 (31.3%)	17 (8.6%)	12 (18.5%)	13 (10.2%)	13 (14%)
	General hospital	16	10	11	10	8	10
	Asylum	3	2	4	2	5	2
	Children's/maternity	6	3	2	0	0	1

[a] These are percentages of those working in the respective countries.
Source: *Medical Directory.*

returning after the war. However, it is also probable that there simply were no longer positions available for doctors in hospitals because the market had been saturated.

As Table 6.11 demonstrates, there does not appear to have been any great discrepancy between the numbers of women gaining hospital appointments in Ireland compared with those attaining hospital appointments in England with regard to the pre-1918 cohort. Nor were women more likely to attain posts in children's or maternity hospitals than in general hospitals. Five years after graduation, 32 per cent of the women graduates who remained in Ireland had succeeded in gaining hospital appointments, while 43 per cent of those who went to England had achieved the same. Ten years after graduation, nearly 41 per cent of Irish women medical graduates in Ireland had attained hospital appointments while almost the same figure (42 per cent) of those in England had achieved the same. This seems to suggest that while it was easier for new graduates to attain hospital appointments in Britain than in Ireland, by ten years after graduation women doctors had the same chance of attaining a hospital appointment in both countries. This does not necessarily mean that Britain was more favourable towards women wishing to acquire hospital appointments but suggests that perhaps it was easier to attain a hospital appointment there, as there were more hospitals. Strikingly, however, for the post-war graduates, opportunities for hospital work were severely diminished. Whereas 32 per cent of pre-war graduates had been successful in attaining hospital appointments in Ireland within five years of graduation, only about 9 per cent of the post-war cohort succeeded in doing the same. Likewise, a smaller percentage of women were successful in attaining hospital appointments in England.

In contrast, opportunities for hospital work did not decrease to the same extent in England: 43.3 per cent of pre-war graduates based in England attained hospital appointments within five years of graduation, compared with 31.3 per cent of the post-war graduates. It is possible that the lack of hospital appointments in Ireland after the war was due to the emergence of a more conservative Irish state after 1922, or that more women were choosing to work in general practice rather than trying to obtain hospital employment.

As Table 6.12 shows, post-war graduates were much more likely to work in general practice than pre-war graduates. This is likely to have been a result of the lack of hospital appointments available due to the huge increase in numbers of women qualifying as doctors and the lack of a corresponding increase in hospital posts in Ireland and England after the war. It is likely that the pre-1918 graduates filled the available hospital posts and that there were then fewer opportunities available for the post-1918 graduates, many of whom were forced to work in general practice soon after graduation. It may

Table 6.12 Numbers of pre-1918 and post-1918 women medical graduates thought to be working in general practice five to fifteen years after graduation, c.1891–1949

	5 years	10 years	15 years
Pre-1918	33 (36.3%[a])	21 (27.6%)	18 (25.0%)
Post-1918	267 (79.0%)	202 (71.4%)	139 (56.7%)

[a] These are percentages of traceable graduates only.
Source: *Medical Directory.*

also have been a result of women returning to medicine when their husbands left for war, as in the cases of three of the women who will be discussed in the next chapter. Or, as stated above, it is possible that more women were now choosing to go into general practice rather than attempting to secure a career in a hospital or the public health sector because general practice meant that women doctors could combine family life more easily with their careers. Also, it is likely that, by the post-war period, the lady doctor was so well established that pursuing a career in general practice was more straight-forward than it had been for the pre-war graduates. However, opportunities for general practice were also restricted, with it being commented that it was more difficult to attain assistantships in practices after the war.[39]

Using Table 6.13, if we compare numbers of pre-1918 graduates in Ireland presumed to be working as general practitioners with numbers in England

Table 6.13 Comparison of the numbers of women medical graduates presumed to be working as general practitioners in Ireland and England, pre-1918 and post-1918 cohorts, five to fifteen years after graduation, c.1891–1949

	5 years		10 years		15 years	
	Ireland	England	Ireland	England	Ireland	England
Pre-1918	26 (49.0%[a])	5 (16.7%)	13 (40.6%)	8 (22.2%)	10 (38.5%)	8 (22.9%)
Post-1918	238 (85.3%)	27 (56.3%)	155 (78.3%)	40 (61.5%)	79 (62.2%)	52 (56.0%)

[a] These are percentages of those working in the respective countries.
Source: *Medical Directory.*

doing the same, it is clear that there are significant differences. Five years after graduation, 49 per cent of those still in Ireland were probably working as general practitioners, compared with only about 17 per cent of Irish women medical graduates in England. This again implies that women who went to England were more likely to secure an appointment in a hospital or in public health than those who remained in Ireland, which is likely to be because there were more opportunities for hospital and public health work in England than in Ireland. Of the post-1918 graduates who remained in Ireland five years after graduation, 85 per cent were probably working as general practitioners, compared with 56 per cent of those who migrated to England. This implies that, by the 1920s, more Irish women doctors who had emigrated were working as general practitioners, in comparison with the earlier period, when such women doctors tended to work in hospital posts or public health.

Public health was also an area in which there were significant differences in opportunities for both the pre- and post-war cohorts (Table 6.14). Nearly 9 per cent of pre-1918 graduates were successful in attaining posts in the public health sector five years after graduation, while just 4 per cent of post-1918 graduates succeeded in doing the same. Certainly, in Britain, women doctors found a special niche for themselves within the public health movement, working initially as assistant medical officers of health and, after 1907, as school medical officers. This was despite claims by the Irish medical profession that there was greater urgency for medical inspection of school-children within the country, as the general death rate in Ireland was higher than that in England or Scotland. Nonetheless, it was not until 1919 that school health inspection and treatment services were introduced to Ireland, under the Public Health: Medical Treatment of Children Act.[40]

Five years after graduation, nearly 4 per cent of the pre-1918 graduates who remained in Ireland were working in public health appointments, while

Table 6.14 Numbers of pre-1918 and post-1918 women medical graduates working in public health five to fifteen years after graduation, c.1891–1949

	5 years	10 years	15 years
Pre-1918	8 (8.8%[a])	12 (15.8%)	17 (23.6%)
Post-1918	14 (4.1%)	28 (9.9%)	53 (21.6%)

[a] These are percentages of traceable graduates only.
Source: *Medical Directory*.

Table 6.15 Comparison of the public health careers of pre-1918 and post-1918 women medical graduates who remained in Ireland with those who emigrated to England, five to fifteen years after graduation, c.1891–1949

	5 years		10 years		15 years	
	Ireland	England	Ireland	England	Ireland	England
Pre-1918	2 (3.8%[a])	6 (20.0%)	3 (9.4%)	9 (25.0%)	4 (15.4%)	12 (34.4%)
Post-1918	9 (3.2%)	5 (10.4%)	17 (8.6%)	10 (15.4%)	29 (22.8%)	23 (24.7%)

[a] These are percentages of those working in the respective countries.
Source: *Medical Directory*.

20 per cent of those who had migrated to England were being employed in the same field. Ten years after graduation, the figures are just as striking, with 9 per cent of women doctors who remained in Ireland being employed in public health, compared with 25 per cent in England. And, fifteen years after graduation, 15 per cent of those who remained in Ireland were employed in public health, compared with 34 per cent of those who went to England. There were more opportunities for women in Ireland to work as doctors in the public health sector following the 1919 Public Health: Medical Treatment of Children Act, as it created opportunities for women doctors to work as medical inspectors of schools. Table 6.15 shows a rise in the number of posts available for the post-1918 cohort in Ireland but not a rise in the percentage of women working in the public health sector, because the number of graduates had, by this point, risen so much. The pre-1918 graduates had taken three posts in the public health sector ten years after graduation, whereas the post-1918 cohort took seventeen such posts. Likewise, fifteen years after graduation, just four of the pre-1918 graduates (15 per cent) were working in public health in Ireland, while twenty-nine of the post-1918 graduates (nearly 23 per cent) were doing the same. For those who went to England, there was little change in the number of posts available in the public health sector after the war, but a significant change in the percentage of women doctors working in the sector. For the pre-1918 graduates, 20 per cent of women doctors based in England were working in the public health sector five years after graduation; however, of the post-1918 graduates just 10 per cent were doing the same. This is similar to the statistics shown for hospital appointments

and, again, it is likely that this decrease in percentages is a result of increased numbers of Irish women graduates in England deciding to work in general practice rather than in hospital or public health appointments.

Conclusion

EVIDENTLY, women medical graduates who emigrated to England were more likely to attain a hospital appointment or position in public health than their counterparts who remained in Ireland. This, however, is likely to have been a result of increased opportunities for these appointments in England rather than it being a case of discrimination against women doctors in Ireland. And it is possible that women who remained in Ireland were more likely to work in general practice because it was easier to set up a practice in Ireland.

It has been claimed that the First World War resulted in new opportunities for women in the workplace and society. Certainly, it seems that the war resulted in a more positive attitude towards women doctors within the contemporary press. And it has been argued that, in England, the war gave women doctors the opportunity to run large general hospitals in a way they had been unable to previously.[41] Doctors such as Lily Baker, whom we will discuss further in Chapter 7, found themselves promoted in their medical careers as a result of vacancies which opened up due to medical men leaving to fight in the war. Likewise, several teaching hospitals in London opened their doors to women medical students. This success was short-lived, however, with many of these hospitals closing their doors again to women a few years later.[42] Although Irish hospitals continued their tradition of allowing women medical students on their wards, the numbers of women medical students matriculating at Irish universities decreased dramatically after the war, although they did not return to the low numbers of the 1880s and 1890s. Irish universities, like British universities, no longer had the same space for women students wishing to study medicine. Likewise, there was increased competition for posts in hospitals and public health considering the large number of women graduates from Irish and British medical schools after the war.

The war does not appear to have resulted in extra vacancies and career opportunities for women doctors. Rather, it appears that women graduating after the war had a far more difficult task than their predecessors in trying to find employment. This, however, may have been because of the lack of vacancies for the huge number of women graduating after the war (as a result of the great intake of women medical students to institutions in the United Kingdom during the years of the First World War). Although there were more opportunities for women in the Irish public health sector after the war, this was a result of the Irish Public Health: Medical Treatment of Children Act 1919 rather than the war. However, it must be stated that the differences in career opportunities may not have all been due to the war but, rather, to other changes over time. In particular, the turbulent political events in Ireland after 1916 and the divisions which these exacerbated may have created an atmosphere which encouraged more women doctors to leave Ireland for England. There is certainly potential for further research on this question.

After 1918, it seems that the medical marketplace became completely saturated. By 1922, the Irish medical journal the *Dublin Medical Press* reported that the number of women medical students had greatly increased over the years of the First World War and that competition for resident posts in hospitals, infirmaries, sanatoria and asylums was now much keener than it had been during the war. In addition, the journal questioned whether women would continue to be as successful at securing appointments as they had been during the war and pointed towards the demand for medical women in India as a possibility for those unable to secure careers within Ireland and the United Kingdom.[43] Just two years previously, the same journal had claimed that the prejudice against women doctors had long since died out and public appointments for women doctors, for example as inspectors of schools and factories, were increasing every year.[44] Thus, it was more likely for the post-1918 women graduates to enter into general practice than their predecessors, as a result of the lack of alternative posts available to them. Despite the fears concerning opportunities for women medical graduates after the war, the drop-out rates for students who matriculated prior to the start of the war and those who matriculated after its end were similar, with 41 per cent of those who matriculated before the war not making it to graduation while 39.5 per cent of those who matriculated after the war did not qualify.

In the next chapter, I will examine the lives of five medical women and the choices they made with regard to career, emigration and marriage. Examining these women's lives provides a deeper insight into the challenges which faced women who graduated in medicine both before and after the war.

Notes

1 Penny Summerfield, 'Women and war in the twentieth century', in June Purvis (ed.), *Women's History: Britain, 1850–1945* (London: Routledge, 1995), pp. 307–332, on p. 307.
2 Penny Summerfield, 'Gender and war in the twentieth century', *International History Review*, 19:1 (1997), pp. 2–15, on p. 4.
3 Gail Braybon, 'Women, war and work', in Hew Strachan, *The Oxford Illustrated History of the First World War* (Oxford: Oxford University Press, 1998), pp. 149–63, on p. 162.

4 Greta Jones, "'Strike out boldly for the prizes that are available to you": medical emigration from Ireland, 1860–1905', *Medical History*, 54:1 (2010), pp. 55–74, on p. 55.
5 *Ibid.*, p. 74.
6 Only seven women out of the 452 graduates appear to have moved to Australia or the United States.
7 Bethel Solomons, *One Doctor in His Time* (London: Christopher Johnson, 1956), pp. 34–5.
8 'Women doctors', *Irish Times*, 23 November 1921, p. 5.
9 'Not a matter for politics', *Irish Times*, 19 August 1925, p. 5.
10 Mary Putnam Jacobi, 'Shall women practice medicine?', *North American Review*, 134:302 (1882), pp. 69–70.
11 'Our daughters' future: women doctors' families', *Times*, 17 April 1922, p. 6.
12 *Ibid.*
13 Pat Jalland (ed.), *Octavia Wilberforce: The Autobiography of a Pioneer Woman Doctor* (London: Cassell, 1994), p. 93.
14 Calculations based on women listed as 'Mrs' or with a changed surname in the *Medical Directory* as well as biographical information gleaned from sources such as the Kirkpatrick Archive (part of the Royal College of Physicians' Archives, Dublin), obituaries and contemporary newspapers.
15 The newspaper commented on the 'curious fact' that 'the young women-doctors are at once snapped up in marriage by practitioners of the opposite sex, they being eligible as partners for life in a double sense'. 'What the world says', *Freeman's Journal*, 24 May 1877, p. 2.
16 Humphrey Rolleston, 'An address on the problem of success for medical women', *BMJ*, 6 October 1923, pp. 591–4, on p. 591.
17 Joyce Delaney, *No Starch in My Coat: An Irish Doctor's Progress* (London: Cox and Wyman, 1971), p. 108.
18 *Ibid.*, p. 109.
19 Deborah Thom, *Nice Girls and Rude Girls: Women Workers in World War I* (London: I. B. Tauris, 1998), p. 45.
20 J. F. Geddes, 'The doctors' dilemma: medical women and the British suffrage movement', *Women's History Review*, 18:2 (2009), pp. 203–18, on p. 211.
21 'The opportunity for women in medicine', *Lancet*, 13 March 1915, p. 563.
22 'War and professions', *Irish Citizen*, 7 November 1914, p. 194.
23 'Women doctors: enlarged field of service: medical practice in war time', *Times*, 22 January 1915, p. 35.
24 'Women doctors wanted', *Votes for Women: Official Organ of the United Suffragists*, 8:383 (1915), p. 331.
25 'Medical women in war time', *Common Cause of Humanity: The Organ of the National Union of Women's Suffrage Societies*, 6:307 (1915), p. 731.
26 Millicent G. Fawcett, 'Equal pay for equal work', *Economic Journal*, 28:109 (1918), pp. 1–6, on p. 5.
27 'Women doctors: enlarged field of service'.
28 'Careers for boys and girls: the medical profession: the outlook', *Weekly Irish Times*, 20 February 1915, p. 5.
29 'The medical woman's opportunity', *Queen*, 27 February 1915. (Scrapbook relating to the Royal Free Hospital and the medical education of women Royal Free Hospital Archives, London.)
30 Wendy Alexander, *First Ladies of Medicine: The Origins, Education and Destination of Early Women Medical Graduates of Glasgow University* (Glasgow: Wellcome Unit for the History of Medicine, University of Glasgow, 1988), p. 59.
31 *Ibid.*, p. 57.
32 'Women and the medical profession', *Votes for Women*, 9:418 (1916), p. 186.

33 'Obituary: Dr Elizabeth Gould Bell', *BMJ*, 21 July 1934, p. 146.
34 Miscellaneous obituaries for Dr Isobel Addy Tate, Kirkpatrick Archive, Royal College of Physicians, Dublin.
35 'Obituary: Miss Lily Baker: pioneer woman surgeon', *Times*, 11 August 1956, p. 11.
36 *Medical Directory.*
37 'Obituary: Dr Elizabeth Budd', *Irish Times*, 22 May 1962, p. 7.
38 'Medical women and the war', *DMP*, 21 June 1915, p. 385.
39 'General practice from the inside', *Magazine of the London School of Medicine for Women and Royal Free Hospital*, 20:90 (1925), p. 7.
40 Sir William J. Thompson, 'Medical inspection of school children', *Dublin Journal of Medical Science*, 136:3 (1913), pp. 161–73, on p. 163, and Finola Kennedy, *Family, Economy and Government in Ireland* (Dublin: Economic and Social Research Institute, 1989), p. 133.
41 Alexander, *First Ladies of Medicine*, p. 59.
42 For example: the London Hospital Medical College first admitted women to its wards in 1918, before closing admission in 1922; St Mary's Hospital admitted women in 1916 but closed admission in 1925; Westminster Medical College admitted women in 1916, before discontinuing admission of women in 1926; and St George's Hospital Medical College admitted women in 1916 and discontinued admission in 1919. Letter giving dates of first women medical students at UK institutions, Medical Women's Federation Archives, Wellcome Library, London (SA/MWF/C.10).
43 'Medical appointments for women', *DMP*, 13 September 1922, p. 212.
44 'Medical women', *DMP*, 28 January 1920, p. 65.

Medical lives: case studies of five Irish women medical graduates

THIS BOOK has examined the backgrounds, educational experiences and careers of women doctors in Ireland who began their university careers between 1885 and 1922. The risk of examining the history of the women in a purely statistical manner, however, is that we may lose sight of the personal stories involved. It is also difficult to gain a sense of the trajectory of individual careers. This chapter, therefore, takes the form of case studies which allow us to examine in detail the lives of five women medical practitioners from the 1890s to the 1940s and beyond.

The first case study is of Emily Winifred Dickson (RCSI, 1891), who was an Irish pioneer woman doctor. There is a rich supply of material available on Dickson, ranging from family papers, including a short autobiographical memoir about her career and life, accounts written by family members and personal papers, to the many newspaper reports relating to her early career, and obituaries. Dickson is the woman for whom we have the fullest picture. The second case study is Emma Martha Crooks (QCB, 1899), who studied at Queen's College Belfast and went on to work as a medical missionary. I have chosen Crooks because, although as a missionary she was not typical of the cohort of women doctors in this study more broadly, her life and career are representative of what certain advocates of women in medicine claimed that women doctors would go on to do. I will draw on missionary magazines, her own personal letters and writings and newspaper reports in order to depict Crooks' life and career. Thirdly, I will examine the life of Lily Baker (TCD, 1906), who represents one of the many Irish women doctors who went to England following graduation. Baker is exceptional in that she had a remark-able hospital career while there and, as a result, there was a wide variety of source material available for the study of her life and career, such as reports in medical journals, newspaper articles and obituary material. Finally, the joint case study of Mary McGivern (UCD, 1925) and Jane D. Fulton (TCD, 1925) represents the many women who worked in general practice following graduation, at a time when the lady doctor was no longer a unique phenomenon in Irish and British society. McGivern remained working in Ireland as a general practitioner, while Fulton worked in England, but there are many parallels between their two stories. I conducted an oral history interview with McGivern's daughter, Mary Mullaney, while information about Fulton's experiences as a doctor in the Yorkshire Dales was gleaned from correspondence with her son, Brian O'Connor, and an account she wrote of her career in the *Yorkshire Dalesman* magazine.

These studies are more than just biographical accounts of the lives of these five women. Because each case study also introduces friends, sisters and colleagues of the women doctors, they are the stories of far more than five women and they open up vignettes of different types of female medical lives. Because Dickson, Crooks and Baker were more exceptional and not exactly representative of the body of women medical graduates more generally (Dickson and Baker having notably successful early careers, while Crooks was a medical missionary), there is more archival material on all three of these women doctors. Despite being untypical, they are nonetheless interesting and worthwhile case studies which give us an insight into the tensions and themes discussed earlier. McGivern and Fulton are the most typical of the women medical graduates. Their stories are worth telling because they are representative of a large number of women doctors who lived and worked in Ireland and England as general practitioners after graduation while simultaneously rearing their families. Taken together, these case studies illuminate the statistics of the previous chapters and, unlike traditional case studies in the history of medicine in Ireland, which tend to highlight the lives of 'great men' and 'great women', they give us an insight into the lives and careers of women doctors who might be classed as 'ordinary'.

Emily Winifred Dickson (RCSI, 1891)[1]

EMILY WINIFRED DICKSON was born in Dungannon, Tyrone, in 1866, the daughter of the Ulster Liberal MP Thomas A. Dickson and his wife Elizabeth Greer McGeagh. Winifred was the second youngest of seven children, three boys, James, John McGeagh and Thomas, and four girls, Sarah Louise, Mary, Emily and Edith. Her sister Mary died in infancy, while her other two sisters, Edith and Sarah Louise, did not go on to university education. Of her brothers, only John McGeagh went on to university education. He studied law at Trinity College Dublin, graduating in 1883 and

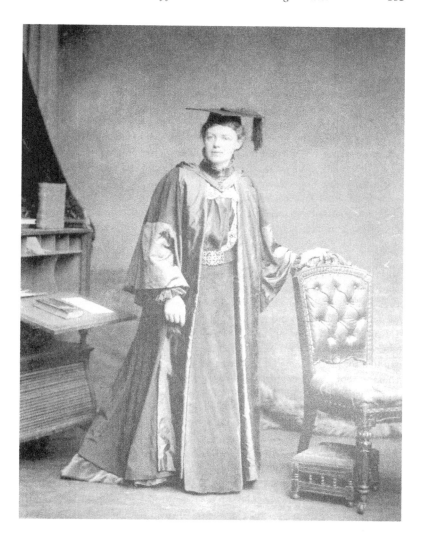

Plate VI Graduation photograph of Emily Winifred Dickson (RCSI, 1891).

qualifying for the bar in 1885 and with a doctorate of laws in 1889.[2] Winifred
Dickson was educated at the Ladies Collegiate School in Belfast and Harold
House School in London.[3] The Ladies Collegiate School had been founded in
1859 by Margaret Byers, a pioneer in women's education in Ireland, and the
school was attended by middle-class Protestant girls. After nursing her sick
mother for a year and with the encouragement of her father, Dickson decided
to pursue a medical education. Her younger sister Edith shared her interest
in caring and later became a nurse and moved to Bombay with her husband,
who was a missionary. Winifred initially attempted to follow her brother and
enrol at Trinity College Dublin for the 1887/88 term. Trinity College was
not at this time open to women students, however. Although Dickson was
supported by the medical faculty, her application was successfully opposed by
the theologians of the university. As a result, she enrolled in the Royal College
of Surgeons in Ireland in the autumn of 1887, where she was the only female
medical student attending lectures.

Winifred Dickson gained her hospital experience at a variety of institutions between 1889 and 1892. She trained at Sir Patrick Dun's Hospital
(post-mortems, medico-chirurgical experience, clinical clerkship, surgical
dressership, diseases of childhood, fever cases), the Rotunda Lying-In hospital
(practical midwifery and diseases of women), the National Eye and Ear
Infirmary (ophthalmology and otology), Donnybrook Dispensary (practical
pharmacy, vaccination) and Richmond Lunatic Asylum (psychiatry).[4] She
studied for her licence and MB degree at the College of Surgeons, achieving
them in 1891 and 1893 respectively. Her latter qualification she achieved with
first-class honours and an exhibition. Also in 1893, Dickson was elected the
first female fellow of the Royal College of Surgeons in Ireland, an important
honour considering that the young doctor was only just beginning her career,
but also indicative of the College's favourable attitude towards women in
medicine.[5] In contrast, there was no female licentiate at the London Royal
College of Surgeons until 1911 and no female fellows until 1920.

In 1893, after graduation, Dickson won a travelling scholarship from
the Royal University of Ireland which permitted her to spend six months
in Vienna and Berlin. Her time in Vienna proved valuable, but in Berlin she
found herself unable to gain admission to many of the clinics. When Dickson
arrived at one of the classes for which she had enrolled by letter, the professor
looked her over, declared she had cheated, that 'Winifred' was a man's name
and that he would not allow her to take his class.[6]

Upon her return to Dublin in 1894, Dickson put up her plate first in her
father's house in St Stephen's Green. In 1895, after he moved to Drogheda,
she moved practice to 18 Upper Merrion Street in Dublin and was appointed
gynaecologist to the Richmond, Whitworth and Hardwick Hospital, where

she worked for four years until her marriage. A photograph taken of the medical staff at the Richmond Hospital during Dickson's time there shows an all-male staff with the exception of Dickson.[7] She was also appointed assistant master to the Coombe Lying-In Hospital, Dublin, for which she became supernumerary assistant in 1894. Dickson took her doctorate in medicine in 1896, in addition to a mastership in obstetrics, both of which she gained with honours. She was then appointed examiner in midwifery to the Royal College of Surgeons. In 1898, she applied unsuccessfully for the position of professor of obstetrics there.[8] Nevertheless, her high standing in the Dublin medical community is apparent from an anecdote told by her friend Mary Griscom. Griscom commented that on one occasion in 1896, she was introduced by Dickson to a medical man on the street who asked Griscom, 'Do you know the best gynaecologist in Dublin?' Griscom racked her brain but could not answer and then the man said, 'She stands by you'.[9] Dickson's early career seems to indicate a great amount of support from the hierarchy of the Irish medical profession, as is testified by the number of favourable letters of recommendation that she received from her former lecturers in Dublin. These letters survive in the family archive and were presumably written following her graduation, when Dickson was applying for hospital posts.

Dickson was part of a very small group of pioneer women doctors in Dublin in the 1890s. Two other women doctors practising in the city at this time were Katharine Maguire (CU, 1891) and Elizabeth Tennant (RCSI, 1894). According to Dickson's memoirs, Maguire was the first woman doctor to practise in Dublin. She initially did so at Upper Mount Street, before moving to 67 Merrion Square, where she practised until at least 1926.[10] Maguire appears to have taken an active role in philanthropy and working among the poor in Dublin throughout her career. Like Dickson, she believed in the necessity of women as Poor Law guardians.[11] Like many other Irish women doctors, she became involved with the Irish Women's National Health Association and gave lectures in Dublin.[12] The Women's National Health Association was established by Lady Aberdeen as a voluntary and charitable organisation with the aim of improving maternity and child welfare, in addition to helping to combat tuberculosis, Ireland's most serious health problem.[13] Fundamentally, the Association had one major aim: 'to reach the women of the country' and to educate them about questions of health and sanitary medicine.[14]

Tennant, who would have been in the year behind Dickson as a medical student at the Royal College of Surgeons, worked as a medical officer to St Catherine's School and Orphanage in Dublin while also running a busy general practice in the city. She became a member of staff at St Ultan's Hospital from its foundation in 1919. Tennant's obituary claims that she 'did a great deal to overcome the prejudices which female practitioners had to meet in the days when their numbers were very few' but that her 'keenness and energy put her on a level with her male colleagues'.[15] She also appears to have played a role in the Irish suffrage movement, attending meetings of the Irishwomen's Suffrage and Local Government Association.[16]

By 1911, there were forty-two female medical practitioners in Dublin.[17] Some of these women doctors met under the auspices of the Irish Association of Registered Medical Women. Katharine Maguire became the first president of this organisation in 1908. As well as providing a community, the Association of Registered Medical Women campaigned for the vote for women, arguing that women had demonstrated that they were equal to men through the employment of medical women in connection with prisons, schools, public health and the Post Office.[18] Winifred Dickson does not appear to have taken part in the meetings of the Association, presumably because at this point she was married and had largely withdrawn from medical society. The very first meeting of this organisation was held at Maguire's house and practice on 29 October 1908 and Lily Baker, whom we will discuss below, was elected honorary secretary.[19] Maguire also hosted the third meeting of the organisation, on 9 November 1911, by which time Everina Massey (RUI, 1890) had become the president and Kathleen Lynn (CU, 1899) had become the secretary, following Baker's resignation after her decision to move to England. Despite the infrequency of its meetings, the fact that such an organisation existed seems to suggest that there was a sense of community or network among these early women doctors in Dublin.

The Association appears to have been active until at least 1915, at which point Lynn was still honorary secretary. The organisation met in November of that year to elect a committee which appointed Marion Andrews (QCB, 1901) as delegate for Ulster, Lucy Smith (QCC, 1898) as delegate for Munster and Florence Condon (RCSci, 1905) as delegate for Leinster. However, because no member of the Association was practising in Connaught, there was no election of a delegate for that region.[20]

All of these 'pioneer' Irish women doctors were deeply interested in philanthropic issues and Dickson was no exception. In her early career, she appears to have been strikingly active within the public sphere and her activities were widely reported in the Irish press. In 1893, the year she graduated with her MD degree, at a meeting of the Dublin Health Society, she gave a lecture on the topic of 'Health and dress'.[21] A version of the paper was published later that year.[22] The following year, while studying in Vienna, she wrote to the *British Medical Journal* about the treatment of women patients in workhouses, arguing that women patients with gynaecological problems generally preferred to be treated by women doctors and that there was a need for women as workhouse doctors.[23] She took an active interest in professional issues, attending, participating and presenting at meetings of the Royal Academy of Medicine in Ireland.[24] Dickson's attendance at these meetings is further indicative of the Irish medical hierarchy's favourable attitudes towards the incorporation of women into the medical profession.

Dickson was not just interested in professional issues. In 1895, at a meeting of the Irish Suffrage Association in Dublin, she urged 'the necessity of well-to-do women taking an interest in questions which affected working women'.[25] She was also involved in the National Society for the Prevention of Cruelty to Children[26] and the Irish Association for the Prevention of Intemperance.[27] In 1895, at a meeting of the Royal Academy of Medicine in Ireland which took place in Dublin, she gave a paper on the need for women as Poor Law guardians in Ireland, with all of her male colleagues present supporting her views.[28] The paper was published.[29] Likewise, in 1895, in a letter to the *Irish Times*, Dickson wrote again of the desperate need for reform within the Irish workhouse system, where the majority of inmates were women and children.[30]

In a letter written in 1942, Dickson commented that women's emancipation was the only worldwide movement she took an interest in, although she was insistent that she did not agree with militant suffrage.[31] Likewise, she was interested in the rights of women within the medical profession. Her obituary claims that it was her correspondence with the secretary of the British Medical Association which helped to get its membership open to women, and Dickson then became one of its first women members when the Association opened membership to women in 1892.[32] Additionally, Dickson was supportive of young women medical students and was the honorary secretary of a committee in Dublin set up to advise women students with regard to their work and also to help them find suitable lodgings.[33]

In April 1899, Dickson gave a paper at a meeting of the Alexandra College Guild entitled 'Medicine as a profession for women', in which she outlined how a woman might go about undertaking medical education, the necessary personal qualities and the career paths a woman could take. Dickson was asked about the issue of combining marriage with a medical career:

> Dr. Dickson, in the course of her reply, said it was impossible to make any general rules to marriage. That was a question that every person had to settle for herself. (Laughter.) If a woman who had spent the best years of her life in preparing for a medical degree was bound on entering the married state to give up the medical profession it would tend to lower the status of the married state. For her part she thought a woman should not give up the medical profession for the profession of marriage unless she liked the latter profession better. (Laughter.)[34]

The question of marriage must have been on Dickson's mind at the time of this address, as, later that year, she married Robert Martin, an accountant.[35]

Despite the implication of her comments above, she decided to give up her career upon marriage. In the same year, she published a version of her paper 'Medicine as a profession for women' in the *Alexandra College Magazine*, the magazine of the Dublin girls' school which contained educational advice for students, news relating to school events and information on 'old girls'. Here, she equated a career in medicine to a government appointment in the civil service, in which a woman had to vacate her position upon marriage:

> Marriage and motherhood will always be the most important professions a woman can engage in, and that if carried out in a proper spirit they will leave no time for medical work ... a doctor's first duty is her patients – she must be at their beck and call at any hour of the day or night. But a married woman's first duty is to her home, and if she tries to combine a doctor's work with her own, to which will she give prominence? One must be first in her heart, and whichever it be, the other will suffer.[36]

Following her own advice, Dickson gave up her promising career on her marriage and went on to have five children, four boys, Russell, Kenneth, Alan and Colin, and one girl, Elizabeth ('Betty'), from 1901 to 1910. The family remained in Dublin and in 1911 were living at 8 Burlington Road. Winifred was listed as 'Medical Doctor Retired', while her husband, Robert, was now the managing director for a textile manufacturer.[37] The family then moved to Castlewarden, Co. Kildare, where they lived from 1912 to 1913. Dickson appears to have withdrawn completely from medical society at this point and does not seem to have been involved in the foundation of the Irish Association of Registered Medical Women. Robert Martin enlisted in the British Army in London on 22 December 1914, in the 2nd Sportsman's Battalion of the Royal Fusiliers (the 24th Battalion) and was posted as a private to Mansfield, Nottinghamshire. He was posted to Burma from 1917 to 1919. He allocated to Winifred 6*d* per day (just over £9 a year) from his pay and she decided to return to work to supplement this income.[38] Winifred Dickson effectually became the sole breadwinner for the family. She and the family moved to England in 1915 and she sent her children to English preparatory and public boarding schools such as Mostyn House, Cheshire, and St Bees in Cumberland, which her son Russell and possibly some of her other children attended.[39] She secured a post first as an assistant superintendent at Rainhill Mental Hospital in northern England. She chose that post on account of the hospital being close to where her children were attending boarding school, and also because the hours off duty would enable her to study in order to bring herself up to date after sixteen years' absence from the practice of medicine.

From 1917, she worked as a war locum in Ellesmere, Shropshire, for a Dr Scott, so that, in her words, she would 'have a home for you all [her children] during the holidays'.[40] In addition to working in general practice, she also acted as the local medical officer of health. She bought the practice in Ellesmere and took on a male assistant but had to give up her rural general practice in 1919, due to bronchial pneumonia brought on by Spanish influenza and the return of her husband from military service. Instead, she bought a practice in Wimbledon, London, and continued to supervise her children's higher education and university careers. She and Robert Martin separated and Dickson became solely responsible for her children. For the rest of her life she undertook peripatetic medical work, moving frequently and dogged by illness. In 1926, as a result of a bout of rheumatoid arthritis, she was forced to give up her practice in Wimbledon and moved to Siena, Italy, to practise. By 1928, she was back in Britain, working in a small general practice at Tunbridge Wells but two years later was forced to give up practice again as a result of pernicious anaemia. However, she undertook locum work for another female doctor and, every winter for the next ten years, undertook a part-time assistantship in a South Wales mining community during the rush months for ten years.[41] In 1940, twenty-five years after her first locum appointment there, she returned to Rainhill Mental Hospital, where she continued to work up until two months before her death in 1944 at the age of seventy-seven.[42] Two years before her death, looking back on her life, she wrote:

> I don't regret anything, even the foolish things, but I see in countless ways that I missed many priceless chances and opportunities, not from wilfulness but from sheer blind stupidity of not appreciating how much they might mean and lots of things I thought I knew all about and didn't know there were worlds unknown that I was unaware existed.[43]

Winifred Dickson was one of the few pioneer women doctors working in Ireland in the 1890s. She was deeply interested in philanthropic and women's issues as well as having a very successful early career. Her future career looked set to be promising. However, upon her marriage in 1899, she sacrificed her career to take care of her family. It was only when her husband was away on war service in 1915 that Dickson began to work again and for the rest of her working life she managed to work her career around her family commitments and illness. She became the sole breadwinner for her family, succeeding in sending her children to boarding school and later university. She died in 1944 from an incurable carcinoma; however, strong-minded and unselfish as she had been throughout her life, she made no mention of it to her family but continued with her work until within a few weeks of her death.

Emma Crooks (QCB, 1899)

I N THE LATE NINETEENTH and early twentieth centuries, women doctors
were regularly encouraged to enter the medical missions. As we learnt
in Chapters 1 and 5, it was claimed that there was a great need for women
doctors in countries such as India, where local religious customs meant that
women patients could be treated only by women doctors. In this section, I will
focus on the career of Emma Crooks, an early woman medical missionary.
Crooks was part of a group of four classmates at Queen's College Belfast
who qualified in 1899 and joined the Presbyterian Missionary Society. Emma
Crooks (QCB, 1899) and Elizabeth Beatty (studied at QCB but LRCP LFPS
Edinburgh/Glasgow, 1899) were sent to China; their classmates Ina Huston
(QCB, 1899) and Annie Crawford (QCB, 1899) went to India. Although, as I
have shown, missionaries were a minority in the overall body of Irish women
medical graduates, they exemplify the type of work that was expected of them.
    Crooks was the daughter of a teacher, while her classmates Beatty and
Huston were the daughters of Presbyterian ministers, and Crawford's father
was a merchant. All were Ulster Presbyterians. The four women attended
the Zenana Mission Conference held in June 1900 at the Adelaide Lecture
Hall, Dublin, a few months before Huston, Crawford and Beatty were due
to depart for India and China. Crooks would not be sent to China until two
years later. There is certainly a sense from the speeches of these women at
the conference, reported in *Woman's Work*, the magazine of the Presbyterian
Missionary Society, that they viewed the opportunity to work in the missions
as a privilege and a vocation. Huston assured the audience that they should
not view the women as heroines because it was the 'greatest delight' for
them to go abroad and 'evangelise the world'. Likewise, Crawford said that
she felt it was a great privilege to be going to Manchuria and that, when she
thought of the suffering of Chinese women there, she realised it would be a
tremendous sacrifice to stay at home in Ireland. Crooks and Beatty expressed
similar sentiments and requested that people would pray for them while they
were away.[44] The women went on to document their work and experiences
in *Woman's Work*. Crawford and Huston disappear from both that magazine
and the *Medical Directory* ten years after graduation, so it is difficult to
determine whether they remained in the missionary field. They did work
as missionaries until at least 1905 in Crawford's case and 1908 in Huston's
case, which is when they last appear in *Woman's Work*. Beatty retired from
her missionary work after eleven years due to ill-health and died seven years
later.[45] Crooks had the longest service in the missionary field, working for
some thirty-two years, retiring briefly in 1933, and then working in Peking
until her death in 1937.

For Crooks, writing in 1912, medical missionary work had two strands:

> Medical work does not mean merely trying to cure the sick in heathen lands; it has a far greater outlook than that. Medical work and mission work are intimately connected. The medical part consists of seeing dispensary patients, having a hospital with in-patients, and doing operations. The missionary part consists in teaching and training native helpers, especially dispensers, teaching Bible classes on Sabbath and teaching and preaching to the patients, both in hospital and at their homes.[46]

Clearly, Crooks fully accepted this dual purpose: to help the sick and poor in less fortunate countries while at the same time attempting to 'evangelise' 'heathen' countries. Crooks passed her final medical examinations in 1899 and the Zenana Committee initially decided that she should not set sail until the autumn of 1900 because they considered it advisable that she should first obtain additional hospital experience and take a course at the new Tropical Diseases Hospital in Dublin.[47] The Boxer uprising broke out in China before the autumn of that year, so Crooks was advised to wait further. She attained a temporary job as house surgeon at the Children's Hospital, Temple Street in Dublin, the first woman to be given that post. She had just begun work at the hospital when the Committee asked if she would leave for India at once rather than waiting indefinitely. She replied: 'My appointment at Temple Street is only for a year. Had I got this offer before, I should only have been too delighted to accept it, but it is the first time they have ever had a Protestant here, so I do not want to give the impression that I think lightly of a promise.' Her contract as house surgeon ended in October 1901 and letters from China advised her not to come until the spring. Crooks stayed on in her post at Temple Street for a few months longer. She wrote to the Committee: 'I feel very pleased that the Committee still think I can go to China. The Sisters here are very pleased to have me for some time longer. They have been very kind to me indeed. It is better to have some experience both of a different religion and of medical work before going abroad.'[48]

In 1902, she was sent from Belfast to Kirin in Manchuria, where she remained for almost her whole life. A meeting was held by the Belfast branch of the Zenana Committee in February to say goodbye to her. The Reverend J. McGranahan told how Crooks had from her early years been deeply interested in missions and had been a bright and willing worker in the Church. Crooks herself spoke of how, during all the years of preparation for her missionary life, she had been stimulated and sustained by the Saviour's words, 'Lo, I am with you always'.[49] This is an apt quotation for her to have chosen, since missionary life often involved personal sacrifice and loneliness. Writing to a friend from Kirin, in 1904, Crooks revealed that she had been in love with a man but could not marry him due to her vocation to be a missionary.[50] Crooks found her work as a missionary to be quite lonely, writing that she was compensated for this by the work she had to do and her Sunday school class.[51] Three years later, she again wrote of her loneliness: 'It is lonely I need not say it – I just have to trust more and that keeps one from feeling loneliness too much'.[52]

According to a 1937 report of the Irish Presbyterian Mission Hospital in Manchuria, Crooks was the first woman doctor to undertake work in the city of Kirin.[53] Speaking in 1921, she stated that the remembrance of the different farewell meetings at which she had been present and the support of the people who attended these often helped her in times of loneliness.[54] She found life in China difficult and commented on the harsh conditions: 'We are working in a very bad dispensary – the walls are damp almost to the roof and the floor (bricks) never dries. We get thoroughly chilled. When it rains, the water pours through the roof, although it has been mended times without number. We never before had greater numbers.'[55]

During the winter months, Crooks' women's hospital was always full and she was convinced that it was the combination of medical skill and Christian faith which drew patients to her. In 1912 she wrote:

> I have been struck by the way one patient brings in another. It is the almost invariable answer, 'I heard from so-and-so of our village; you know she had treatment. How skilful the doctor is, and *how good the doctrine is*, and how well cared for the patients are. This religion is good'. And that story is spread north, south, east and west.[56]

Sometimes, the waiting room of the hospital had to be used to accommodate patients and patients were being turned away because of the lack of beds. The conditions at her dispensary were inadequate, with damp walls and a leaky roof.[57] Her old classmate Ina Huston shared similar experiences. Writing in 1902, Huston spoke of the dispensary that she had just set up in Broach, India. The dispensary had formerly been a shop and contained two rooms upstairs: the larger one was where patients waited to be seen and where a Bible woman spoke to them about the gospel, while the other, smaller room was used for seeing patients.[58] As a result of the steadily growing number of patients, Huston predicted that they would soon need to establish a mission hospital to cater for the demand. By 1906, she and the other missionaries at Broach had established such a hospital to treat women from various castes. She described the medical work being conducted by herself and the other missionaries as incorporating three branches: the dispensary, where women would come to seek medical assistance and where they would be educated about the gospel; the hospital; and visiting the houses of sick people, where oftentimes Huston would come across female patients who had been treated by native doctors without being examined.[59]

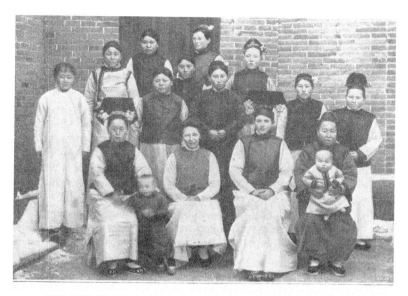

OUR LADY MISSIONARIES IN KIRIN AND SOME OF THE CHRISTIAN WOMEN.
Miss M'Mordie is in centre, and on her left is Miss Crooks, a sister of Dr. Emma, whom she has been helping in the Hospital. Dr. Emma Crooks stands with her back against the door. Most of the Chinese women are dispensers. Mrs. Liu is at the extreme right of the picture. The young woman on her right is Miss Liu, the former nun spoken of by Miss M'Mordie. The mother who has the nice fat baby on her knee is Mrs. Dwan, a Bible-woman. Some of the girls are teachers who assist Miss M'Mordie in the girls' school.

Plate VII The staff of Mission Hospital, Kirin. Emma Crooks (QCB, 1899) is pictured at the back, centre. From the July 1911 issue of *Woman's Work* (p. 156).

There appears to have been a sense of community among the women doctors, with occasional reports in *Woman's Work* of women medical missionaries working in the same country meeting up with each other, such as Lillie Dunn (QCB, 1904), who met with Huston and Elizabeth Montgomery, another medical missionary, in India in 1907.[60] Likewise, Eva (Mary Evelyn) Simms (QCB, 1904) was working in Chinchow, Manchuria, China, fifty miles from Elizabeth Beatty, in 1909.[61]

Annie Crawford had similar experiences to Emma Crooks with her work in Ahmedabad, India. She worked in a dispensary in the afternoons and visited the local orphanage in the evenings.[62] Working with the orphans appears to have been a trying career for Crawford, with outbreaks of pneumonia, the plague and malaria being commonplace. She still managed to find some light in the darkest situations, however, writing, for example, in 1902:

After the two deaths, the other children got quite alarmed and could scarcely be got to go to the little room that we use as a hospital. My stethoscope was an object of special terror. One child, in her wanderings, called it a 'sap' (a snake); and another, who seemed very frightened when I went to examine her, gave as the reason afterwards that she thought it (the stethoscope) would kill her as it had killed little Nathi![63]

For Crooks, life in Kirin was similarly treacherous. There were often outbreaks of infectious diseases such as scarlatina, diphtheria, tuberculosis and erysipelas to contend with. Crooks also found herself being discouraged when former patients who had converted to Christianity returned to 'heathendom'.[64] It was claimed in the 1937 report on the work of the Kirin hospital that Crooks experienced difficulties not only as a woman doctor but also as a foreigner attempting to carry out medical work in Kirin.[65] In 1911, she had to abandon her dispensary because of the unsuitable conditions. She wrote that it would cost £150 to build a new dispensary but that she did not want to place a burden on the missions committee at home, so she would try to find a way to raise the money herself.[66]

Elizabeth Beatty, working in Kwangning, China, also experienced problems. In 1911, she wrote about the threat of the plague that had affected the area she worked in. She stated that the disease had disorganised all of her work and that she had to explain to her patients that it was not the Lord who had sent the disease. Beatty, like Crooks, proved herself capable of dealing with such challenges. She set about inoculating locals in the area against the disease and stated that, in spite of the stress of the outbreak, she 'never was as peaceful in [her] life'.[67] Beatty was forced to leave the missions in 1917, after eleven years' work, owing to poor health, and moved to live in Berkley, California, where she died in 1924.[68]

In July 1911, a great fire attacked Kirin, leaving 30,000 locals homeless. Luckily, Crooks' hospital was unaffected.[69] Other dangers faced the missionaries: on one occasion, Crooks and some friends were captured by robbers en route to Chaoyangchen, a nearby city. She described them as 'real mounted highwaymen armed with rifles and revolvers' but her party was luckily set free, to their surprise, having heard stories from other missionaries working in nearby areas.[70]

Crooks frequently commented on the great assistance she received from the Chinese women helpers at her hospital.[71] As the years passed, she felt that she had gained the confidence of the local people:

We have had many interesting cases: some shot by robbers, some of attempted suicide, with the usual history of unhappy homes, others coming in to get rest and quiet during their illness, a few brought in to die, because it was unlucky to die at home, and quite a number of small children were left with us to look after and care for while they were ill. Such a thing would have been quite impossible only a few years ago. It is very encouraging that people now trust us in this way. Even the small precious sons are left in the hospital alone, so we know that it must have a good reputation amongst non-Christians.[72]

Crooks remained working in Kirin, Manchuria, for thirty-two years, retiring in 1933 and returning to Ireland. She resigned from her post on account of ill-health. The Zenana Committee commented as follows on the occasion of her resignation:

No one who has known her in her thirty-two years of service has failed to be impressed by her sympathy with suffering humanity. Her skill, her time, her thought, and her means have been continually at the disposal of those in need. No one could have given more freely of her very best for the sick in Kirin. Her name is known far and wide in Kirin and is a passport to the good wishes of every section of the community. The Church members feel that they are losing their best friend, and have come, group after group, imploring her to reconsider her decision.[73]

It was remarked that at the time of her leaving, 'not only had she built up a flourishing medical work but her name had become a synonym for love and kindness and it now bids fair to become legendary in the district'.[74] Following her retirement, Crooks returned to China, but to Peking, where she helped at the American Presbyterian Mission Hospital. The Zenana Committee urged her to come home but she refused, stating that although her health was failing, she did not feel inclined to go home while she could still contribute to China's need. She died in October 1937, following a severe heart attack.[75] Upon her death, two of her Bible students composed the following poem, of which the English translation is below:

Alas, Dr. Crooks has suffered sickness and died in Peking,
For this the people of Kirin and Ireland are sorrowing,
When one thinks of your thirty years in Kirin it seems as one day,
By your labours were saved and healed numberless women and children,
All are grateful, all admire when they think of your kind face,
Your labours and loyalty overcame even the waves of the Atlantic and Pacific,
Your heart is broken and your spirit is tired,
But one desire has not been fulfilled,
Tired to death in Kirin, in Kirin to be buried with your wish,
By your spirit Ireland and Kirin have been brought together as one,
Your body may be dead but your spirit and works will live in Christ after you
    forever.[76]

This poem illustrates the tireless efforts on Crooks' part among the poor in Manchuria and the sense that she was valued very much within the community of Kirin. Following her death, her place in Manchuria was occupied for some time by a doctor called Rachel Irwin. However, after Irwin left, there was no

female doctor in Kirin and the author of a 1936 account of the work of the
hospital commented that 'Mere men doctors are a poor substitute in the eyes
of our women patients, accustomed for decades to being cared for in our
hospital by women doctors'.[77] This statement suggests that women doctors
such as Crooks and her contemporaries who worked as medical missionaries
provided valuable, indeed irreplaceable work in the missionary field. They
worked in largely female-dominated environments and undertook responsibility for taking charge of entire hospitals and dispensaries. Through working
as medical missionaries, these women doctors found their own special niche
in the medical marketplace and were able to exercise more authority and
responsibility than they might have had they secured appointments in other
fields of medical work.

Lily Baker (TCD, 1906)

LILY BAKER was one of the many Irish women doctors who emigrated
to England after qualification to seek employment. Baker was born in
South Africa in 1879 and was a member of the Church of Ireland. We know
little of her family background but, in 1911, she and her elderly aunt were
living together in Dublin.[78] At the age of nineteen, she had matriculated at
the Royal College of Science in Dublin, but transferred to Trinity College
when it admitted women in 1904 and became the College's first female
medical graduate, in 1906. Her sister Madeline matriculated two years later
at the Catholic University[79] and qualified in 1907. Lily initially worked as a
clinical clerk and external assistant at the Coombe Hospital, Dublin, and
afterwards as a house surgeon at the Drumcondra Hospital.[80] In 1907, the
two sisters established a dispensary for women and children in Drumcondra.
They were said to be the only women doctors then working on the north side
of Dublin.[81] Lily was also working as a demonstrator in anatomy to women
medical students at Trinity College at this time and she remained in this
position for three years.[82] This appointment would not have come about if it
were not for the separation of men and women medical students for anatomy
dissections at the College, as discussed in Chapter 4. According to one article
in *TCD: A College Miscellany* in 1905, while Baker was still a student, this
dissecting room had been a favourite haunt of a male demonstrator 'who,
tired of demonstrating to the mere male, wished to while away a pleasant
little interval of an hour or so' but the board of the College had now enforced
a rule that only the 'head of the battalion' (presumably the professor of
anatomy) could demonstrate to the women medical students.[83] Clearly, two
years later, by the time of Baker's appointment, the board had decided that

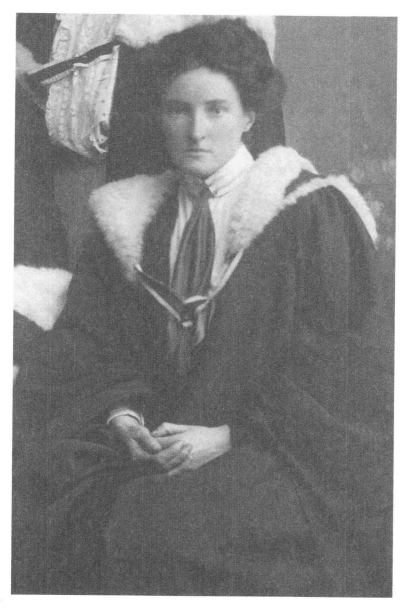

Plate VIII Graduation photograph of Lily Baker (TCD, 1906).

women should be taught by female demonstrators only. At this point, there had been no other female medical graduates from Trinity, so Baker did not face competition for the post. Madeline moved to England in 1908, where she worked as a physician at a private hospital in London.[84]

While working at Trinity College, Baker was involved with the establishment of the Dublin University Voluntary Aid Detachment, an organisation set up in conjunction with St John's Ambulance.[85] In the event of war or a national emergency, the members of the organisation agreed to act as army nurses in their own country. They were most commonly women who were trained in first aid and nursing. Baker gave the preliminary course of lectures to women students and graduate members of the Detachment.[86] At this time she was concurrently practising as a general practitioner from an address at 18 Merrion Street, Dublin.[87]

Like Winifred Dickson and the pioneers we met earlier in the chapter, Baker became involved in other medical and philanthropic activities from an early stage of her career. Just a year after graduation, she was on the committee for the Tuberculosis Exhibition, organised by the Women's National Health Association in 1907.[88] This travelling exhibition in 1907 had the aim of educating women on health matters relating to tuberculosis. The exhibition visited between eighty and ninety places in Ireland and attracted large crowds.[89] The exhibition committee, led by Lady Aberdeen as president, comprised twelve members: two lady doctors, Ella Ovenden (later Webb, CU, 1904) and Lily Baker; two other women, Lady Matheson and Mrs Nugent Everard; six male members of the medical profession, Sir William J. Thompson, Professor E. J. McWeeney, Professor Mettam, D. Edgar Flinn, P. Dunne and Michael F. Cox; as well as two honorary secretaries, Mrs Rushton and Dr Alfred E. Boyd.[90]

Ovenden and Baker were placed in charge of the 'domestic science' display at the exhibition, while their male counterparts in the medical profession were involved in more medical and scientific displays, such as the 'literary section', organised by Boyd, which included municipal and Poor Law exhibits such as tables and diagrams for tuberculosis death rates in major cities in Britain and Ireland.[91] This illustrates the organisation's belief that facts relating to public health could be 'driven home better still by individual speaking to individual, by woman speaking to woman, by mother speaking to mother'.[92]

In 1911, Lily followed Madeline to England, moving to Bristol, where she worked as an assistant surgeon to the Bristol Private Hospital for Women and Children and subsequently as a gynaecologist at the Walker Dunbar Hospital at Clifton and its associated out-patient dispensary. Baker was at this point the first female doctor to be appointed to the staff of a teaching hospital outside London. In addition, Baker worked for several antenatal clinics and acted as the physician in charge of infant welfare clinics, in the days when these were financed and largely run by voluntary organisations. She also opened a voluntary gynaecological clinic for working mothers. As a result of her involvement in all of these institutions, Baker became very well known in Bristol.[93]

Despite moving to England earlier, Madeline does not appear to have attained the same career success as her sister. In 1917, she was living at the same address as her sister in Clifton, Bristol, while working as a company doctor to the Welsh National Memorial Association. Five years later, she was back in London, working as a medical officer to the Church Army Dispensary for Women and Children and the Given Wilson Health Centre for Infants in Plaistow. She later moved to Bath, where she worked as a medical officer at the West Dispensary until the end of her career.[94] In the previous chapter, we learnt that women doctors who emigrated to Britain had a higher chance of attaining posts within the public health sector: this was certainly the case for Madeline Baker. Like Madeline, of the pre-war graduates, 25 per cent of those in England ten years after graduation were working in public health, in contrast with 9 per cent of those who remained in Ireland.

In contrast, Lily Baker had a series of hospital appointments, like 42 per cent of women doctors based in England ten years after graduation. Despite not living in Ireland but clearly as a result of her excellent reputation in Bristol, she, like Winifred Dickson before her, was elected a fellow of the Royal College of Surgeons in Ireland in 1912. Baker was the eighteenth female fellow of that College, so, at this point, female fellows were still uncommon.[95] In 1914, she became acting obstetric registrar at the Bristol Royal Infirmary while the male registrar was away on military service in the First World War. When he returned, Baker joined the medical branch of the Royal Air Force and served in France and Germany until the end of 1919. A photograph from 1919 depicts Baker in Maresquel, France, at the base of the Women's Royal Air Force in her role as honorary medical officer in charge of the force.[96] One female doctor, Letitia Fairfield, in a speech in 1927 referring to Baker's work during the war, commented that 'Her speciality then was the management of the colonels, who were hard to please ... for one thing, in the RAF the colonels were not long past their twenty-first birthday, and they regarded women appointed to the force as one of the minor horrors of war'.[97]

In 1921, an antenatal clinic was established in the department of obstetrics at the Bristol Royal Infirmary and Baker took charge of this. Under her care, the clinic developed so rapidly that, by 1926, around 1,250 new cases were attending annually.[98] In October 1926, the board of governors of the Infirmary, with the unanimous support of the honorary medical staff, elected Baker to the newly created post of honorary assistant physician in charge of the antenatal department, with the Medical Women's Federation giving a dinner in her honour to mark the occasion. The Federation had been founded in 1917 as a network for women doctors in Britain, but its origins lay in the earlier Association of Registered Medical Women, which had been established in 1879 (with only nine members).[99] As we saw above, Baker had been involved in the Irish branch of the Association as honorary secretary prior to moving to England. At the dinner, Lady Barrett, MD MS, the vice-president of the Medical Women's Federation, proposed a toast to Lily Baker, commenting that her success had been won through the value of her work and that 'the ante-natal work in a hospital staffed by men, put into the hands of a woman, was a great compliment'. Professor Winifred Cullis shared similar sentiments, stating that 'Dr. Baker's appointment was open proof of the capacity of women and the generosity of men. She was helping to break down the feeling that there were things which men could do and which women could not.'[100]

Baker held this post until the end of her career, while concurrently holding the posts of medical examiner and lecturer on the obstetrics board at Bristol Royal Infirmary. According to her obituary: 'Miss Baker was a skilled and experienced gynaecological surgeon and obstetrician, and was much loved by her patients. She was noted for her kindness to young women doctors who were starting out in practice at a time when this was unusual and something of an adventure.'[101] This is somewhat reminiscent of Dickson, who was the honorary secretary to a committee set up to aid women medical students in finding accommodation upon arrival in Dublin. However, unlike Dickson, Baker never married and this clearly had an important bearing on her career. It is surely possible that, had she married, she might not have achieved the same level of career success.

Baker's career and that of her sister, Madeline, proved to be very different. Lily had a very successful hospital career, while Madeline worked in the public health sector all her life. Both women are representative of women doctors in the cohort who migrated to England for work and the opportunities they attained in Britain were ones which may not have been open to them had they remained in Ireland. Likewise, if either of the two sisters had married, it is questionable whether they would have achieved the same career success.

Mary McGivern (later Connolly) (UCD, 1925) and Jane D. Fulton (later O'Connor) (TCD, 1925)[102]

MARY McGIVERN AND JANE D. FULTON could be said to be typical of the post-1918 cohort of women medical graduates from Irish institutions. Approximately 79 per cent of these women graduates were listed in the

Medical Directory with an address but no specific post, suggesting that they were likely to have worked in general practice.

Mary McGivern was born in Banbridge in 1900, the daughter of a publican and grocer, Peter McGivern, and Agnes O'Brien from Limerick. McGivern was the only daughter of five children and, like many of the other Catholic women graduates in this study, she attended a convent school, the Siena Convent in Drogheda, Co. Louth. She is the only Catholic in this chapter and is representative of the rising numbers of Catholic women students from the 1900s. Her reasons for deciding to study medicine were personal: the excitement of the prospect of being away from home for six or seven years and living in Dublin was what encouraged her to undertake medical education. Like Winifred Dickson's father, Peter McGivern was supportive of his daughter's decision to study medicine. She matriculated at University College Dublin in the 1918/19 term. At this point, there were fifteen other women medical students in her class.[103] Of these women students, twelve (75 per cent) succeeded in graduating.

Jane Fulton, who graduated the same year as McGivern, was born in Strabane, Co. Tyrone, in 1901, the second child in a large Presbyterian family of five sons and five daughters and two orphan cousins. She was the first in her family to attend university and she matriculated at Trinity College in the 1919/20 term, a year after McGivern.[104] She was one of twenty female medical students in her year, of whom just nine succeeded in qualifying. While at university, she resided at Trinity Hall, the halls of residence for Trinity College, and played hockey for the university team.

McGivern, on the other hand, resided at the Dominican hostel for female students in Dublin while attending university. With regard to her experiences at university, she later said she had enjoyed herself, noting that because women were in the minority within their class, they received a great deal of attention from the male students. However, because of the Civil War in Dublin and the presence of English soldiers, students' social life in the evenings was restricted and it was not so common for them to go out at night. She did not experience discrimination during her time at University College Dublin, with the exception of one occasion when a Benedictine monk did not allow her into the dissecting room, although the reason for this is unclear. She made lifelong friends during her time at university, who would later visit McGivern's house and reminisce about their experiences.

McGivern's future husband was also a medical graduate of University College Dublin. His name was J. J. Connolly, from Ballybay in Co. Monaghan, and was one or two years ahead of her in medical school. He went to her native town of Banbridge to do a locum in late 1924 and they were married after her graduation in 1925. They settled in Banbridge and her husband

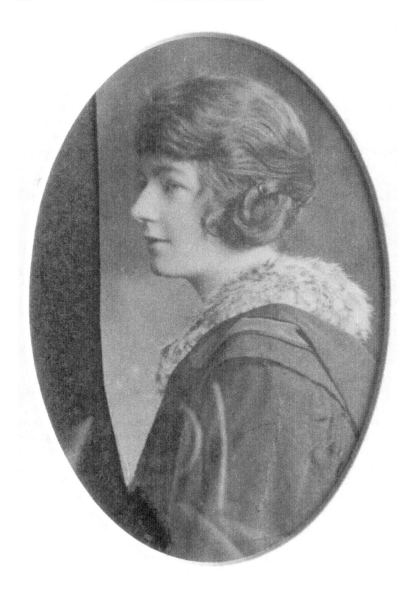

Plate IX Graduation photograph of Mary McGivern (UCD, 1925).

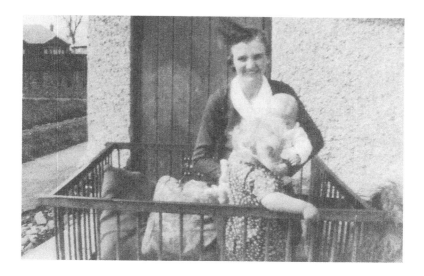

Plate X Jane D. O'Connor (née Fulton) (TCD, 1925) with her children Maeve and Brian, in Catterick, Yorkshire, 1932.

opened his own practice there in 1933. Mary initially gave up practice on marriage. Their first child was born in 1926, with four more following.

In contrast, following graduation, Fulton emigrated to Pontefract, Yorkshire, for employment and she worked in general practice. In 1928, she married her husband, Leo, who was a medical officer in the Royal Air Force at Catterick, in north Yorkshire. She had previously met him while gaining her clinical experience at Baggott Street Hospital, Dublin. Her two children were born in 1930 and 1931, and thereafter she decided to give up medical practice. Her husband bought a practice in 1933 in the Yorkshire Dales and, despite her decision to give up practice because her children were still young, they 'optimistically had [her] name put on the brass plate at the gate'.[105] In Fulton's words: 'The country folk had scarcely even heard of a woman doctor. Worse, we weren't even Yorkshire, but complete foreigners – it takes at least 10 years to become a local in those parts.' Even though her children were still young, Fulton worked part time in the practice, gaining the trust of the female patients in the area. She recounted two anecdotes of her time as a general practitioner:

> I did a week's locum once in another dale even more remote than ours. My first visit
> there was to an old lady of 80 who greeted me with: 'We did hear that our doctor
> was ill and he had a woman doctor doing his work, but we've got to be thankful for
> anyone these days'. In the same practice a man aged over 70 with bronchitis asked
> 'Are you married?' 'Yes' 'Is your husband alive?' 'Yes' 'Oh well, in that case you can
> look at my chest.'[106]

At first, before she learnt to drive, she would walk into the town to visit
patients, with her faithful mongrel dog with one leg shorter than the others
following her everywhere on these trips; for patients who lived further away,
her husband would drive her.

McGivern, despite having decided to give up practice upon marriage,
helped in her husband's practice with the dispensing of medicines. According
to her daughter:

> Yeah, she was bringing up that family and they were all close enough in age and
> she was quite happy bringing up her family and there was, my father at that time
> had a dispensary; he used to be dispensing his own medicine, and certainly, she
> used to help with that.[107]

Like Dickson during the earlier war, McGivern returned to work when her
husband joined the Army. He joined up in 1939 and was initially posted in
Holywood, Co. Down. His wife took a refresher course in a Dublin hospital
before he moved away and took over his entire practice, which at the time
was small. Initially, the majority of patients were Catholics but, as the practice
grew, people of other religions came to it too. At first, some patients did not
want to go to a female doctor. Some even remarked, 'I don't want to see the
lady doctor, I want to see the doctor himself'. However, the practice began to
grow under her care and she had to employ an assistant female doctor, Olivia
Clarke. McGivern appears to have managed very well while her husband was
away on war duty. Her daughter said that there was always someone in the
house to look after the children, in the form of neighbours or friends. The
work was difficult, however, with McGivern often being called out in the
middle of the night to attend to women in labour. Her daughter stated:

> And it was always difficult at night when the telephone rang and you had to say
> to your mother, 'someone wants you out' and she'd be tired … I used to feel really
> sorry for her at times … and even during the night when she would answer the
> phone herself at night and, I'm not saying all deliveries are at night but they seem
> to be, a lot in late … and she, she had a good capacity of being able to get back to
> sleep and when they were delivering, there was always a consultant … he would
> come from Newry if they were in trouble, when I say in trouble, I mean if some
> difficulty arose with the patient. So yes. And he would come over and she got on
> very well with him. But it was an anxious time and you'd be thinking 'oh will she
> ever get back to bed?'[108]

In spite of such difficulties, Mary McGivern enjoyed working, with maternity being her favourite area of medicine, and she did not want to give up her career upon her husband's return. It appears also that she was able to make a good living from her work in general practice and was able to afford to send her children to boarding school for their secondary education. Although McGivern's husband returned to the practice in 1945, he became ill and retired, but Mary kept it going. Clarke had left her post and a male assistant was employed to help out. At the time, the family lived in what were two houses joined together. In one side of the house was the waiting room, dispensary and surgery and an upstairs bedroom where the assistant, if and when there was an assistant, slept. The family lived in the other house.

With regard to philanthropic work, McGivern does not appear to have taken part in associations like the women in the earlier case studies, presumably because she was living and working in a rural town with fewer opportunities for such activities. However, she clearly took a great interest in the welfare of her patients. Her patients in the late 1940s often experienced discrimination in relation to housing matters on account of the fact that they were Catholics and she would often call to council members personally and plead on behalf of her patients. In addition, McGivern served on the board of the local hospital, where she campaigned for it to be promoted from cottage hospital status. Along with her husband, she would carve the turkey for the Christmas dinner at the hospital each year.

War also brought Fulton back to full-time practice, upon her husband's return to the Royal Air Force in 1940. She was taught to drive by locals in the area and lorry drivers would recognise her car and give her a wide berth on the road. Working during wartime, Fulton also found that, as a doctor, she had other uses within the community. She wrote that she took the daily papers to the distributors in some villages, as well as medicines and sometimes groceries to outlying farms and towns. Like Baker before her, Fulton involved herself in philanthropic work, teaching first aid to members of the St John's Ambulance. Like McGivern, she arranged for her children to go to Catholic boarding schools, which suggests that both women were earning enough from their general practice to be able to do this. After her husband's return in 1945, Fulton continued working in general practice alongside him.[109] Working as a country doctor, she encountered many difficulties. She later wrote of one occasion in 1947 when the Dales experienced the worst snowfall for many years:

> One afternoon at the beginning of this I was called to an emergency in a village six miles away. I had to dig three times to get the car out of drifts and was rather shaken when I finally got to the house. The husband of the patient offered to drive back with me but I said: 'I may not be able to get home but you certainly would not

get back' so I set off alone. To my relief after a short distance I saw in the mirror the snowplough behind me. I pulled into a cutting that had been dug to allow cars to meet or pass, thinking I would have an easy run home behind the plough. But the plough itself soon got stuck in a huge snowdrift. As the men shovelled the snow out the blizzard blew it back and things looked hopeless. Then the men from the quarries began to arrive on their way home from work. They took shovels from their cars (everyone carried a shovel at that critical time) and fell to work cheerfully in spite of the adverse conditions. Eventually a track was cleared and the snowplough started. The rest of the cars followed slowly and carefully, taking the easier road back to the town. No car, no pedestrian went up that road for the next nine weeks.[110]

Fulton retired from practice in 1964, and she and her husband moved to Killiney, Co. Dublin, and later to Sligo, where they lived until her death in 1986. Mary McGivern retired from general practice at the age of seventy and one of her sons, who trained in medicine at University College Galway, then took over the practice. She died in 1990.

Conclusion

THIS CHAPTER has discussed the lives of five medical women in order to give a more thorough insight into the themes and tensions discussed in previous chapters. Around the time of Dickson's entry into medical school, advocates of medical education for women were claiming that there was a distinct need for women to work in the missionary field. Crooks, who graduated six years after Dickson, became a medical missionary, thus entering into a career which women doctors were encouraged to choose. Although only a small number of Irish women actually worked as missionary doctors, Crooks' life and career suggest an overwhelming philanthropic desire to use her medical skills to help others, and she is representative of women doctors who worked in largely female-dominated environments, where they, like Crooks, took charge of entire hospitals, in careers where they were given far more authority and responsibility that they might have enjoyed had they remained in Ireland.

In Chapter 3, I examined some of the factors that might have influenced a woman's decision to take up medical education and her choice of university. Evidently, all five women in this study were typical of the cohort generally, as they came from well-to-do middle-class backgrounds. Their choices of university appear to reflect their religious sensibilities: Dickson, as a Protestant, attempted to gain access to Trinity College Dublin initially, but then was admitted to the Royal College of Surgeons. Crooks, a Presbyterian, attended Queen's College Belfast. Lily Baker, a Protestant, gained her degree from

Trinity College Dublin. It is unclear why her sister, Madeline, attended the Catholic University, although we do not know for certain what her religion was. If Madeline was a Protestant, her attendance at the Catholic University gives validity to claims that there were a number of Protestant women attending the medical school there. Finally, McGivern, a Catholic, attended the Catholic University, while Fulton attended Trinity College Dublin. Economic factors proved to be important here: all the women appear to have had the financial and personal support of their families, which allowed for them to attend medical school. Similarly, most of the women attended their local university, where possible. Clearly, in the case of McGivern her closest university, Queen's College Belfast, did not match her religious persuasion, so she went to Dublin.

In Chapter 4, I examined women's experiences of medical education at Irish universities from the 1880s to 1920s. Unfortunately, I was able to find very little material relating to these women's time at medical school, which highlights the difficulty that exists in finding out about student experience.

In Chapter 5, I suggested that Irish women doctors did not necessarily end up in the careers that were deemed most suitable for them by advocates of women in medicine, such as in women's hospitals and as missionaries. Emigration to England was also an important part of the stories of early women doctors and this may be seen in the stories of Dickson, Baker and Fulton. In their professional careers, three of the five women worked, at least initially, in the spheres of obstetrics and paediatrics, conforming to expectations of what women doctors would do in their careers. However, in doing so, they are not typical of women doctors in the overall cohort. Evidently, the majority of women doctors, like Fulton and McGivern, worked in general practice. Less common were women who worked solely in the spheres of women's health or the missionary field, like Baker and Crooks. Dickson's career is more varied: she initially started out working as a gynaecologist but later worked in a mental hospital and in general practice, returning to work at the mental hospital later in her career. The careers of Dickson, Fulton and McGivern were certainly shaped by their marriages but they demonstrate the effect of the war, as depicted in Chapter 6. Dickson gave up her early brilliant career upon marriage but returned to work after her husband left for army service. Similarly, Fulton and McGivern returned to work full time, managing their husbands' practices after their husbands went to war.

Taken together, these narratives provide us with an insight into the experiences of ordinary women doctors. In a field of historical study which tends to favour stories of men, in particular men who were 'extraordinary', these case studies demonstrate the importance of the personal narrative and show that the stories of ordinary women doctors can be just as engaging.

Notes

1   Dickson will be referred to by her maiden name, as this is the name she retained when practising.
2   'John McGeagh Dickson in the words of one of his granddaughters, Mrs Leslie Lucas and delivered by Evan Powell-Jones', private collection of Niall Martin, Edinburgh.
3   Correspondence with Niall Martin and Martin family papers.
4   Matriculation record for Emily Winifred Dickson, Matriculation albums of students matriculating through Royal/National University of Ireland from 1890 to 1922, National University of Ireland Archives, Dublin.
5   Roll of fellows of the College, in Royal College of Surgeons in Ireland, *Calendar, October 1923 to September 1924* (Dublin: Dublin University Press, 1923–24), pp. 83–95.
6   Dr Mary Griscom, 'Obituary for Winifred Dickson Martin', *Medical Women's Federation Quarterly Review*, July 1944, private collection of Niall Martin, Edinburgh.
7   Emily Winifred Dickson papers, private collection of Niall Martin, Edinburgh.
8   Typed memoir, Emily Winifred Dickson papers, private collection of Niall Martin, Edinburgh.
9   Griscom, 'Obituary for Winifred Dickson Martin'.
10 *Medical Directory* entries for Katharine Maguire.
11 'Letter. Condition of workhouses', *Irish Times*, 5 June 1895, p. 6.
12 'Women's National Health Association: lecture by Dr Katharine Maguire', *Irish Times*, 12 March 1908, p. 7.
13 Greta Jones, *'Captain of All These Men of Death': The History of Tuberculosis in Nineteenth And Twentieth Century Ireland* (Amsterdam: Rodopi, 2001), p. 101.
14 Countess of Aberdeen (ed.), *Ireland's Crusade Against Tuberculosis. Vol. 1: The Plan of Campaign: Being a Series of Lectures Delivered at the Tuberculosis Exhibition, 1907, Under the Auspices of the Women's National Health Association of Ireland* (Dublin: Maunsel, 1908), p. 5.
15 'Dr. Elizabeth A. Tennant', *Irish Times*, 19 February 1938, p. 6.
16 'Women's suffrage movement', *Irish Times*, 16 September 1907, p. 9.
17 Irene Finn, 'Women in the medical profession in Ireland, 1876–1919', in Bernadette Whelan (ed.), *Women and Paid Work in Ireland, 1500–1930* (Dublin: Four Courts Press, 2000), pp. 102–19, on p. 103.
18 'Memorials: medical women', *Votes for Women: Official Organ of the United Suffragists*, 6:255 (1913), p. 241.
19 'Medical news', *BMJ*, 21 November 1908, p. 1575.
20 Letter from Kathleen Lynn to Medical Women's Federation secretary, dated 1915, Medical Women's Federation Archives, Wellcome Library, London (SA/MWF/C.80).
21 'Dublin Health Society', *Freeman's Journal*, 22 February 1893, p. 6.
22 E. Winifred Dickson, 'The distribution of weight in clothing', *Aglaia: The Journal of the Healthy and Artistic Dress Union*, no. 1 (1893), pp. 9–13, private collection of Niall Martin, Edinburgh.
23 Emily Winifred Dickson, 'Women as workhouse doctors', *BMJ*, 14 April 1894, p. 839.
24 See, for example, 'Royal Academy of Medicine in Ireland: obstetrics section', *Dublin Journal of Medical Science*, 108:1 (1899), pp. 63–73.
25 'Women's suffrage: conference in Dublin', *Freeman's Journal*, 28 January 1895, p. 3.
26 'National Society of Prevention of Cruelty to Children: annual general meeting', *Freeman's Journal*, 17 June 1896, p. 2.
27 'Irish Association for the Prevention of Intemperance', *Freeman's Journal*, 15 January 1897, p. 2.

28 'Royal Academy of Medicine in Ireland: state medicine section', *BMJ*, 9 March 1895, pp. 536–7.

29 E. Winifred Dickson, *The Need for Women as Poor Law Guardians* (Dublin: John Falconer, 1895).

30 'Conditions of workhouses', *Irish Times*, 3 June 1895, p. 7.

31 Letter from Emily Winifred Dickson to her son, Russell, dated Rainhill, 24 November 1942, Emily Winifred Dickson papers, private collection of Niall Martin, Edinburgh.

32 D. Margaret Wilkinson, 'Winifred Dickson Martin', *Medical Women's Federation Quarterly Review*, July 1944, private collection of Niall Martin, Edinburgh, and 'Admission of women to the British Medical Association', *Irish Times*, 25 August 1892, p. 5.

33 Clara L. Williams, 'A short account of the school of medicine for men and women, RCSI', *Magazine of the London School of Medicine for Women and the Royal Free Hospital*, no. 3 (January 1896), p. 107.

34 'Alexandra College Guild', *Irish Times*, 24 April 1899, p. 6.

35 Correspondence with Niall Martin.

36 E. Winifred Dickson, 'Medicine as a profession for women', *Alexandra College Magazine*, 14 (1899), pp. 368–75, on pp. 374–5.

37 1911 census record for Martin Family, 8 Burlington Road, Dublin, National Library, Dublin.

38 Information on Robert Martin courtesy of Christopher Dickson and Niall Martin.

39 Correspondence with Niall Martin.

40 Typed memoirs of Emily Winifred Dickson.

41 'Obituary: E. Winifred Dickson', *BMJ*, 26 February 1944, pp. 308–9.

42 'Obituary: D. Margaret Wilkinson', reprinted from the *Medical Women's Federation Quarterly Review* (July 1944), private collection of Niall Martin, Edinburgh.

43 Letter from E. Winifred Dickson to her son, Russell.

44 'Zenana mission conference', *Woman's Work*, no. 35 (July 1900), pp. 242–3.

45 'Obituary: Dr Elizabeth Beatty', *Irish Times*, 13 August 1924, p. 6.

46 E. Crooks, 'Medical work in Kirin: an address at the annual meeting in June', *Woman's Work*, no. 84 (1912), pp. 273–4.

47 Marion F. Hilton, *Dr. Emma Crooks*, Highway series no. 5 (Belfast: Presbyterian Church in Ireland Foreign Mission, c.1937), p. 2.

48 *Ibid.*, p. 3.

49 'Farewell to Dr Emma Crooks', *Woman's Work*, no. 42 (1902), p. 127.

50 Letter from Emma M. Crooks, Presbyterian Mission, Kirin, Manchuria, to 'Ned' (nickname for a female friend), dated 9 February 1904, Public Record Office of Northern Ireland, Belfast (D1727/2/1).

51 *Ibid.*

52 Letter from Emma M. Crooks to Ned, dated 15 November 1907, Sunshine Cottage, Irish Presbyterian Mission, Kirin, Manchuria, N. China, Public Record Office of Northern Ireland, Belfast (D1727/2/2).

53 Irish Presbyterian Mission Hospital, Kirin, Manchuria, Report 1937, Public Record Office of Northern Ireland, Belfast (D2332/3).

54 'Farewell meeting', *Woman's Work*, New Year number (January 1921), p. 243.

55 Hilton, *Dr. Emma Crooks*, p. 13.

56 Crooks, 'Medical work in Kirin', p. 275.

57 'Kirin', *Woman's Work*, no. 75 (1910), p. 63.

58 'Broach: more dispensary work', *Woman's Work*, no. 44 (1902), pp. 179–80.

59 'Annual meeting', *Woman's Work*, no. 59 (1906), p. 247.

60 'Letter from Lillie Dunn', *Woman's Work*, no. 62 (1907), p. 34.

61 'Medical work in Manchuria', *Woman's Work*, no. 71 (1909), p. 251.

62   'Ahmedabad', *Woman's Work*, no. 39 (1901), p. 65.
63   'Ahmedabad', *Woman's Work*, no. 43 (1902), p. 155.
64   'Kirin', *Woman's Work*, no. 77 (1911), p. 110.
65   Irish Presbyterian Mission Hospital, Kirin, Manchuria, Report 1937.
66   'Kirin', *Woman's Work*, no. 78 (1911), pp. 127–8.
67   'Kwangning', *Woman's Work*, no. 78 (1911), pp. 124–5.
68   'Obituary: Dr. Elizabeth Beatty', *Irish Times*, 13 August 1924, p. 6.
69   'News from China', *Woman's Work*, no. 79 (1911), p. 155.
70   'Kirin', *Woman's Work*, summer number (1915), p. 85.
71   'Teaching kindness', *Woman's Work*, New Year number (1916), p. 152.
72   Hilton, *Dr. Emma Crooks*, p. 28.
73   *Ibid.*, p. 29.
74   Irish Presbyterian Mission Hospital, Kirin, Manchuria, Report 1937.
75   Hilton, *Dr. Emma Crooks*, p. 30.
76   Irish Presbyterian Mission Hospital, Kirin, Manchuria, Report 1937.
77   *Forty Years of the Kirin Manchuria Hospital, 1896–1936*, Public Record Office of Northern Ireland, Belfast (D2332/2).
78   1911 census record for Lily Baker, 18.1 Merrion Street, Dublin.
79   *Medical Students' Register* for 1898/99 (London: General Medical Council, 1899).
80   'Obituary: Lily A. Baker', *BMJ*, 7 July 1956, p. 48, from file on Lily A. Baker, Kirkpatrick Archive, Royal College of Physicians, Dublin.
81   'College news', *Alexandra College Magazine*, no. 30 (1907), p. 56.
82   'College news', *Alexandra College Magazine*, no. 31 (1907), p. 55.
83   'News from the schools: the Medical School', *TCD: A College Miscellany*, 11:196 (1905), p. 156.
84   'College news', *Alexandra College Magazine*, no. 33 (1908), p. 66.
85   'Dublin University Voluntary Aid Detachment', *BMJ*, 29 November 1913, p. 1462.
86   *Ibid.*
87   1911 census record for house 18.1 Merrion Street (upper), South Dock, Dublin.
88   'Tuberculosis Exhibition', *Irish Weekly Times*, 19 October 1907, p. 7.
89   'Tuberculosis Exhibition in Bray', *Irish Times*, 27 March 1909, p. 11.
90   Countess of Aberdeen, *Ireland's Crusade Against Tuberculosis*, p. 153.
91   *Ibid.*, pp. 153–67.
92   *Ibid.*, p. 7.
93   'Obituary: Dr Lily A. Baker', *BMJ*.
94   *Medical Directory* entries for Madeline Baker.
95   Roll of the fellows of the College.
96   Photograph of Lily Baker and Miss Chauncey, in Diana Condell and Jean Liddiard (eds), *Working for Victory? Images of Women in the First World War, 1914–18* (London: Butler and Tanner, 1987), p. 53.
97   'Complimentary dinner to Dr. Lily Baker', *BMJ*, 12 February 1927, p. 804, from file on Lily A. Baker, Kirkpatrick Archive, Royal College of Physicians, Dublin.
98   'Ante-natal work at the Bristol Royal Infirmary', *BMJ*, 6 November 1926, p. 851.
99   'History of the Medical Women's Federation', www.medicalwomensfederation.org.uk/new/about/History.html, consulted on 10 May 2010.
100   'Complimentary dinner to Dr Lily Baker', *BMJ*, 1927.
101   'Obituary: Lily A. Baker', *BMJ*.
102   Because the married surnames of these two women are similar, I will refer to each by their maiden names in this case study to avoid confusion.
103   *Medical Students' Register* for 1917/18.
104   *Medical Students' Register* for 1919/20.
105   J. D. O'Connor, 'Doctor in the dales', *Yorkshire Dalesman*, December 1983, pp. 750–1, private collection of Brian O'Connor, Sligo.

106 *Ibid.*
107 Oral history interview with Mary Mullaney.
108 *Ibid.*
109 Correspondence with Brian O'Connor, Sligo.
110 O'Connor, 'Doctor in the dales'.

8

Conclusions

The results of the recent examination for medical degrees in London University furnish further proof to the extent to which women are entering the profession. Twenty of the forty-eight successful candidates are women, one of whom was awarded the University medal. This feminine invasion of medicine is deplored by nobody except, perhaps, the oldest of old fogeys.[1]

BY 1922, women doctors had firmly established themselves within the Irish medical profession. Additionally, the above quotation from the *Irish Times*, from 1921, suggests that numbers of women qualifying with medical degrees in Britain were similarly high. Indeed, one article in the student magazine *QCB* in 1911 commented that future historians writing about the history of Queen's College Belfast would write about a time when men and women students at the College were in equal numbers.[2] The *Irish Times'* phrase 'feminine invasion' seems to imply that women doctors had conquered the medical profession using force against opposition, while those who were opposed to women working in medicine were deemed to be old-fashioned in their views. This is comparable to those modern historians on women in the higher education movement who refer to women's admission to universities as a 'struggle'. The road to this 'feminine invasion' in the Irish context had proved itself surprisingly straightforward. The Irish medical hierarchy of the King and Queen's College of Physicians of Ireland had welcomed the admission of women to take its licence examinations from 1877 and, after that decision, most of the Irish universities soon followed suit, forming a contrast with how we have usually perceived the British situation.

The Irish medical profession, unlike that in Britain, demonstrated liberality of thought with regard to the issue of the admission of women to Irish medical schools, in spite of the mixed attitudes to women's study of medicine in Britain and Ireland which existed at the time. The issue of admitting women to medical education was complex, yet it could be said that it was part of wider trends within the women's higher education movement in the United Kingdom. However, it is clear that the question of women's admission to study medicine was distinctive with regard to the particular arguments that were made against it.

These issues and the history of British women's struggle to enter the medical profession have been well documented.[3] However, the role of the King and Queen's College of Physicians of Ireland in allowing women's entry to the medical profession has been seriously underplayed by historians of women in medicine, who have tended to focus on the heroic efforts of Sophia Jex-Blake and her cohort to gain admission to medical training.[4] Likewise, there are important differences between the story of women's admission to the medical profession in Britain and women's admission to the medical profession in Ireland. I have drawn attention to the decision of the King and Queen's College to allow women to take its licence examinations. Evidently, that decision was based around several factors: the social context of the period, the liberal Irish medical profession and College finance. The context differs from that in Britain, where there was a greater emphasis on gendered segregation in medical education. In Ireland, there existed equal opportunities for women doctors in the medical societies, again in contrast with Britain. Women doctors such as Katharine Maguire and Emily Winifred Dickson attended and participated at meetings of the Royal Irish Academy of Medicine, suggesting that they were seen as equals in the professional sphere by the male medical hierarchy.

This book has provided a collective biography of the lives of ordinary women medical students and doctors, rather than focusing on the 'great women' within this cohort of Irish medical graduates. It would have been very easy to write a narrative that focused on the first women medical graduates as pioneers and failed to take the wider issues into account. Through the use of statistics, the study has provided a snapshot of the life of the average female medical graduate in the period, of her social background, experiences and career. The 'Biographical index' provides basic details of over 450 individual women who successfully graduated, to assist future research. Chapters 1, 4 and 7 supplemented the statistical chapters of the book and gave an insight into the story behind women's admission to study medicine in Ireland, as well as their experiences as students and doctors.

The main primary sources used in this book were official documents relating to the universities such as matriculation records, minute books and calendars, professional publications such as the General Medical Council's annual *Medical Students' Register* and the *Medical Directory*, and contemporary material such as newspaper reports, student guides, the publications of suffrage and missionary societies, medical journals and student newspapers. In order to gain a more personal insight into the stories of Irish women doctors in the period, I have examined obituary material, personal letters, autobiographical accounts and memoirs, in addition to correspondence and oral history material kindly provided by the children and grandchildren of these women doctors. All of these sources combined to give a clear picture of women in medical education from the 1880s to the 1920s and in the medical profession from the 1880s to the ends of the careers of the final graduates in the cohort. However, the book would have been significantly strengthened by further personal material. It is unfortunate that we do not possess equivalent statistics relating to numbers of male medical students, their social and geographical backgrounds, careers and destinations. Also lacking are equivalent statistics for women medical students in other countries. Such statistics would provide a useful comparative basis for this book.

The women who studied medicine in the period tended to come from middle-class backgrounds and their choice of medical school hinged on which schools were open to women, their religious persuasion, financial factors and the type of qualification they wished to obtain. Clearly, these factors are not distinctive to female medical students but may be related to male medical students and female students in general. However, it is possible that women medical students may have required more family support for their chosen career than their male counterparts, for whom a medical education would have been viewed as more acceptable.

In the same way that an egalitarian attitude was shown towards women with regard to their admission to the medical schools, Irish educational institutions proved themselves to be favourably disposed towards women students with regard to medical education. Women were treated fairly and were educated alongside men at Irish universities. This contrasts greatly with Britain, where men and women were separated for both hospital classes and lectures. There was one particular exception in the case of Irish medical education: for anatomy dissections, women were separated from the men, through the construction of separate dissecting rooms. It seems that the problem Irish universities had was with women dissecting the male corpse, in particular in the company of men.

Nevertheless, in spite of the almost complete integration of women, it is clear that, in the context of Irish universities, women medical students came to occupy a world which was very much separate from the men. In common with their British and American sisters, who experienced a sense of separatism, Irish women medical students had an identity of their own.[5] Lady medicals reconciled this level of distinction between themselves and the men students through their self-identification as a cohort. Thus, women medical students provided a network of support for each other through their years of medical study and friendships formed in university often lasted through their professional careers, with Dublin women doctors in the early twentieth century meeting under the auspices of the Irish Association of Registered Medical Women.

Chapter 5 examined what happened to women medical students after graduation. Contrary to the career paths that were expected of them, as outlined in Chapter 1, such as missionary work and work in women's hospitals, this chapter revealed that Irish women graduates tended to work primarily in general practice, hospital appointments in general hospitals and within the field of public health. Women graduates were more likely to work in hospitals and the public health sector if they emigrated to Britain for work; however, this is likely to have been because there simply did not exist the same quantity of job opportunities for women doctors in Ireland. Because of this, women doctors in Ireland generally chose to go into general practice. Certainly, the majority of women graduates who remained in Ireland, particularly the post-1918 graduates, appear to have worked in general practice. The fact that the majority of Irish women graduates worked in general practice is likely to have had more to do with a lack of appointments in hospitals and public health in Ireland than with any discrimination against women doctors. The large number of women who appear to have remained working in general practice for their entire careers suggests that women doctors found a niche in this area of work, rather than in the areas that were expected of them in the nineteenth century, such as women and children's health and the missionary field. This may also have been down to personal preference, as general practice would have allowed women doctors a means of balancing work and family life. The fact that these women were able to maintain careers in this field indicates that the 'lady doctor' had become an accepted part of Irish society.

It has often been claimed that the First World War opened up new opportunities to women in the workplace. Indeed, it appears to have resulted in increased opportunities for women doctors in Ireland but these were short-term gains, and after the war there was a shortage of posts for the huge numbers of women graduating in medicine from Irish institutions and the medical marketplace became saturated. As a result, women who graduated after 1918 cohort were more likely to go into general practice than their predecessors; however, this may also have been a result of increased acceptance of the lady doctor as general practitioner.

Chapter 7 demonstrated the importance of the personal story within the social history of medicine, something which is often lost through an over-reliance on statistics. Through examining the lives of Emily Winifred Dickson,

Emma Crooks, the Baker sisters and Jane D. Fulton and Mary McGivern, I have illuminated the different career choices discussed in Chapter 5 that were open to women doctors and shown how these Irish women navigated these in their own lives.

Potential for future research

THIS STUDY has been limited to the experiences of women doctors matriculating from 1885 to 1922, so there is certainly scope for future research into the history of women in medicine in Ireland after this period. With the establishment of the Irish Free State in 1922 and a more conservative society in Ireland which emphasised the importance of the woman's role in the home, we must ask how this might have affected the numbers of women entering medical schools and university courses generally and how later generations of women doctors juggled family life and a career through changing social and economic climates. It is likely that some themes outlined in this book also have relevance for the next generation of women graduates. Emigration was certainly one, with Joyce Delaney (TCD, 1949) commenting:

> it was every doctor's ambition to become a medical 'all-rounder' and for this it was necessary to get as much experience as possible. We were, like the eggs, for export to England. America, as a place of employment didn't enter most of our minds. It was associated with 'wild colonial boys' and tin trunks. Middle-class Dublin in that era rather looked down its nose at any suggestion of an American accent.[6]

Sheena Scanlon (RCSI, 1949) emigrated to Manchester after graduation, where she said she experienced discrimination as a woman doctor.[7] Certainly, the experiences of doctors, both male and female, who emigrated from Ireland to Britain in the twentieth century is a topic which could be further researched.

Likewise, there is scope for work on the roles of women doctors outside the medical profession, in particular in philanthropic work and the suffrage movement. Some women doctors, such as Eliza Gould Bell (QCB, 1893), were ardent supporters of extending the franchise to women. Bell herself was close friends with the Pankhursts and Lady Betty Balfour.[8] Other graduates in the cohort, such as Mary Strangman, took a more direct role in the Irish suffrage movement. In February 1912, she was part of a deputation of five Irish women who met with Augustine Birrell, the Chief Secretary for Ireland. At the meeting with Birrell, Strangman asked for the parliamentary franchise for women. In her view, women had already proven their suitability to take part in the legislation of the country through their work on district councils and voluntary work in charitable associations. She felt that 'to make a good nation, they must have good women, and they could not have good women while they were in subjection'.[9] She was also one of six delegates at a 'historic mass meeting' of Irish suffragettes on 1 June 1912, to demonstrate their determination to secure the vote.[10] She also spoke at a meeting of the Irish Suffrage Federation in October of the same year.[11] Lucy Smith (QCC, 1898) was the honorary secretary of the Munster branch of the Irish Association of Women Graduates and Candidate Graduates.[12] There is much scope for research into the involvement of women doctors within these female communities.

One obvious area which could also be examined is the history of medical students and medical education more generally in Ireland. We still do not possess statistics relating to the backgrounds and careers of male medical graduates in Ireland in the nineteenth and twentieth centuries.

We now know more not only about Irish women in medicine but about the experiences of medical students and doctors of both sexes. Fundamentally, the book shows that the study of students' experience of Irish medical education gives deeper insights into the history of the Irish medical profession, which, rather than being stuffy and conservative as one might have assumed, showed itself to be forward-thinking and liberal. The egalitarian nature of Irish medical education led to women's incorporation into the Irish medical profession. Likewise, women doctors were readily accepted into learned societies such as the Royal Academy of Medicine from the 1880s.

This study has shown that medical women, with regard to their admission to medical school, experiences and careers, were treated fairly by the Irish medical hierarchy. This is important, because it encourages us as historians to think about Ireland as having a distinctive history of medical education and, indeed, history of medicine from that of Britain. It challenges us to reconsider the way that we think about the history of women in higher education and in the professions in Ireland and, indeed, the history of medical education in Ireland.

Notes

1 'Women doctors', *Irish Times*, 23 November 1921, p. 4.
2 'Five years at Queen's: a retrospect', *QCB*, 7:8 (1911), p. 14.
3 For example: Caitriona Blake, *Charge of the Parasols: Women's Entry into the Medical Profession* (London: Women's Press, 1990), and Thomas Neville Bonner, *To the Ends of the Earth: Women's Search for Education in Medicine* (Cambridge, MA: Harvard University Press, 1992).
4 For example: Edythe Lutzker, *Women Gain a Place in Medicine* (New York: McGraw-Hill, 1969), and Shirley Roberts, *Sophia Jex-Blake: A Woman Pioneer in Nineteenth Century Medical Reform* (London: Routledge, 1993).
5 See, for example, Virginia G. Drachman, 'The limits of progress: the professional

lives of women doctors, 1881–1926', *Bulletin of the History of Medicine*, 60:1 (1986), pp. 58–72.

6 Joyce Delaney, *No Starch in My Coat: An Irish Doctor's Progress* (London: P. Davies, 1971), p. 22.

7 Oral history interview with Dr Sheena Scanlon, August 2009.

8 'Obituary: Elizabeth Gould Bell', *BMJ*, 21 July 1934, p. 146.

9 'Deputation to Mr Birrell', *Votes for Women: Official Organ of the United Suffragists*, 5:207 (1912), p. 320.

10 'Irishwomen meet', *Irish Weekly Times*, 8 June 1912, pp. 12–13.

11 'Coming events', *Irish Times*, 25 October 1912, p. 5.

12 'Irish Association of Women Graduates and Candidate Graduates', *Irish Times*, 23 November 1910, p. 9.

Biographical index

THIS INDEX and the statistics for this book are based on the information from the databases I compiled as part of my research. The first database, of women medical students matriculating at Irish institutions from 1885 to 1922, is based on the matriculation registers of Queen's College Belfast, Queen's College Galway and Queen's College Cork, in addition to the *Medical Students' Register* (for students from the other colleges), the 1911 census and the matriculation registers of the National University of Ireland, for students of the Queen's Colleges who did not provide adequate information in the university registers. This database records each student's name, age/date of birth, year of matriculation, religion, birthplace; father's name; father's occupation, religion and whether the student succeeded in qualifying.

This information also appears in the second database, which concerns the women who successfully graduated. The second database is mostly based on the *Medical Directory* and contains information regarding the qualifications attained by graduates, the length of time taken to achieve their qualification, and their post and location five, ten, fifteen, twenty-five and thirty-five years after graduation. The database also contains additional biographical details which have been gleaned from obituary material or the Kirkpatrick Archive (held at the Royal College of Physicians of Ireland) concerning the women's publications, additional career information, husbands and death dates if known.

The index compiles this information for all the graduates, who are listed by their maiden name.

Issues with dates of birth and death

IN SOME CASES, graduates' dates of birth and death were unknown, so 'fl.' has been given to signify their earliest and last known dates of activity, which are usually their date of matriculation and year of last known entry in the *Medical Directory*. In some cases, graduates' birth dates are listed as 'c.[year]'. This is because only their age was listed in the matriculation records or the 1911 census rather than date of birth, so their year of birth has been worked out by subtracting their age from the year of matriculation (if age was gleaned from the registers) or from 1911 (if age was gleaned from the census). For graduates whose death dates were unknown, I have given the year of their last entry in the *Medical Directory*. 'Later' designates a married name.

Abbreviations

See pp. xv–xvi for a list of abbreviations used for medical institutions and medical degrees. In addition, DPH is diploma in public health.

Asst	assistant
Clin	clinical
GP	general practitioner
Ho	house
Hon	honorary
Jun	junior
Med	medical
MO	medical officer
MOH	medical officer of health
Phys	physician
Res	resident
Sch MO	school medical officer
Sen	senior
Supt	superintendent
Surg	surgeon

ADAMS, Martha (?–1936), from Armagh; father Andrew Adams, country gentleman. Religion unknown. Matriculated QCB 1906/07; qualified MB BCh BAO (Glasgow) 1901; DPH, Dublin, 1908. Worked as Sch MO in Blackpool c.1906–26.

ADDERLEY, Clara (fl. 1909–30), background unknown. Matriculated TCD 1909/10; qualified MB BCh BAO 1915. Worked in India with Dublin University Mission after graduation. Not listed from 1930.

ADDERLEY, Esther (?–29 May 1948), background unknown. Matriculated TCD 1909/10; qualified MB BCh BAO 1916. Worked in India with Dublin University Mission. Not listed from 1931.

ALEXANDER, Marion Cameron (1898–post-1955), from Belfast; father James Alexander, solicitor. Religion Presbyterian. Matriculated QCB summer 1915; qualified MB BCh BAO 1920; diploma in psychiatry (Edinburgh) 1928. Worked as MO at Argyll and Bute Asylum, Scotland, 1925, then, 1935 was MO at West Riding Asylum, Somerset. Listed, 1945 as District MO and Public Vaccinator in Milverton and factory doctor, 1955.

ALLEN, Anna Margaret Emily (c.1903–post-1927), from Fermanagh; father Robert Allen, barrister. Religion Church of Ireland. Matriculated RCSI 1918/19; qualified LRCPI & LM, LRCSI & LM 1925; DPH (Dublin) 1927. Married Edward Durand, Asst Secretary of Commerce, Washington, DC. No career details known.

ALLMAN, Dora Elizabeth (c.1871–1955), from Bandon, Cork; father Samuel Allman, schools inspector. Religion Church of Ireland. Matriculated QCC 1890/91; qualified MB BCh BAO 1898. Worked as MO at Armagh Asylum until at least 1933.

ANDERSON, Dorothy Margaret (1899–post-1936), from Cookstown, Tyrone; father James Dickson Anderson, merchant. Religion Presbyterian. Matriculated QCB 1916/17; qualified MB BCh BAO 1921; DPH 1923; MD 1925. Living in Peacehaven, Sussex, 1926; from 1936 Casa Figallo, Via Dante, Rapallo, Italy (no post listed at either address); then not listed. Published on 'Scrons meningitis – repeated lumbar puncture recovery', *British Medical Journal*, 1926.

ANDERSON, Helen (?–15 June 1937), from Galway; father Alexander Anderson, president of Queen's College Galway. Religion Presbyterian. Matriculated QCG 1919/20; qualified MB BCh BAO 1925. Married Francis Lydon, doctor. Practised in London until death.

ANDREWS, Marion Braidfoot (c.1873–post-1936), from Belfast; father unknown. Religion Church of Ireland. Matriculated QCB 1896/97; qualified MB BCh BAO 1901; MD 1910; DPH 1914. Working as Gynaecological Surg at Ulster Hospital for Women and Children, 1906–11; 1916 was Hon Commander QUB Women VAD Red Cross and Certified Surg Wellington Park Home. By 1926 Sch MO and Asst MOH, Worcester. Listed as retired, 1936. Published on 'Nephrectomy and ovariotomy during different pregnancies of the same patient', *Journal of Obstetrics and Gynaecology*, 1909.

ARMOUR, Bessie McCammon (fl. c.1901–post-1959), from Antrim; father William Armour, farmer. Religion Presbyterian. Matriculated QCB 1919/20; qualified MB BCh BAO 1924. Lived in Suffolk for entire career, 1934–49, presumed GP. Listed as retired, 1959.

ARMSTRONG, Henrietta (c.1895–post-1941), from Tipperary; father Simon Carter Armstrong, Church of Ireland clerk in holy orders. Matriculated TCD 1920/21;

qualified MB BCh BAO 1926. In 1936 based in Fukien, China, with Dublin University Mission. In 1941, address given in Tempo, Fermanagh, then not listed.

ARMSTRONG, Margaret Mary (29 September 1898–post-1929), from Tubercurry, Sligo; father Luke Armstrong, merchant. Religion Catholic. Matriculated QCG 1918/19; qualified MB BCh BAO 1924. Address in Tubercurry, Sligo, given, 1929, then not listed.

ATKINSON, Sybil (?–26 July 1939), from Tyrrelspass, Westmeath, background unknown. Married to Hector Atkinson, captain. Matriculated RCSI 1920/21; qualified LRCPI & LM, LRCSI & LM 1926. Address in Dublin given, 1931, then Westmeath, 1936, then not listed.

AUGHNEY, Honoria (13 September 1900–post-1959), from Tullow, Carlow; father Patrick Aughney, farmer. Religion Catholic. Matriculated UCD 1919/20; qualified MB BCh BAO 1924; DPH 1933. Listed in Carlow, 1929–34. Working in public health offices, 1939. Kildare. Chief MOH Wexford, 1949–59. Published on 'Production and distribution of milk in Wexford', *Irish Journal of Medical Science*, 1956; 'Some aspects of fluoridation', *Irish Journal of Medical Science*, 1957.

AUSTIN, Barbara Joyce (c.1900–post-1930), from Antrim; father unknown. Religion Church of Ireland. Matriculated RCSI 1919/20; qualified LRCPI & LM, LRCSI & LM 1925. Working as GP in Altringham, 1930, then not listed.

BAILE, Enid (?–03 July 1932), from Kilkenny; adoptive father J. J. McQuade. Religion unknown. Matriculated RCSI 1918/19; qualified LRCPI & LM, LRCSI & LM 1922; DPH (Liverpool) 1932. Working as Res MO, Clapham Maternity Hospital, 1927; Asst MO, Maternal and Child Welfare, Burnley, 1932, then not listed.

BAKER, Alfreda Helen (1893–post-1956), from Belfast; father Alfred Baker, art master. Religion Church of England. Matriculated QCB summer 1915; qualified MB BCh BAO 1921. Worked as Ho Surg, Royal Victoria Hospital, Belfast, 1926; Res Surg, Hounslow Hospital, England, 1931; Consultant Surg, Hounslow Hospital, 1936; Surg at Elizabeth Garrett Anderson Hospital from 1946 until at least 1956. Published on 'Granulosa-cell tumours of the ovary', *Proceedings of the Royal Society of Medicine*, 1932; 'Series of cases of duct papilloma of the breast', *British Medical Journal*, 1934; 'Diffuse intraduct carcinoma of breast', *British Journal of Surgery*, 1935.

BAKER, Lily Anita (c.1879–1956), born in South Africa; father unknown. Religion Church of Ireland. Matriculated RCSI 1898/99; qualified MB BCh BAO from TCD 1906; FRSCI 1912. Worked in Dublin initially after graduation, in practice with sister, Madeline, then moved to Bristol, 1911, and worked at Bristol Royal Infirmary until at least 1941.

BAKER, Madeline (fl. 1900–42), born in South Africa; father unknown. Religion Church of Ireland. Matriculated Catholic University 1900/01; qualified MB BCh BAO 1907. Worked in Dublin initially in practice with sister Lily, then moved to England, 1910. In 1917, was working as a company doctor to the Welsh National Memorial Association. In 1922, in London, working as a MO to the Church Army Dispensary for Women and Children and the Given Wilson Health Centre for Infants in Plaistow. Later moved to Bath, where she worked as MO at the West Dispensary, Bath, until at least 1942.

BALDWIN, Monica Mary (5 December 1900–post-1960), from Macroom, Cork; father Samuel Baldwin, merchant. Religion unknown. Matriculated UCD 1921/22;

qualified MB BCh BAO 1925. Listed in Macroom, 1930–35, then moved to England. Working as Asst MO, Durham County Mental Hospital, 1940, and Asst Psychiatrist at Winterton Hospital, 1950–60.

BALL, Kathleen Mary (fl. 1921–60), background unknown. Matriculated TCD 1921/22; qualified MB BCh BAO 1925. By 1940 working as Asst MOH in Shrewsbury, England. Working as Asst MOH, Salop County Council, 1950–60.

BALL-DODD, Henrietta Clery (c.1894–post-1947), from Cork; father Henry C. Ball, shopkeeper. Religion Catholic. Matriculated RCSI 1917/18; qualified LRCPI & LM, LRCSI & LM 1922. Married Edward Ball-Dodd, doctor, year unknown. Worked as MO for an assurance company, York, until at least 1947.

BAMBER, Maggie (later listed Mrs McCall) (c.1901–post-1960), from Antrim; father John Bamber, horse dealer. Religion Presbyterian. Matriculated QCB 1918/19; qualified MB BCh BAO 1925. Listed in Ballymena, 1930–35, then Staffordshire, England, 1940–60, no post given until 1960, when Sch MO.

BARRY, Catherine Mary (later Barry-McKenna) (4 July 1898–post-1959), from Kilkenny; father John Barry, vet. Religion Catholic. Matriculated UCD 1917/18; qualified MB BCh BAO 1924. Working in Kenya, 1939, then London, 1949 (address but no post) and Essex, 1959 (address but no post).

BEAMISH, Henrietta O'Donoghue Martin (1880–post-1932), from Clonakilty, Cork; father George Beamish, Church of Ireland clergyman. Religion Church of Ireland. Matriculated QCC 1900/01; qualified LRCPI & LM, LRCSI & LM 1907. Listed address but no post in Clonakilty, 1912–32.

BEATTIE, Mary Frances Robina (c.1898–post-1958), birthplace unknown; father Presbyterian clergyman. Religion Presbyterian. Matriculated QCB summer 1916; qualified MB BCh BAO 1923. Worked as GP (Beattie and Beattie) in St Leonards-on-Sea, England, from 1928 until at least 1958.

BEATTY, Lizzie (?–1924), birthplace unknown; father Presbyterian minister. Religion Presbyterian. Matriculated QCB 1894/95; qualified LRCP LRCS Edin, LFPS Glas 1899. Worked as GP initially at 18 Upper Merrion Street (1904), then became medical missionary in China with Irish Presbyterian Society, 1906–17, then retired to California due to ill-health.

BEATTY, Myra Kathleen (1901–post-1934), birthplace unknown; father Presbyterian minister. Religion Presbyterian. Matriculated QCB 1919/20; qualified MB BCh BAO 1924; MD 1927; BSc 1928. Working, 1934 as Musgrave Research Student in Biochemistry and Demonstrator of Physiology at QUB, then not listed. Published on 'Muscle enzymes', *Journal of Physiology*, 1926.

BEIRNE, Elizabeth ('Betty') (1894–1979), born in Montmellick; father Patrick Beirne, member of the Royal Irish Constabulary. Matriculation date unknown; qualified MB BCh BAO 1919. Worked in India. Information courtesy of great-niece, Anne Beirne.

BELL, Eliza Gould (?–9 July 1934), from Belfast; father Hugh Bell, occupation unknown. Religion unknown. Matriculated QCB 1888/89; qualified MB BCh BAO 1893. Married Hugh Fisher, doctor. Worked as GP in Belfast until at least 1928.

BELL, Frances Elizabeth (fl. 1917–56); father farmer (father's name and birthplace unknown). Religion unknown. Matriculated QCB summer 1917; qualified MB BCh BAO 1921; DPH 1922. Worked as MO, Lisburn, 1926–36; Anaesthetist, Armagh

County Infirmary, 1946 until at least 1956. Published on 'Hypersensitiveness to quinine', *British Medical Journal*, 1923.

BELL, Margaret Smith (?– August 1906), from Belfast; father Joseph Bell, union clerk. Religion unknown. Matriculated QCB 1889/90; qualified LRCPI & LM, LRCSI & LM 1894. Worked in Manchester as GP and Asst at 'The Grove', Fallowfield, until death. Married Douglas Boyd, doctor.

BERGIN, Margaret (29 January 1899–post-1959), from Brosna, King's County; father John Bergin, farmer. Religion unknown. Matriculated UCD 1918/19; qualified MB BCh BAO 1924; DPH 1927. Worked as Asst MOH Borough, Southwark, 1934–49; 1959 was working as Asst MOH London County Council.

BINGHAM, Norah Eileen (1902–post-1950), birthplace unknown; father solicitor's clerk. Religion Church of Ireland. Matriculated QCB 1919/20; qualified MB BCh BAO 1925. Listed at 'Ardneagh', Ardenlee Avenue, Ravenhill Rd, Belfast, until 1950, presumably GP.

BLACKLAY, Helen (1895–post-1958), birthplace unknown; father seedsman. Religion Presbyterian. Matriculated QCB summer 1917; qualified MB BCh (Edin) 1923. Listed in Derry 1928–33, then MO, Durham County Council, 1938–48. Living in Scotland, 1958.

BLUMBERG, Sarah (1902–post-1937), background unknown; father draper. Religion Jewish. Matriculated QCB 1920/21; qualified MB BCh BAO 1927. Address in Down, 1932–37, then not listed.

BODDIE, Flora Mabel (1903–post-1962), birthplace unknown; father civil engineer. Religion Church of Ireland. Matriculated QCB 1921/22; qualified MB BCh BAO 1927. Address but no post in Bushmills, Antrim, 1932–37, then listed MO, Bushmills Dispensary District, from 1942; listed address but no post in Bushmills again from 1952–62.

BOLAND, Mary (fl. 1915–56), background unknown. Matriculated RCSI summer 1915; qualified LRCPI & LM, LRCSI & LM 1921. Address in Blackrock, Dublin, until 1936, when in London, listed address but no post until 1946. In 1956, address in Sussex given.

BOLAND, Winnifred W. (1896–post-1956), birthplace unknown; father merchant. Religion unknown. Matriculated QCB 1913/14; qualified MB BCh BAO 1921. Address in Newry, 1926–31, then Bootle, Liverpool, 1936–56.

BOUCHIER-HAYES, Margery (?–15 April 1931), from Rathkeale; father Stephen Bouchier-Hayes, doctor. Religion unknown. Matriculated TCD 1916/17; qualified MB BCh BAO 1922. Address in London, 1927–32, then not listed.

BOYD, Catharine Laura (fl. 1896–1938), birthplace unknown; father merchant. Religion unknown. Matriculated QCB 1896/97; qualified MB BCh BAO 1903. Ho Surg, Children's Hospital, Dublin, initially, then moved to England by 1913, working as Sch MO, Yorkshire Education Committee. By 1918, working as Sch MO, Enfield Education Committee, then 1928 until at least 1938 was Clin Asst at West Royal Ophthalmological Hospital and at St Mary's Hospital, London.

BOYD, Eileen Agnes (c.1889–post-1958), from Dublin; father Samuel Parker Boyd, wholesale druggist. Religion Presbyterian. Matriculated TCD 1918/19; qualified MB BCh BAO 1923. Listed at address in London, 1928–33, then was Asst Pathologist at the

Seamen's Hospital, Greenwich, 1938–48. Retired by 1958. Published on 'Investigation of sweat in rheumatic subjects', *Irish Journal of Medical Science*, 1934; 'Urea nitrogen content of blood before and after spinal anaesthesia', *British Journal of Anaesthesia*, 1936.

BRADY, Ita Dympna (27 March 1895–post-1958), from Meath; father Phillip Brady, farmer. Religion Catholic. Matriculated UCD 1917/18; qualified MB BCh BAO 1923; DPH 1926. Listed address in Kildare, 1928, and Dublin, 1933–38, then Asst MOH, Co. Dublin, 1948–58.

BRANGAN, Eileen (c.1901–post-1934), from Meath; father John Brangan, physician and surgeon. Religion Catholic. Matriculated TCD 1918/19; qualified MB BCh BAO 1924. Address but no post in Kells, Meath, 1929–34, then not listed.

BRENNAN, Jane Anne (later Coghlan) (9 December 1897–post-1958), from Mayo; father William Brennan, farmer. Religion unknown. Matriculated QCG 1917/18; qualified LRCPI & LM, LRCSI & LM 1923. Dispensary MO and MOH, Foxford, from 1933 until at least 1958.

BRERETON, Annie Genevieve (1 January 1900–post-1928), from Dublin; father Michael Brereton, grocer and publican. Religion Catholic. Matriculated UCD 1918/19; qualified MB BCh BAO 1923. Listed in Fitzwilliam St, Dublin, 1928, then not listed.

BRIDGFORD, May Ethel (?–1917), background unknown. Matriculated RCSI 1895/96; qualified LRCPI & LM, LRCSI & LM 1901. Working at London Medical Mission, Lambeth St, London, 1911, then listed Australia, 1916, then not listed.

BRITTAIN, Mabel Elizabeth (fl. 1919–61), background unknown. Matriculated TCD 1919/20; qualified MB BCh BAO 1926. Listed address but no post in Dublin, 1931–61.

BRODERICK, Henrietta (fl. 1920–60), background unknown. Matriculated RCSI 1920/21; qualified LRCPI & LM, LRCSI & LM 1925. Working as MO, Grosvenor Sanatorium, Ashford, England, 1940, and Asst Chest Phys, Dartford area, 1950–60.

BRODERICK (later Magner), Mary Florence (5 August 1898–post-1957), from Roscommon; father Francis Broderick, teacher. Religion unknown. Matriculated UCD 1916/17; qualified MB BCh BAO 1922. Address but no post in Sligo, 1927, then address but no post in London, 1932–57.

BROWN, Ann Jane (fl. 1917–36), birthplace unknown; father clerk. Religion unknown. Matriculated QCB summer 1917; qualified LRCP LRCS Edin and LRFPS Glas 1926. Address in Cregagh Rd, Belfast, given 1931–36, then not listed.

BROWNE, Julia Marcella (c.1895–post-1932), from Ballyhooley; father Patrick Brown, Sergeant Royal Irish Constabulary. Religion Catholic. Matriculated QCC 1912/13; qualified MB BCh BAO 1917; DPH (RCSI) 1920. Worked as MOH, Stepney Borough, England, c.1922–32, then not listed.

BUDD, Elizabeth (c.1885–1962), from Maryborough Town; father William Budd, general secretary of the Methodist Mission House. Religion Methodist. Matriculated RCSI 1911/12; qualified LRCPI & LM, LRCSI & LM 1916. In 1921, listed as 'late demonstrator in anatomy, RCSI, and Recruit. Med. Controller, Queen Mary's, AAC Irel.' From 1926 to 1951, address at Dartmouth Square, Dublin, given.

BURKE (later Hughes), Cecilia Elizabeth Gertrude (20 November 1895–post-1956), from Tubbercurry, Sligo; father Patrick Burke, merchant. Religion unknown.

Matriculated UCD 1916/17; qualified MB BCh BAO 1921. Listed in Tubbercurry, Sligo, address but no post, 1926, then not listed again until 1946 and 1956 in Cork, presumably GP.

BURNS, Elsie Anna (c.1895–post-1955), birthplace and father unknown. Religion Methodist. Matriculated TCD 1915/16; qualified MB BCh BAO 1920. In 1925 working as Asst Res MO, City Hospital, Fazakerly Annexe, Ho Surg, Liverpool, Stanley Hospital, then Asst Res MO, City Hospital, 1930. MO, City Hospital, Fazakerley, Visiting Phys, City Hospital East and South, 1935–45. In 1955, listed as Deputy Med Supt, City Hospital, Fazakerley.

BURT, Alida Charlotte (fl. 1917–26), background unknown. Matriculated TCD 1917/18; qualified MB BCh BAO 1921; DPH (England) 1923. In 1926 listed as late Ho Surg, Queen's Hospital for Children, Hackney, London, then not listed.

BYRNE, Kathleen Rose (fl. 1918–47), background unknown. Matriculated TCD 1918/19; qualified MB BCh BAO 1932. Listed at North Circular Road, Dublin, 1937–47, then not listed.

BYRNE, Lucretia Helena Hastings (fl. 1915–56), background unknown. Matriculated RCSI 1915/16; qualified LRCPI & LM, LRCSI & LM 1921. Working as medical missionary, Med Supt, Church of England Zenana Missionary Society Hospital, Dongkau, China, from 1931 until at least 1946. In 1956 listed at address in London. Published 'Case of puerperal tetanus', *China Medical Journal*, 1927.

CALWELL, Isobel (1904–post-1962), from Belfast; father William Calwell, doctor. Religion Presbyterian. Matriculated QCB 1921/22; qualified MB BCh BAO 1927. Addresses in Belfast, 1932–62.

CALWELL, Sarah Elizabeth (c.1886–post-1927), from Antrim; father Robert Calwell, builder. Religion Presbyterian. Matriculated QCB 1904/05; qualified MB BCh BAO 1912. Address in Duncairn Gardens, Belfast, 1917–27, then not listed.

CANDON, Attracta (6 September 1897–post-1926), from Roscommon; father Bartholemew Candon, egg and butter exporter. Religion Catholic. Matriculated QCG 1915/16; qualified MB BCh BAO 1921. Address in Ballaghadereen, Roscommon, 1926, then not listed.

CAREY, Catherine (fl. 1920–60), background unknown. Matriculated UCD 1920/21; qualified MB BCh BAO 1925. Working as Asst MO, Farnham Hospital, Finglas, 1930–35, then Cork, address but no post, 1940–50. Listed as Sen MO, Cork Mental Hospital, 1960.

CARLISLE, Charlotte Christiana (c.1895–post-1960), from Down; father Hugh Carlisle, vet. Religion Presbyterian. Matriculated QCB summer 1917; qualified MB BCh BAO 1925. Worked at Mission Hospital, Mandagadde, Shimoga, Mysore, India, 1930 until at least 1935. Listed as Med Supt, Bridgman Memorial Hospital, Johannesburg, 1940 and 1950; then address in Down, 1960.

CARROLL, Eileen Clare (c.1900–post-1957), from Dublin; father John Augustine Carroll, first-class clerk at estate duty office. Religion Catholic. Matriculated UCD 1917/18; qualified MB BCh BAO 1922. Address in Dublin, 1927–47; 1957, listed as Asst MO, Mental Hospital, Monaghan.

CARROLL, Hanora (later Sheehan) (c.1899–post-1939), from Limerick; father James Carroll, farmer. Religion Catholic. Matriculated QCC 1918/19; qualified MB BCh BAO 1924. In 1934–39 was working as MO, Infant Welfare Centre, Kent Road, London, then not listed.

CARROLL, Mary Kate (c.1886–1967), from Donoughmore, Cork; father John Carroll, occupation unknown. Religion Catholic. Matriculated QCC 1907/08; qualified MB BCh BAO 1915. Address in Cork given, 1920, then address but no post in Walkden, near Manchester, 1925–50. Listed as MOH, Worsley, 1950.

CARROLL, Norah Angela (20 April 1902–post-1960), from Clontarf; father John A. Carroll, civil servant. Religion unknown. Matriculated UCD 1919/20; qualified MB BCh BAO 1925. Listed at Drumcondra Rd, Dublin, 1930–40, then, 1950 and 1960 listed as Asst MO, Farnham House, Finglas.

CARSON, Henrietta (fl. 1921–36), from Waterford, background unknown. Matriculated RCSI 1921/22; qualified LRCPI & LM, LRCSI & LM 1926. Listed at address in Devon, 1936 then not listed again. Husband Alistair McKendrick, details unknown.

CATHCART, Kathleen Margaret (c.1901–post-1960), from Belfast; father Thomas Cathcart, physician and surgeon. Religion Presbyterian. Matriculated QCB 1919/20; qualified MB BCh BAO 1925. Listed at Newtownards Rd, Belfast, 1930 and 1935, then listed as MO, Maternal and Child Welfare, Belfast Corporation, 1940, 1950 and 1960.

CHAMBERS, Catherine Wilson (c.1895–post-1957), born in Scotland; father John Chambers, engineer. Religion Presbyterian. Matriculated QCB 1918/19; qualified MB BCh BAO 1922. Listed in Belfast for entire career, then Lancashire, England, 'retired', 1957.

CHAMBERS, Gladys Eileen (c.1896–post-1933), from Leitrim; father Joseph Chambers, senior inspector of national schools. Religion Church of Ireland. Matriculated QCB summer 1913; qualified MB BCh BAO 1918. Working as Asst Sch MO, Education Committee, Liverpool, 1923–33, then not listed.

CHAMBERS, Winifred (c.1899–post-1932), birthplace unknown; father vet. Religion unknown. Matriculated QCB summer 1917; qualified MB BCh BAO 1922. Address at Newry Street, Banbridge, 1927 and 1932, then not listed.

CHANCE, Alice Bury (later Carleton) (c.1892–1979), from Dublin; father Arthur Chance, surgeon. Religion Catholic. Matriculated UCD 1912/13; qualified MB BCh BAO 1917. Working as anatomy demonstrator, University of Oxford, 1922–32. In 1942, not listed. Working as Phys, Dermatology Department, Radcliffe Infirmary, Oxford, 1952. Published 'Skin disease', *British Journal of Dermatology*, 1943.

CHAPMAN, Marjorie (c.1889–post-1947), from Donegal; father Robert Chapman, chemist and optician. Matriculated TCD 1907/08; qualified MB BCh BAO 1912. Listed at address Diamond, Donegal, 1917 until at least 1947, presumed GP.

CLARKE, Ina Marion (c.1885–post-1944), from Dublin; father unknown. Religion Church of Ireland. Matriculated RCSI 1904/05; qualified LRCPI & LM, LRCSI & LM 1909; FRCSI 1910. Working as Demonstrator in Anatomy, TCD and RCSI, 1914, 1924 was Asst at Out-patient Department, Grosvenor Hospital for Women and Elizabeth Garrett Anderson Hospital, and Phys, Women's Workers Dispensary and St Marylebone Dispensary, Welbeck St, London. In 1934 was Phys to the Women Workers Department, St Marylebone Dispensary. In 1944, address in Surrey but no post.

COFFEY, Bridget (24 February 1897–post-1955), from Limerick; father John Coffey, farmer. Religion unknown. Matriculated UCD 1915/16; qualified MB BCh BAO 1920. In Limerick, 1925, then MO at The Manor, Epsom, Surrey, 1930 and 1935, then Sen Hospital MO, Tooting Bec Hospital, London, 1945 and 1955.

COGHLAN (later Conway), Josephine Mary Benedicta (1900–90), from Wicklow; father unknown. Religion Catholic. Matriculated UCD 1921/22; qualified MB BCh BAO 1925; DPH 1928. Married Stephen Conway, vet, 1926. Worked as GP in Salem, Wicklow, for entire career.

COGHLAN, Margaret Mary (fl. 1905–20), background unknown. Matriculated Catholic University 1905/06; qualified LRCPI & LM, LRCSI & LM 1910. Address at Claremorris 1915 and 1920, then not listed.

COGHLAN, Sarah Mary (30 August 1896–15 June 1929), from Foxford, Mayo; father Michael Coghlan, farmer and commercial traveller. Religion unknown. Matriculated UCD 1916/17; qualified MB BCh BAO 1925. Based in Foxford, presumably GP, until death.

COLLERAN, Delia (later Colleran-Begley) (30 December 1898–post-1958), from Moylough, Co. Galway; father James Colleran. Religion unknown. Matriculated QCG 1918/19; qualified MB BCh BAO 1923. Worked as dispensary MO in Lennane, 1933 until at least 1958.

COLLIER, Georgina (later Harvey) (fl. 1893–1937), birthplace unknown; father Wesleyan clergyman. Religion Wesleyan. Matriculated QCB 1893/94; qualified LRCP LRCS Edin 1897. Married Joseph Harvey, GP in London, in practice with husband 1902 until at least 1937.

COLLINS, Annie (c.1901–post-1965), from Cork; father farmer. Religion Catholic. Matriculated QCC 1920/21; qualified MB BCh BAO 1930. Listed address in Kent, 1935, Temp Asst MO, Heston and Isleworth, 1945, and Asst MOH, 1955 and 1965.

CONDON, Florence Maude Mary (c.1870–15 September 1921), born in Burma; father Major Edward Condon, in army armoured marine division. Matriculated RCSci 1895/96; qualified LRCPI & LM, LRCSI & LM 1905.

CONNOLLY, Evelyn Elizabeth (c.1896–post-1961), from Donegal; father unknown. Religion Church of Ireland. Matriculated TCD 1921/22; qualified MB BCh BAO 1926. Based in Castlerea, Roscommon, until at least 1951, presumably GP; address in Sligo given, 1961.

CONNOLLY, Evelyn Mary (fl. 1914–54), background unknown. Matriculated UCD 1914/15; qualified MB BCh BAO 1919; diploma in tropical medicine (Liverpool) 1920. Worked in Uganda as Res MO, Nsambya Mission Hospital, Kampala, for entire career, until at least 1954.

CONNOLLY, Mary Frances Josephine (fl. 1917–57), background unknown. Matriculated RCSI 1917/18; qualified LRCPI & LM, LRCSI & LM 1922. Based at Fitzwilliam St, 1927–57; worked as Asst Surg at Royal Victoria Eye and Ear Hospital, Dublin, and Ophthalmic Surg, Dr Steevens' Hospital, Dublin.

COPES, Jane (later Mrs S. G. Johnston) (c.1894–post-1956), from Down; father Thomas Copes, farmer. Religion Presbyterian. Matriculated QCB 1912/13; qualified LRCP LRCS Edin, LRFPS Glas 1921. Worked as Dispensary MO and MOH in Banbridge, Co. Down, for whole career, until at least 1956.

COTTER, Mary (c.1903–post-1930), from Cork; father John Cotter, farmer. Religion Presbyterian. Matriculated QCC 1921/22; qualified MB BCh BAO 1925. Address but no post in Clare, 1930, then not listed.

COTTER (later Flynn), Mary Josephine (1902–post-1962), from Cork; father Patrick Cotter, draper. Religion Catholic. Matriculated QCC 1920/21; qualified MB BCh BAO 1927. Listed in Coachford, Cork, 1932 and 1937, then London, 1942, address but no post, then Asst Sch MO in Kent, 1952 and 1962.

COTTER, Nora (5 April 1894–post-1957), from Cork; father Eugene Cotter, national school teacher. Religion Catholic. Matriculated QCC 1917/18; qualified MB BCh BAO 1922. In London from 1932 or earlier working as MO for Public Health Department of London County Council and Child Welfare Centre until at least 1957.

COULSON, Dorothy May (fl. 1917–48), birthplace unknown. Religion Church of Ireland. Matriculated RCSI 1917/18; qualified LRCPI & LM, LRCSI & LM 1923. Based in London, 1933–48, presumably GP.

COVENEY (later Horgan), Mary Kate (23 April 1897–post-1937), from Kinsale; father B. Coveney, farmer. Religion unknown. Matriculated QCC 1917/18; qualified MB BCh BAO 1922. Listed at address in Nottingham, 1927–37, presumably GP.

COWAN, Margaret Lucretia (fl. 1918–28), background unknown. Matriculated TCD 1918/19; qualified MB BCh BAO 1923. Address in Derry, 1928, then not listed.

COWHY, Mary (?–8 April 1951), background unknown. Matriculated Catholic University 1902/03; qualified MB BCh BAO 1908. Listed in Buttevant, Cork, until at least 1943, possibly GP.

COX, Mary Violet (c.1901–post-1954), from Roscommon; father Arthur Cox, farmer. Religion Church of Ireland. Matriculated QCB 1919/20; qualified MB BCh BAO 1929. Worked at Ruberry Hill Hospital, Birmingham, as MO and later Deputy Med Supt, 1939 until at least 1954. Retired to Ballygally, Antrim.

COYNE, Angela Gertrude (15 November 1893–post-1926), from Tralee; father John Coyne, inspector of national schools. Religion unknown. Matriculated UCD 1916/17; qualified MB BCh BAO 1921. Listed at Waterloo Rd, Dublin, 1926, then not listed.

CRAIG, Gladys Lilian (c.1902–post-1931), from Derry; father David Craig, dental surgeon. Religion Presbyterian. Matriculated TCD 1919/20; qualified MB BCh BAO 1926. Listed at address in Derry, 1931, then not listed.

CRAWFORD, Annie Helen (fl. 1894–1904), birthplace unknown; father merchant. Religion unknown. Matriculated QCB 1894/95; qualified MB BCh BAO 1899. Worked in India as medical missionary at Zenana Mission House, Bombay, after graduation, not listed after 1904.

CRAWFORD, Bridget (fl. 1918–32), background unknown. Matriculated RCSI 1918/19; qualified LRCPI & LM LRCSI & LM 1927. Listed in Cork, 1932, then not listed.

CRAWFORD, Caroline Joanna (fl. 1903–13), birthplace unknown; father teacher. Religion unknown. Matriculated QCB 1903/04; qualified MB BCh BAO 1908. Working at Bennett Hospital, Wuchang Hankow, Central China, 1913, then not listed.

CRONIN (later Philpott), Elizabeth Mary (1896–post-1931), from Cork; father William Cronin, farmer. Religion Catholic. Matriculated QCC 1917/18; qualified MB BCh BAO 1921. Listed in Mallow, Cork, 1926 and 1931, then not listed.

CRONIN, Elizabeth Mary (c.1894–post-1956), from Butteraut, Cork; father John Cronin, farmer. Religion Catholic. Matriculated QCC 1915/16; qualified MB BCh BAO 1921. Listed in Buttevaut, Cork, presumably GP, 1926–56.

CROOKS, Emma Martha (?–1937), background unknown; father teacher. Religion Presbyterian. Matriculated QCB 1894/95; qualified MB BCh BAO 1899. Worked in China for entire career until 1937 as medical missionary with Presbyterian Missionary Society.

CROSS, Mary Christina (c.1900–post-1933), from Cork; father Thomas Cross, carriage builder. Religion Catholic. Matriculated QCC 1917/18; qualified MB BCh BAO 1923. Hon Surg, Bon Secours Hospital, Cork, 1928; address in Cork given, 1933, then not listed.

CULLEN, Annie (4 May 1899–post-1929), from Dungannon; father Terence Cullen, pork merchant. Religion Catholic. Matriculated UCD 1917/18; qualified MB BCh BAO 1924. Listed in Dungannon, 1929, then not listed.

CULLEN (later O'Meara), Louisa Mary (fl. 1903–61), birthplace unknown; father Laurence Cullen, justice of the peace. Religion Catholic. Matriculated UCD 1921/22; qualified MB BCh BAO 1926; DPH 1928. Married Richard O'Meara, doctor. Listed in Wicklow, 1931, and Wolverhampton, 1936, then working as psychiatrist, General Hospital, Jersey, until at least 1961.

CUMMINS, Lilian Maude Cunard (fl. 1892–1902), born in London; father William Cummins, gentleman. Matriculated RCSI 1892/93; qualified LRCPI & LM, LRCSI & LM 1897. Working as Surg and Med Registrar and Clin Asst, Out-patient Department, London Homeopathy Hospital, 1902, then not listed.

CUNNINGHAM, Teresa Genevieve (6 March 1895–post-1959?), from Monaghan; father P. Cunningham, occupation unknown. Religion unknown. Matriculated UCD 1917/18; qualified MB BCh BAO 1924. Working as MO and public vaccinator and MO, child welfare and antenatal centres, London, 1934–39, then listed as Ophthalmic Surg, Monaghan Hospital, 1949 and address in Buckinghamshire, 1959.

CUSSEN, Eileen (fl. 1919–63), background unknown. Matriculated RCSI 1919/20; qualified LRCPI & LM, LRCSI & LM 1928. Address in Dundrum 1933–53, then Macclesfield, Cheshire, 1963.

DALTON, Catherine (fl. 1903–41), from Cork; father Patrick Dalton, shopkeeper. Religion Catholic. Matriculated QCC 1920/21; qualified MB BCh BAO 1926. Address in London, 1931–41, then not listed.

DALY, Dorothy Alice (c.1896–7 March 1927), from Dublin; father Robert Daly, civil servant. Religion Church of Ireland. Matriculated TCD 1916/17; qualified MB BCh BAO 1921. Listed in Birmingham, 1926.

DAVIDSON, Victoria (fl. 1897–1938), from Cork; father Robert Davidson, occupation unknown. Religion Wesleyan. Matriculated QCC 1914/15; qualified LRCPI & LM, LRCSI & LM 1923. Working as MO, Hahnemann Hospital, Liverpool, 1933, listed at address in Liverpool, 1938, then not listed.

DEALE (later Deale-Ross), Violet (1891–1926), from Ranelagh; father unknown. Religion Methodist. Matriculated TCD 1910/11; qualified MB BCh BAO 1916. Working as Med Supt, Portsmouth Municipal Maternity Hospital and child welfare centres, 1921, listed at address in Southsea, 1926, then not listed. Married George Ross, doctor.

DELANY, Alice Evelyn Sylvia (24 January 1893–post-1943), from Portarlington, King's County; father Dennis Delany, gentleman farmer. Matriculated RCSI 1917/18; qualified LRCPI & LM, LRCSI & LM 1923; DPH 1928. Listed at Portarlington, 1933, and Sheffield, 1938–43, then not listed.

DELANY, Mary (fl. 1897–1920), from Cork; father Joseph Delany, builder. Religion Catholic. Matriculated QCC 1915/16; qualified MB BCh BAO 1920. Not listed.

DENGEL, Anna (1892–1980), from Steeg, Tyrol, Austria; father Edward Dengel, merchant. Religion Catholic. Matriculated QCC 1914/15; qualified MB BCh BAO 1919. Worked as medical missionary in India, then founded Medical Missionary Sisters. Remained in America fundraising and as editor for the *Medical Missionary*.

DEVLIN (later Townsend), Cecilia Columba (c.1900–post-1957), from Cork; father Michael Devlin, bandmaster. Religion Catholic. Matriculated QCC 1917/18; qualified MB BCh BAO 1922. Working at Mental Hospital, Cork, 1927, then listed address in Felixstowe, England, 1932–47. Listed as MO, South Cerney Infant Welfare Centre, 1957.

DICKSON (later Martin), Emily Winifred (1866–1944), born in Tyrone; father Thomas Dickson, MP. Religion Presbyterian. Matriculated RCSI 1887/88, graduated LRCPI & LM, LRCSI & LM 1891, MB BCh BAO 1893, FRCSI 1893, MD 1896. Practice at 18 Upper Merrion Street, 1895, and Phys to the Richmond Hospital, Dublin. Married Robert Martin, 1899. Gave up practice on marriage. Returned to work, 1915, at Rainhill Asylum, Lancashire, then 1917 was locum for GP in Ellesmere, Shropshire. Practising in London in the 1920s, then Siena, Italy, 1928. In 1930, was working in practice in Tunbridge Wells. In 1940 returned to work in Rainhill Asylum until death, 1944.

DILLON-LEETCH, Margaret (fl. 1916–32), background unknown. Matriculated TCD 1916/17; qualified MB BCh BAO 1922. Working as GP in Macclesfield (Dillon-Leetch and Lomas) 1932, then not listed.

DILWORTH (later Ryan), Catherine (c.1896–post-1935), from Cork; father Timothy Dilworth, occupation unknown. Religion Catholic. Matriculated QCC 1919/20; qualified MB BCh BAO 1925. Listed at address in York, 1935, then not listed.

DIXON, Eileen Mary (5 June 1896–post-1956), from Sandymount; father Martin Dixon, surveyor. Religion Catholic. Matriculated UCD 1915/16; qualified MB BCh BAO 1921. Working as MO, Manorcunningham Dispensary District, 1926–31, then address in Dublin, 1936–56. Published 'Sir Dominic Corrigan: genius and ill-health', *Irish Digest*, 1943.

DOBBIE, Mina (?–23 November 1949), background unknown. Matriculated TCD 1889/90; qualified MB BCh BAO 1896; MD 1899. Working in London: Sen Ho Surg, Clapham Maternity Hospital, Asst Ho Surg, Battersea Maternity Hospital, Clin Asst, New Hospital for Women, 1901–06, Asst Sch MO, London County Council, 1911, lecturer at Physician Training College, Chelsea, MO, Askes' Girls' School, 1921, and MO, Chelsea College of Physical Education, MO, Aske's Girls' School, 1931. Published 'Prevention and treatment of spinal curvature', *Journal of the Royal Institute of Public Health*, 1909.

DOBBIN, Dorothy Isobel (c.1894–post-1942), birthplace unknown; father merchant. Religion unknown. Matriculated QCB summer 1912; qualified MB BCh BAO 1917. Working as Asst Sch MO, London County Council, and Clin Asst, Elizabeth Garrett

Anderson Hospital, London, 1922–27, then Asst Sch MO, 1932–42. Address but no post in Middlesex, 1952.

DOBBIN (later Crawford), Mabel (c.1891–1917), born in India; father unknown. Religion Church of Ireland. Matriculated TCD 1908/09; qualified MB BCh BAO 1913; MD 1914. Worked as Hon Asst Surg, Liverpool Hospital for Women, and Registrar, Liverpool Maternity Hospital, 1923–28, then not listed. Published 'Spasmodic stricture of uterus', *British Medical Journal*, 1922.

DOBSON, Mary (c.1900–post-1959), birthplace unknown; father farmer. Religion unknown. Matriculated QCB summer 1918; qualified MB BCh BAO 1924. Working, presumably as a GP, in Belfast/Down/Lurgan until 1959.

DOCKRELL, Anne Dorothy (fl. 1918–59), birthplace unknown; father Maurice Dockrel. Religion unknown. Matriculated TCD 1918/19; qualified MB BCh BAO 1924. Address in Dublin, 1929, Cheshire, 1934. Then in Dublin until 1959 at least, listed as barrister-at-law, King's Inn, and Dermatologist, Royal City Hospital, 1949.

DOHERTY, Mary Kate (19 September 1898–post-1930), from Crossmolina; father Dominic Doherty, teacher. Religion unknown. Matriculated UCD 1916/17; qualified MB BCh BAO 1925. Listed in Mayo, 1930, then not listed.

DONAGHY, Mary Margaret (c.1901–post-1937), birthplace unknown; father solicitor. Religion unknown. Matriculated QCB summer 1918; qualified MB BCh BAO 1922. Addresses in Belfast until at least 1937, presumably working as a GP.

DONALDSON, Margaret Hazel (fl. 1921–61), background unknown. Matriculated TCD 1921/22; qualified MB BCh BAO 1926. Anaesthetist at Drumcondra Hospital, 1931–36, then Phys at the National Orthopaedic Hospital, Dublin, 1941 until at least 1961.

DOOLEY, Pauline Mary (c.1899–post-1936), from King's County; father Edward Dooley, farmer. Religion Catholic. Matriculated RCSI 1918/19; qualified LRCPI & LM, LRCSI & LM 1926. Listed at address in Birr, 1931–36, then not listed.

DORAN, Winifred Mary (fl. 1906–38), birthplace unknown; father teacher. Religion unknown. Matriculated QCB 1906/07; qualified LRCP LRCS Edin, LFPS Glas 1913. Ho Surg, West Sussex General Hospital, 1923, later Res MO, Borough General Hospital, Warrington, 1928 and 1938.

DORMAN, Dorothy Charlotte Hobart (c.1910–post-1938), from Armagh; father Henry Dorman, GP, a member of the Golden Age. Matriculated TCD 1917/18; qualified MB BCh BAO 1923; DPH 1925. Listed in Armagh, 1928, and London, 1933 and 1938 (addresses but no posts given), then not listed.

DOUGLAS (later Benson), Dorothy Herbert (fl. 1917–47), background unknown. Matriculated RCSI 1917/18; qualified LRCPI & LM, LRCSI & LM 1922. Address c/o Lloyds Bank, Pall Mall, Dublin, 1932–47.

DOWNING, Alice Mary Angela (c.1901–post-1928), from Kerry; father Eugene Downing, solicitor. Religion Catholic. Matriculated TCD 1918/19; qualified MB BCh BAO 1923; DPH 1924. Listed as MO, West African Medical Service, 1928, then not listed.

DOWNING, Lena (c.1901–post-1940), from Cork; father shopkeeper. Religion Catholic. Matriculated QCC 1919/20; qualified MB BCh BAO 1925. Address in Kenmare, 1930–35, then Dublin, 1940, then not listed.

DOWSE, Eileen Hilda (c.1896–post-1955), from Belfast; father William Dowse, Church of Ireland clergyman. Religion Church of Ireland. Matriculated TCD 1915/16; qualified MB BCh BAO 1920; DPH 1921. Worked as Asst Sch MO, Belfast Education Authority, until at least 1955.

DOWSON, Mary Emily (fl. 1886–1901), background unknown, trained at the London School of Medicine for Women; qualified LRCPI & LM, LRCSI & LM 1886. Working as lecturer on forensic medicine and hygiene at the London School of Medicine for Women, 1891–1901, then retired.

DOYLE, Honoria (15 September 1899–post-1928), from Sligo; father James Doyle, farmer. Religion unknown. Matriculated QCG 1918/19; qualified MB BCh BAO 1923; DPH 1925. Listed in Sligo, 1928, then not listed.

DUFF, Alice Mary (28 August 1902–22 February 1951), from Dunleary, Dublin; father John Duff, clerk. Religion Catholic. Matriculated UCD 1920/21; qualified MB BCh BAO 1926. Listed at 51 Dartmouth Square, Dublin, 1931 and 1936, then registrar, Wolverhampton Eye Infirmary, 1941, and Ho Surg, Ear and Throat Hospital, Wolverhampton, 1951.

DUFF, Sara Geraldine (5 September 1897–post-1956), from Dublin; father John Duff, retired civil servant. Religion Catholic. Matriculated UCD 1916/17; qualified MB BCh BAO 1921. Listed in Dublin, 1926 and 1931, Meath, 1936–56 (address but no post).

DUNLOP, Agnes Joyce (c.1899–post-1952), birthplace unknown; father engineer. Religion unknown. Matriculated QCB summer 1917; qualified MB BCh BAO 1927. MO, Islington Dispensary, London, 1932–37, then address but no post in south-east London, 1942–52.

DUNLOP, Martha Lyons (c.1898–post-1957), from Antrim; father William Dunlop, farmer. Religion Presbyterian. Matriculated QCB summer 1916; qualified MB BCh BAO 1922. Antrim, 1927, address in Kent, 1932, then listed as Asst MOH, Gillingham, Kentin 1937 and 1947, then MOH, Gillingham, 1957.

DUNN, Lillie Eleanor (c.1879–post-1939), birthplace unknown; father farmer. Religion Presbyterian. Matriculated QCB 1898/99; qualified MB BCh BAO 1904. Worked at Zenana Mission Hospital, Broach, with Irish Presbyterian Missionary Society for entire career, until at least 1939.

EBERLE, Emily Elizabeth (?–12 September 1908), background unknown. Matriculated RCSI 1889/90; qualified MB BCh BAO 1894; FRCSI 1898. Worked as Phys and Surg, Bristol Private Hospital for Women and Children, from 1899 until at least 1904.

ELLIOT, Rachel Anna (c.1902–post-1960), birthplace unknown; father retired merchant. Religion unknown. Matriculated QCB summer 1919; qualified MB BCh BAO 1925. Ho Surg, Royal Victoria Hospital, Belfast, 1930, MO, Ministry of Health, London, 1940–60, at least.

ENGLISH, Adeline (1878–27 January 1944), from Mullingar; father Patrick English, pharmacist. Religion unknown. Matriculated RCSI/Catholic University 1896/97; qualified MB BCh BAO 1903. Worked as Asst MO, District Asylum, Ballinsloe, 1908–38, also lectured in mental diseases at UCG, 1918–38.

ENRIGHT, Margaret Anne (c.1888–post-1953), born in Paighton, Devonshire; father Daniel Enright, collector of customs and excise. Religion Catholic. Matriculated QCC

1913/14; qualified MB BCh BAO 1918; DPH 1920. Asst in Bacteriology and Pathology at UCC, 1923, Bacteriologist, St Ultan's Hospital, Dublin, 1928–53.

ENTRICAN, Dorothy Isabel (c.1900–post-1961), birthplace unknown; father Presbyterian minister. Religion Presbyterian. Matriculated QCB summer 1919; qualified MB BCh BAO 1926. Worked in China at London Mission Hospital, Wuchang, 1936–51, then address in Bengal, India, 1961.

ERSKINE, Frances Mary (c.1879–post-1958), from Tyrone; father John Erskine, feltmaker. Religion Presbyterian. Matriculated QCB summer 1918; qualified MB BCh BAO 1923; DPH 1924. Sch MO, Co. Antrim Health Committee, 1933–48, listed as retired, 1958.

EVANS, Nancy (c.1897–post-1962), from Cork; father Richard Evans, occupation unknown. Religion Catholic. Matriculated QCC 1918/19; qualified LRCPI & LM, LRCSI & LM 1927. Listed in Swansea, Wales, 1937–62, presumably GP.

EVOY (later Barter), Mary (c.1897–post-1957), from Cork; father Patrick Evoy, farmer. Religion Catholic. Matriculated QCC 1917/18; qualified MB BCh BAO 1922. Listed address in Douglas, Cork, 1927–57.

FAGAN, Mary Josephine (fl. 1918–39), background unknown. Matriculated RCSI 1918/19; qualified LRCPI & LM, LRCSI & LM 1924. Listed in Mullingar, 1929–39, address but no post.

FAHY, Angela (c.1897–post-1931), from Ballinrobe; father Michael Fahy, merchant. Religion Catholic. Matriculated QCG 1916/17; qualified MB BCh BAO 1921. Worked as dispensary MO, Galway, 1926–31, then not listed.

FAIR, Aileen (c.1901–post-1940), from Galway; father Joseph Fair, farmer. Religion Church of Ireland. Matriculated TCD 1920/21; qualified MB BCh BAO 1925. Address but no post in Galway, 1930, and 1935, then Nairobi, Kenya, 1940, then not listed.

FAIR, Olive Victoria (c. 1899–20 February 1932), from Sligo; father William Fair, fishery manager. Religion Church of Ireland. Matriculated TCD 1917/18; qualified MB BCh BAO 1922. Address in Sligo, 1927 and 1932, presumably GP.

FARRELL (later Adam), Agnes Catherine (9 September 1900–post-1949), from Kells, Meath; father David Farrell, farmer. Religion unknown. Matriculated UCD 1919/20; qualified MB BCh BAO 1924. Address in Chester, England, 1934–49, then not listed. Married James Adam, doctor.

FARRELL, Mary Josephine (19 April 1892–1975), from Longford; father J. P. Farrell, journalist. Religion unknown. Matriculated UCD 1911/12; qualified MB BCh BAO 1916. Worked as a medical referee for the Longford War Pensions Committee, 1921–26, then MO, Longford Dispensary, 1931–51.

FARRINGTON, Mary (9 June 1899–post-1960), from Dublin; father Andrew Farrington, chemist. Religion Catholic. Matriculated UCD 1917/18; qualified MB BCh BAO 1925. Address in Dublin, 1930–35, then pathologist, Children's Hospital, Dublin, and St Ultan's, Dublin, 1940–60.

FERGUSON (later Pearson), May Clemence (c.1899–post-1959), from Cork; father Lawson Ferguson, hairdresser. Religion Catholic. Matriculated QCC 1916/17; qualified MB BCh BAO 1921; DPH 1924. In 1926, listed as Sch MO in Norwich and Clin Asst, Great Ormond Street Hospital, London, then listed in Cork, 1939–59.

FITZGERALD (later Fehily), Clare (c.1897–post-1956), from Ballineen, Cork; father Patrick Fitzgerald, hotel proprietor. Religion Catholic. Matriculated QCC 1916/17; qualified MB BCh BAO 1921. Address at Glencarbery, Ballineen, Cork, 1926–56.

FITZSIMON, Emily Frances Mrs (fl. 1891–1901), birthplace unknown; father minister. Matriculated QCB 1891/92; qualified LRCP LRCS Edin, LFPS Glas 1896. Address but no post at Tralee, 1901, then not listed.

FLAVELLE, Ruth (c.1899–post-1926), from Dublin; father Henry Flavelle, secretary, Grand Lodge. Religion Church of Ireland. Matriculated TCD 1916/17; qualified MB BCh BAO 1921; DPH 1923. Address in Rathmines, 1926, then not listed.

FLYNN, Mary Bridget (1 December 1900–26 September 1939), from Roscommon; father James Flynn, teacher. Religion Catholic. Matriculated QCG 1918/19; qualified MB BCh BAO 1924. Listed in New Jersy, no post, 1934 and 1939.

FOLEY, Bridget M. (c.1897–post-1940), from Sligo; father Edward Foley, mineral water manufacturer. Religion unknown. Matriculated QCG 1915/16; qualified MB BCh BAO 1925. Working as Asst MOH, Lincoln, England, 1935 and 1940, then not listed.

FOLEY (later Foley-Taylor), Elizabeth Mary (24 May 1900–post-1934), from Galway; father Dermot Foley, customs and excise officer. Religion unknown. Matriculated UCD 1918/19; qualified MB BCh BAO 1923. Listed in Ballinasloe, 1928, then Research Radiotherapist, Westminster Hospital, London, 1938–48. Radiologist in Capetown, South Africa, 1958. Published 'Coarctation of the aorta', *British Journal of Radiology*, 1934.

FULTON (later O'Connor), Jane Dick (1901–1986), from Strabane, Tyrone; father farmer. Religion Presbyterian. Matriculated TCD 1919/20; qualified MB BCh BAO 1925. Address but no post in Yorkshire, 1935–64.

FULTON, Jane McGully (fl. 1900–22), birthplace unknown; father farmer. Religion unknown. Matriculated QCB 1900/01; qualified MB BCh BAO 1907. Worked as Asst MO, Hull City Asylum, England, 1912 until at least 1917, then address in England, 1922, then not listed.

GAFFIKIN, Prudence Elizabeth (fl. 1894–1935), background unknown. Matriculated QCB 1894/95; qualified LRCP LRCS Edin, LFPS Glas 1900. Working as Gynaecologist and MO at Children's Ulster Hospital, Belfast, 1905, then Sch MO in Enfield, England, 1910. Based in Dublin, 1915, then MO, East Islington Child Welfare Centre, London, 1925 until at least 1935.

GALLAGHER, Mary Alice (c.1893–post-1950), from Down; father national school teacher. Religion Catholic. Matriculated QCB 1910/11; qualified MB BCh BAO 1915. Working as surgical officer, North Staffs Infirmary, Stoke-on-Trent, 1920, Surg at ear, nose and throat clinics, Derbyshire, 1925, address but no post in Manchester, 1930, then Surg, Ear, Nose and Throat Department, Longton Hospital, Stoke-on-Trent, 1940, and address but no post in Staffordshire, 1950.

GALVIN, Mary Magdalen (c.1897–post-1956), from Cork; father Barry Galvin, solicitor. Religion Catholic. Matriculated QCC 1916/17; qualified MB BCh BAO 1921, DPH 1924. Res MO, North Infirmary, Cork, 1926, then MO, City Dispensary, Cork, 1936–56.

GARDINER, Elizabeth Mary (21 February 1898–post-1955), from Arklow; father C. Gardiner, doctor. Religion unknown. Matriculated UCD 1911/12; qualified MB BCh BAO 1920. Address in Rathangan, Kildare, 1925–35, then Dublin, 1945, and back in Kildare, 1955.

GARDNER, Dorothy Margaret (1899–post-1956), from Down; father George Gardner, designer. Religion Presbyterian. Matriculated QCB summer 1917; qualified MB BCh BAO 1921; DPH 1923. Address but no post in Belfast, 1926–31, then Asst MO, Belfast Mental Hospital, Examiner for Nursing Certificate, Royal Medical Psychiatric Association, 1936, Dep Med Supt, Belfast Mental Hospital, 1946–56.

GLASGOW, Isobel Little (c.1901–post-1958), birthplace unknown; father minister. Religion unknown. Matriculated QCB summer 1918; qualified MB BCh BAO 1923. MO and MOH, Strangford Dispensary District, 1933, MO, Downpatrick Dispensary, 1938, MO, General Hospital, Downpatrick, 1948–58.

GLEESON, Ella (fl. 1913–34), background unknown. Matriculated RCSI 1913/14; qualified LRCPI & LM, LRCSI & LM 1919. Dublin: address but no post, 1924–34.

GLOVER, Agnes (1 November 1899–post-1963), born in India; father Henry Glover, doctor. Religion unknown. Matriculated UCD 1921/22; qualified MB BCh BAO 1928. Working at Main Hospital, Raipur, India, 1933–38, then at Robertson Medical School, Nagpur, 1943–53. Retired in India, 1963.

GLYNN, Sarah Louisa (fl. 1892–1904), background unknown. Matriculated RCSI 1892/93; qualified LRCPI & LM, LRCSI & LM 1899. Listed as late Res MO, Drumcondra Hospital, Dublin, 1904, then not listed.

GOGGIN, Catherine (c.1898–post-1956), from Cork; father John Goggin, draper. Religion Catholic. Matriculated QCC 1916/17; qualified MB BCh BAO 1921; DPH 1923. Address in Cork, 1926–31, then addresses in London, 1936–56.

GOGGIN, Mary (c.1901–post-1959), from Cork; father John Goggin, draper. Religion Catholic. Matriculated QCC 1918/19; qualified MB BCh BAO 1924. In Cork, 1929–34, then England, address uncommunicated, 1939–59.

GOOD, Susanna Hosford (c.1886–post-1949), from Bandon, Cork; father James Good, occupation unknown. Religion Methodist. Matriculated QCC 1906/07; qualified LRCPI & LM, LRCSI & LM 1914. Address but no post in Kinsale, Cork, 1919–49.

GRAHAM, Doris Louisa (fl. 1915–55), background unknown. Matriculated TCD 1915/16; qualified MB BCh BAO 1920. Based at Waterloo Road, Dublin, 1925–30, then Zenana Missions, Bengal, India, 1935 until at least 1955.

GRAHAM, Elizabeth Saunders (fl. 1896–1908), background unknown. Matriculated QCB 1896/97; qualified LRCP LRCS Edin, LFPS Glas 1903. Listed at address in Down, 1908, then not listed.

GROGAN, Amelia (fl. 1888–1920), background unknown. Matriculated Carmichael College 1888/89; qualified MB BCh BAO 1895. Asst at Mullingar Asylum, 1900, then MO, Lawes Road Hospital for Women, Brighton, England, 1910; then in London, address but no post, 1920, then not listed.

GUY, Violet Mary Elizabeth (c.1902–post-1950), from Donegal; father Francis William Guy, national school teacher. Religion Church of Ireland. Matriculated QCB 1920/21; qualified MB BCh BAO 1925. Address but no post in Belfast, 1930–35, then Downpatrick, Down, 1940–50, then not listed.

HADDEN, Winifred Eileen (c.1894–post-1955), from Armagh; father William Hadden, doctor. Religion Methodist. Matriculated QCB summer 1915; qualified MB BCh BAO 1920. Address but no post in Portadown, Armagh, 1925–55.

HALPENNY (later O'Dea), Attracta (fl. 1920–34), birthplace unknown; father farmer. Religion unknown. Matriculated RCSI 1920/21; qualified LRCPI & LM, LRCSI & LM 1924; DPH 1927; MRCPI 1932. Pathologist, Richmond Hospital, Dublin, and St Ultan's, 1929–34, then not listed. Married to Sean O'Dea.

HAMILTON (later Coffey), Ellen (c.1903–post-1961), from Cork; father P. Hamilton, agent. Religion Catholic. Matriculated QCC 1920/21; qualified MB BCh BAO 1926. Based in Cork, 1931–51, then listed at Chingford Hospital, London, 1961.

HANNAN, Mary Josephine (fl. 1890–1905), background unknown. Year of matriculation unknown; qualified LRCPI & LM, LRCSI & LM 1890. Listed as MO, Lady Dufferin's Hospital, Agra, Kotah, India, 1895. Listed address but no post in Dublin, 1900, address uncommunicated, 1905, then not listed.

HARGRAVE, Jeanette Carroll (c.1868–post-1940), from Cork; father Abraham Hargrave, occupation unknown. Religion Church of Ireland. Matriculated QCC 1893/94; qualified LRCPI & LM, LRCSI & LM 1905. Address but no post in Dublin, 1910, then MO. Sanatorium, Bridge-of-Weir, Scotland, 1915, then Dep Sch MO and MO, Maternity and Child Welfare Committee, Lowestoft, England, 1920. Address but no post in Lowestoft, 1930, retired in Dublin, 1940.

HAWKESWORTH (later Shaw), Ethel Dorothy (c.1897–post-1956), from Cork; father Anthony Hawkesworth, solicitor. Religion Church of Ireland. Matriculated QCC 1915/16; qualified MB BCh BAO 1921, Asst Sch MO and Asst MOH, Co. Boro, Dewsbury, 1926, then Asst MOH until 1956.

HEGARTY (later Heape), Anne (c.1893–post-1934), from Carrignavan, Cork; father James Hegarty, farmer. Religion Catholic. Matriculated QCC 1913/14; qualified MB BCh BAO 1919. Listed at address in Cork, 1924–29, then listed in India, c/o Grindlay and Co., Bombay, 1934, then not listed.

HEGARTY, Margaret Josephine (c.1892–post-1963), birthplace unknown; father farmer. Religion Catholic. Matriculated QCB 1921/22; qualified MB BCh BAO 1928. Listed at address in Malone Rd, Belfast, 1933–53, then listed as MOH, Bishop Auckland, England, 1963.

HENRY, Dorothy Isabel (c.1893–post-1934), from Antrim; father James Henry, barrister. Religion Methodist. Matriculated TCD 1917/18; qualified MB BCh BAO 1924. Address but no post at Belgrave Square, Rathmines, Dublin, 1929–34, then not listed.

HENRY, Jeannie Lyle (1900–post-1958), from Antrim; father Thomas Henry, farmer. Religion Presbyterian. Matriculated QCB 1917/18; qualified MB BCh BAO 1923. Address but no post in south-east London, 1928–38, then Asst MO, Child Welfare Centre, London, 1948, and Asst MO, Public Health Service, London County Council, 1958.

HENRY (later Thompson), Mary Elizabeth (fl. 1910–16), background unknown. Matriculated QCB 1910/11; qualified MB BCh BAO 1916. Not listed in *Medical Directory*. Married Archibald William Thompson.

HERON, Margaret Isabel (c.1900–post-1957), birthplace unknown; father clergyman. Religion unknown. Matriculated QCB summer 1919; qualified MB BCh BAO 1932. Address but no post in Tipperary, 1937, then MO, Bootle General Hospital, 1942, then Res MO, Forster Green Hospital, Belfast, 1947–57.

HILL, Kathleen Edna (c.1900–post-1958), from Westmeath; father Thomas Hill, clerk of district asylum. Religion Church of Ireland. Matriculated TCD 1918/19; qualified MB BCh BAO 1923. Address but no post in Westmeath, 1928, then address in Rathmines, Dublin, 1933–58.

HOGAN (later Clery), Mary Gabriella (fl. 1917–37), from Nenagh; father P. Hogan, occupation unknown. Religion unknown. Matriculated RCSI 1917/18; qualified LRCPI & LM, LRCSI & LM 1922; FRCSI 1926. Address but no post in Nenagh, 1927–32, then address uncommunicated, 1937, then Fitzwilliam Street, Dublin, 1937. Married Anthony Clery.

HOLLAND, Doris Elizabeth (fl. 1916–56), from Cork; father unknown. Religion Church of Ireland. Matriculated TCD 1916/17; qualified MB BCh BAO 1921. Address but no post in Birmingham, 1926, then based at Foxrock, Dublin, 1931 until at least 1956.

HONAN, Mary (c.1900–post-1957), from Tipperary; father Patrick Honan, inspector of national schools. Religion Catholic. Matriculated QCB summer 1918; qualified MB BCh BAO 1932. Address but no post in Derby, England, 1937–57, presumably GP.

HORAN, Mary (fl. 1915–56), background unknown. Matriculated TCD 1915/16; qualified MB BCh BAO 1921. Working as Sen Ho Surg, Throat Hospital, Golden Square, London, Ho Surg, Metropolitan Ear, Nose and Throat Hospital, London, 1926, then Clin Asst, Mt Vernon Hospital, London, 1931. Asst Res MO and Ho Phys, London Temperance Hospital, Sen Ho Surg, Throat Hospital, Golden Square, 1936–46, then address but no post in London, 1956. Published 'Extensive hairy pigmented mole', *Proceedings of the Royal Society of Medicine*, 1931; 'Melanotic carcinoma cutis', *Journal of Dermatology*, 1931; 'Psychogenic aspect of dermatology', *Practitioner*, 1931.

HOSKIN, Rosaleen Hilda (16 December 1899–12 September 1975), from Sandymount; father Richard Hoskin, customs officer. Religion Unitarian. Matriculated RCSI 1917; qualified LRCPI & LM, LRCSI & LM 1923; DPH 1924. Address but no post in Cheshire, 1928–32, then address but no post in Dublin, 1932–75. Did not practise. With thanks to Professor Barbara Wright for providing me with this information about her mother.

HUGHES (later Quinn), Madeline (c.1898–post-1957), birthplace unknown; father cattle-dealer. Religion unknown. Matriculated QCB 1917/18; qualified MB BCh BAO 1922. Address but no post in Belfast, 1927, Tyrone, 1932–37, Armagh, 1947–57.

HUSTON, Alexandrina 'Ina' Crawford (fl. 1894–1904), birthplace unknown; father minister. Religion Presbyterian. Matriculated QCB 1894/95; qualified MB BCh BAO 1899. Working in Bombay, India, with Irish Presbyterian Mission, 1904, then not listed.

JACKSON, Ellen (c.1895–post-1957), background unknown. Matriculated QCB summer 1917; qualified MB BCh BAO 1922. Address but no post in Belfast, 1927 and 1932, then Ballymena, Antrim, 1937 until at least 1957.

JOLY (later West), Lucy Mary (c.1900–post-1959), from Dublin; father unknown. Religion Church of Ireland. Matriculated TCD 1919/20; qualified MB BCh BAO 1924.

Address but no post in Dublin, 1929, not listed, 1934, then address but no post in Wales, 1939 until at least 1959.

JONES, Teresa (fl. 1917–32), background unknown. Matriculated UCD 1917/18; qualified MB BCh BAO 1922. Bacteriologist, St Ultan's Hospital, Dublin, 1927, address but no post in Dublin, 1932, then not listed.

JOYCE (later O'Malley), Sarah (10 July 1906–post-1958), from Mountrowen, Leenane, Galway; father Thomas Joyce, farmer. Religion Catholic. Matriculated QCG 1916/17; qualified MB BCh BAO 1923. Address but no post in Galway, 1928–33, then Anaesthetist, Central Hospital, Galway, and Galway School Medical Scheme, 1938, Visiting Anaesthetist, Central Hospital, Galway, 1948, and Lecturer in Anaesthetics, University College Galway, Visiting Anaesthetist, Central Hospital, Galway, 1958.

KEANE (later Balassa), Julia A. (c.1898–post-1955), from Tormevara, Tipperary; father John Keane, ex-sergeant of the Royal Irish Constabulary. Religion Catholic. Matriculated QCC 1915/16; qualified MB BCh BAO 1920. Address but no post in Wolverton, Buckinghamshire, England, 1925–30, then Schools Medical Inspector in Oxford, 1935. Address but no post in Oxford, 1945–55.

KEHOE, Anne Carmelita (15 July 1898–post-1934), from Bridgetown, Wexford; father John Kehoe, national school teacher. Religion Catholic. Matriculated UCD 1917/18; qualified MB BCh BAO 1924. Address but no post at Herbert Place, Dublin, 1929–34, then not listed.

KEIRANS, Mary Margaret (c.1890–post-1951), from Monaghan; father Felix Keirans, manufacturer's agent. Religion Catholic. Matriculated Catholic University 1908/09; qualified MB BCh BAO 1916. Based at Newbliss, Monaghan, presumably GP, 1921 until at least 1951.

KELLEHER, Ellen (c.1898–post-1929), from Cork; father Jeremiah Kelleher, doctor. Religion Catholic. Matriculated QCC 1918/19; qualified MB BCh BAO 1924. Address but no post in Cork, 1929, then not listed.

KELLEHER, Julia Lucy (c.1892–post-1930), from Cork; father Jeremiah Kelleher, civil servant. Matriculated QCC 1911/12; qualified MB BCh BAO 1915. Worked as Asst Med Supt, Townleys Hospital, 1920–30, then not listed.

KELLY, Anne Jane (3 June 1899–post-1948), from Drumkeerin, Leitrim; father Terence Kelly, shopkeeper. Religion unknown. Matriculated QCG 1917/18; qualified MB BCh BAO 1923. Worked as MO, Kiltyclogher Dispensary, 1928–48.

KELLY, Elizabeth (fl. 1910–20), background unknown. Matriculated UCD 1910/11; qualified MB BCh BAO 1915. Working as MO, North Riding Asylum, Yorkshire, 1920, then not listed.

KENNEDY, Aileen Maryjoy (c.1903–post-1935), birthplace unknown; father doctor. Religion unknown. Matriculated QCB 1921/22; qualified MB BCh BAO 1930. Address but no post at University Square, Belfast, 1935, then not listed.

KENNEDY, Kathleen Mary (15 June 1901–post-1960), from Dublin; father Denis Kennedy, doctor. Religion Catholic. Matriculated UCD 1920/21; qualified MB BCh BAO 1925. Asst Res MO, Royal National Hospital for Consumption, Newcastle, 1930, Res Surg, Royal Hospital, Wolverhampton, 1935, then temporary Visiting Phys, Cork Dispensary Hospital, 1940–50, and Visiting Phys, St Finbar's, Cork, 1960.

KENNEDY, Kathleen Olive Moore (fl. 1917–68), background unknown. Matriculated RCSI 1917/18; qualified LRCPI & LM, LRCSI & LM 1923; DPH 1924. Address but no post in Fermanagh, 1928–33, then address but no post in London, 1938–68.

KIELY (later Forrest), Mary Agnes (c.1897–post-1957), from Cork; father Jeremiah Kiely, farmer. Religion Catholic. Matriculated QCC 1915/16; qualified MB BCh BAO 1922. Address but no post in Cork, 1927–57, presumably GP.

KIERNAN (later Malone), Eileen (fl. 1921–61), background unknown. Matriculated RCSI 1921/22; qualified LRCPI & LM, LRCSI & LM 1926. Address but no post in Birmingham, 1931. Not listed, 1936. Part-time MO, Birmingham Public Health Department, 1941. Address but no post in Staffordshire, 1951–61.

KILKELLY, Ethel Rose (11April 1896–post-1954), from Athlone; father Michael Kilkelly, draper. Religion Catholic. Matriculated UCD 1914/15; qualified MB BCh BAO 1919; DPH 1920. Asst MO for the county borough, Wolverhampton, 1924, not listed, 1929, Asst Sch MO and Certified MO, Wolverhampton, 1934, address but no post in Athlone, 1944–54. Published 'Investigation of cholera cases', *School Medical Officers Annual Report*, 1924; 'Rheumatism in school children', *School Medical Officers Annual Report*,1928.

KILLIAN, Elizabeth (c.1894–post-1947), from Roscommon; father unknown. Religion Catholic. Matriculated QCG 1917/18; qualified MB BS (Durham) 1922; DPH 1923. Address but no post in Athlone, 1927, then Ballinasloe, 1932–47.

KING, Catherine Margaret (fl. 1917–48), background unknown. Matriculated RCSI 1917/18; qualified LRCPI & LM, LRCSI & LM 1923. Address but no post in Sandycove, Dublin, 1928–38, retired, 1948.

KING, Ellen (18 October 1894–post-1932), from Dicksgrove, Kerry; father Jeremiah King, custom house officer. Religion unknown. Matriculated UCD 1912/13; qualified MB BCh BAO 1922. Presumed GP in west London, 1927–32, then not listed.

KING, Mary Josephine (fl. 1915–25), background unknown. Matriculated RCSI 1915/16; qualified MB BCh BAO 1920. Working as MOH, Mullingar Dispensary, MO, Mullingar, Consultant Phys, County Hospital, Mullingar, 1925, then not listed.

KIRKER, Arabella (c.1893–post-1921), from Down; father secretary to limited company. Religion Baptist. Matriculated QCB 1911/12; qualified MB BCh BAO 1916. Listed as Asst MOH, Matern and Child Welfare, in Down, 1921, then not listed.

KIRKER, Ida May (c.1896–post-1947), from Down; father secretary to limited company. Religion Baptist. Matriculated QCB summer 1916; qualified MB BCh BAO 1922. Address but no post in Banbridge, Down, 1927–32, then address but no post in Belfast, 1937–47.

KOELLER, Helen (c.1900–post-1933), from Belfast; father Francis Koeller, musician. Religion Church of Ireland. Matriculated QCB summer 1917; qualified MB BCh BAO 1923. Asst Sch MO, London County Council, 1928, Radiologist and MO, Ultraviolet Department, Queen Mary's Hospital, Roehampton, and Asst Sch MO, London County Council, 1933, not listed.

LAWLER, Bertha (c.1900–post-1931), from Wexford, birthplace unknown; father unknown. Religion Church of Ireland. Matriculated TCD 1918/19; qualified MB BCh BAO 1924; diploma in tropical medicine and health, Cambridge, 1926. Address but no post in Essex, England, 1931, then not listed.

LEDLIE, Alexandra Holmes Crawford (fl. 1916–56), background unknown. Matriculated RCSI 1916/17; qualified LRCPI & LM, LRCSI & LM 1921. Certified Factory Surg, Cork, 1926 until at least 1956.

LEMASS (later Lemass-Boland), Alice Mary (31 March 1901–post-1935), from Dublin; father John Lemass, hatter. Religion Catholic. Matriculated UCD 1919/20; qualified MB BCh BAO 1925. Address but no post in Dublin, 1930, then Res MO, City Infirmary, Dublin, 1935, then not listed.

LEMON, Ruth (fl. 1917–57), background unknown. Matriculated TCD 1917/18; qualified MB BCh BAO 1922; DPH 1924. Address but no post in Loughgall, Armagh, 1927–32, then dispensary MO and MOH, Loughall, 1937–47, then address but no post in Loughgall, 1957.

LINEHAN, Bridget (?–12 April 1936), background unknown. Matriculated UCD 1915/16; qualified MB BCh BAO 1921; DPH 1934. Asst MO, County Mental Hospital, Lancaster, 1926–31, then not listed.

LIVINGSTON, Mary Cecilia (c.1903–post-1935), from Armagh; father William Livingston, linen manufacturer. Religion Church of Ireland. Matriculated TCD 1920/21; qualified MB BCh BAO 1925. Address but no post in Lurgan, Armagh, 1930–35, then not listed.

LOGAN, Mary Ellen Margaret (?–12 March 1925), birthplace unknown; father doctor. Religion unknown. Matriculated QCB 1896/97; qualified LRCPI & LM, LRCSI & LM 1902; licentiate of Apothecaries' Hall 1913. Res MO, Infirmary, Lisburn Rd, Belfast, 1907–17, then not listed.

LONG, Mary Anderson (c.1900–post-1959), from Derry; father William Long, farmer. Religion Presbyterian. Matriculated QCB summer 1918; qualified MB BCh BAO 1924. MO, Derry Regional Education Committee, 1929, then MOH and MO, Feeny, 1934–59.

LOWRY, Eleanor (fl. 1899–42), birthplace unknown; father builder. Religion unknown. Matriculated QCB 1899/1900; qualified MB BS (London) 1907. Sen Ho Surg, Victoria Hospital for Children, Hull, 1912, Asst Surg, Women's Hospital for Children, Harrow Rd, Clin Asst, Eye, Ear, Throat Department of the Royal Free Hospital, London, 1917, Throat and Ear Surg, Elizabeth Garrett Anderson Hospital, London, 1922–32, retired in Antrim, 1942. Published 'Throat and ear defects from the standpoint of the elementary school child', *Journal of Oto-laryngology*, 1924.

LUCE, Ethel (fl. 1913–53), background unknown. Matriculated TCD 1913/14; qualified MB BCh BAO 1918; MD 1919. Worked as researcher with Beit Memorial Fellowship in London, 1923, then Sterling Sen Fellow and Lecturer in Paediatrics at Yale University, USA, 1928, Research Fellow in Biology at University of Rochester, 1933, and Professor of Zoology at University of Rochester, 1943 until at least 1953. Published 'Influence of diet and sunlight upon the growth-promoting...', *Bio-Chemistry Journal*, 1924.

LUCEY, Mary Patricia (1892–post-1949), from Cork; father Daniel Joseph Lucey, wool manufacturer. Religion Catholic. Matriculated QCC 1915/16; qualified MB BCh BAO 1924. Address but no post in Cork, 1929–49, then not listed.

LYNCH, Ita Mary (c.1902–post-1936), from Cork; father Timothy Lynch, customs officer. Religion Catholic. Matriculated QCC 1919/20; qualified MB BCh BAO 1926. Address but no post in Sunday's Well, Cork, 1931–36, then not listed.

LYNN, Kathleen Florence (28 January 1874–14 September 1955), from Dublin; father Church of Ireland clergyman. Religion Church of Ireland. Matriculated RCSci 1895/96; qualified MB BCh BAO 1899. Address but no post in Rathmines, Dublin, 1904–09. Clin Asst, Royal Victoria Eye and Ear Hospital, Dublin, 1914. Founded St Ultan's Hospital, Dublin, 1919, worked as Phys at St Ultan's until at least 1934.

LYONS (later Lyons-Thornton), Bridget (13 May 1896–post-1957), from Longford; father Patrick Lyons, farmer. Religion Catholic. Matriculated QCG 1915/16; qualified MB BCh BAO 1922. Address but no post in Longford, 1927, in Dublin, 1932, Asst MOH and Sch MO, Dublin County Borough, 1937–57.

LYSTER, Alexandra Mary (c.1903–post-1929), background unknown. Matriculated QCB 1921/22; qualified MB BCh BAO 1929. Not listed in *Medical Directory*.

MacRORY, Elizabeth (fl. 1894–1935), birthplace unknown; father solicitor. Religion unknown. Matriculated QCB 1894/95; qualified MB ChB (Edinburgh) 1900. Address but no post in Dumferline, Scotland, 1905, address but no post in London 1910, Medical Inspector, London County Council, 1915–25, then Asst MO, London County Council, 1935.

MADDEN, Violet (c.1898–post-1960), from Limerick; father Phillip Madden, farmer and justice of the peace. Religion Catholic. Matriculated QCC 1918/19; qualified MB BCh BAO 1925. Appointment at Ballinacurra Hospital, Knocklong, Limerick, 1930–35, address but no post in Dublin, 1940–50, then Phys, St Ultan's Hospital, Dublin, and Sunshine Home, Stillorgan, 1960.

MAGNER, Josepha Thomasine Mary (21 July 1898–post-1927), from Limerick; father Patrick Magner, rate collector. Religion Catholic. Matriculated UCD 1917/18; qualified MB BCh BAO 1922. Address but no post in London, 1927, then not listed.

MAGNER (later Walsh), Una (c.1892–post-1956), from Cork; father Edward Magner, doctor. Religion Catholic. Matriculated QCC 1915/16; qualified MB BCh BAO 1921; DPH 1927. Address but no post in Cork, 1926, then London, 1931–36, then Cleveleys, Lancashire, 1946–56.

MAGUIRE, Katharine (?–1931), from Boyle, Roscommon; father Reverend John Maguire, minister. Religion unknown. Year of matriculation unknown; qualified MB BCh BAO 1891. Listed address but no post, Dublin, until at least 1926.

MAGUIRE, Wilhelmina Colquhoun (c.1901–post-1959), from Belfast; father William Maguire, occupation unknown. Religion Catholic. Matriculated RCSI 1919/20; qualified LRCPI & LM, LRCSI & LM 1924. Visiting Phys, Court Theatre and Chelsea Palace Theatre, 1929, Asst MO, Camberwell House Mental Hospital, 1934–39, address but no post in London, 1949, Sch MO, Public Health Department, Dagenham, 1959.

MAHER, Nora Bridget (fl. 1920–37), background unknown. Matriculated RCSI 1920/21; qualified LRCPI & LM, LRCSI & LM 1927. Address but no post in Cashel, Tipperary, 1932–37, then not listed.

MARSHALL, Gladys Christeen Mary (c.1900–post-1957), from Tyrone; father David Marshall, Presbyterian clergyman. Religion Presbyterian. Matriculated RCSI 1917/18; qualified LRCPI & LM, LRCSI & LM 1922. Address but no post in Belfast, 1932–57.

MARTIN, Elizabeth Mary (c.1891–post-1956), from Belfast; father Samuel Martin, commission agent. Religion Presbyterian. Matriculated QCB summer 1916; qualified

MB BCh BAO 1921; DPH 1923. Ho Surg, Isle of Wight County Hospital, 1926, Asst Sch MO, Portsmouth, 1931–56.

MARTYN (later Fogarty), Bridget (31 December 1895–post-1954), from Flaskagh, Galway; father John Martyn, landholder. Religion Catholic. Matriculated QCG 1914/15; qualified MB BCh BAO 1919. Med Supt, Holgate, Middlesbrough, 1929 and 1935, later temporary lecturer, University College Galway, 1944, then address but no post in Galway, 1954.

McCAFFREY, Mildred Mary (20 September 1901–January 1950), from Bawnboy, Cavan; father Hugh McCaffrey, merchant. Religion Catholic. Matriculated UCD 1920/21; qualified MB BCh BAO 1926. Address but no post in Swanlibar, Cavan, 1931–41.

McCALLUM, Amy Connellan (c.1886–post-1943), from Belfast; father financial secretary to education board. Religion Church of Ireland. Matriculated QCB summer 1910; qualified MB BCh BAO 1918. Demonstrator in Anatomy at QCB, 1923, Res Med Supt, Rossclare Sanatorium, 1938, address but no post, 1943, then not listed.

McCANN (later Rath), Monica Mary (27 May 1897–post-1956), from Newry, Down; father James McCann, rate collector. Religion unknown. Matriculated UCD 1915/16; qualified MB BCh BAO 1921. Address but no post in Clare, 1926, Armagh, 1931, then dispensary MO, Termonfeckin, 1936–56.

McCARTHY, Ellen (c.1902–post-1961), from Cork; father Cornelius McCarthy, occupation unknown. Religion Catholic. Matriculated QCC 1920/21; qualified MB BCh BAO 1926. Address but no post in Schull, Cork, 1931–36, then address but no post in London, 1951, and MO, North Infirmary, Cork, 1961.

McCARTHY (later McCarthy-Doherty), May (c.1895–post-1952), from Cork; father Florence McCarthy, occupation unknown. Religion Catholic. Matriculated QCC 1918/19; qualified LRCPI & LM, LRCSI & LM 1927. Address but no post in Cork, 1932, then Capetown, South Africa, until 1952.

McCOLGAN, Kathleen Gertrude (17 June 1900–post-1938), from Donegal; father Joseph McColgan, merchant. Religion unknown. Matriculated UCD 1919/20; qualified MB BCh BAO 1923. Address but no post in Donegal, 1928–33, then in Kilkenny, 1938, then not listed.

McCONNON, Eileen M. (c.1901–post-1951), from Cork; father Michael McConnon, national school teacher. Religion Catholic. Matriculated QCC 1918/19; qualified MB BCh BAO 1926. Address but no post at Sundays Well, Cork, 1931–6, then Manchester, 1941–51.

McDANIEL, Eveline (c.1898–post-1956), birthplace unknown; father merchant. Religion unknown. Matriculated QCB summer 1916; qualified MB BCh BAO 1921. MO, Maternity and Child Welfare Scheme, Clin Asst, Children's Hospital, Belfast, 1926, Professor of Therapeutic Pharmacology and Material Medica, UCG, Jun Surg, Central Hospital, Galway, 1931, part-time school medical inspector, Clogher, 1936–46, then address but no post in Clogher, 1956.

McDERMOTT, Jane Mary (19 January 1902–10 March 1929), from Naas, Kildare; father Thomas McDermott, merchant. Religion Catholic. Matriculated UCD 1921/22; qualified MB BCh BAO 1926. Asst to Dr Laverty in Bray Dispensary District.

McDERMOTT, Mary Josephine (fl. 1917–59), background unknown. Matriculated RCSI 1917/18; qualified LRCPI & LM, LRCSI & LM 1924. Address but no post in Westmeath, 1934, then Manchester, 1939–59.

McDONALD, Christina (fl. 1919–63), background unknown. Matriculated TCD 1919/20; qualified MB BCh BAO 1928. Ho Surg, Sunshine Home, Bray, 1933, then London, address but no post 1938–53, then Asst MO, County Borough, West Ham, 1963.

McDOWELL, Margaret Irwin (c.1898–post-1933), from Derry; father Thomas McDowell, butter and egg merchant. Religion Presbyterian. Matriculated QCB 1917/18; qualified MB BCh BAO 1923; DPH 1924. Clin Asst, Eye, Ear and Throat Hospital, Derry, 1928–33, then not listed.

McELROY, Lilian (c.1903–post-1964), born in Lanarkshire, Scotland; father John McElroy, doctor. Religion Presbyterian. Matriculated QCB 1921/22; qualified MB BCh BAO 1929. Address but no post in Belfast, 1939, not listed, 1944, then part-time Asst MO, Child Welfare, Belfast, 1954–64.

McENROY, Margaret (27 December 1902–post-1961), from Newfarngone; father Bryan McEnroy, farmer. Religion Catholic. Matriculated QCG 1920/21; qualified MB BCh BAO 1926. Address in English provinces (precise address uncommunicated), 1931, address but no post in Nottingham, 1941, New Donnington, 1951–61.

McEVOY, Mary Josephine (16 November 1898–post-1958), from Dublin; father W. J. McEvoy, publican. Religion Catholic. Matriculated UCD 1916/17; qualified MB BCh BAO 1923. Address but no post in Dublin, 1928–33, then London, 1938–58.

McGEE, Sarah Anne (c.1896–post-1928), from Fermanagh; father William McGee, farmer. Religion Catholic. Matriculated QCC 1917/18; qualified MB BCh BAO 1923. Address but no post in Leitrim, 1928, then not listed.

McGIVERN (later Connolly), Mary (15 December 1900–March 1989), from Banbridge, Co. Down; father Peter McGivern, merchant. Religion Catholic. Matriculated UCD 1918/19; qualified MB BCh BAO 1925. Married J. J. Connolly (GP), 1925. Worked as GP in Banbridge for entire career after husband left for service in Second World War.

McGLOUGHLIN, Mary Kathleen (fl. 1920–30), background unknown. Matriculated UCD 1920/21; qualified MB BCh BAO 1925. Res MO, Walthamstow UDC Isolated Hospital, Chingford, 1930, then not listed.

McGRATH (later McGrath-Bowen), Anna Mary Pauline (c.1902–2 July 1951), from Carrick-on-Suir, Tipperary; father Thomas McGrath, grocer. Religion Catholic. Matriculated UCD 1921/22; qualified MB BCh BAO 1925. Married W. H. Bowen. MOH, Enniscorthy, 1930–60.

McGUCKIN, Clara Mary (c.1900–post-1928), background unknown. Matriculated QCB 1918/19; qualified MB BCh BAO 1923. Working as Anaesthetist, Mater Infirmary Hospital, Belfast, 1928, then not listed.

McGURK, Sara (c.1897–post-1921), birthplace unknown; father publican. Religion unknown. Matriculated QCB summer 1916; qualified MB BCh BAO 1921. Not listed in *Medical Directory*.

McKERNAN, Hilda Kathleen (24 January 1901–post-1939), from Dublin; father John McKernan, head constable, Royal Irish Constabulary. Religion Catholic. Matriculated UCD 1919/20; qualified MB BCh BAO 1924. Address but no post in Dublin, 1929, address uncommunicated, 1934, London uncommunicated address, 1939, then not listed.

McKNIGHT (later Henry), Maud Warren (c.1898–post-1957), from Belfast; father Robert McKnight, chemist. Religion Church of Ireland. Matriculated QCB summer 1918; qualified MB BCh BAO 1922. Working as Anaesthetist at Royal Victoria Hospital, Belfast, 1927–32, then Nigeria (c/o Public Works Department), 1937–47, and South Africa, address but no post, 1957.

McQUILLAN, Mary Rose (c.1904–post-1969), unknown; father publican. Religion unknown. Matriculated QCB summer 1922; qualified LRCP LRCS Edin 1934. Address but no post in Wales, 1939, Belfast, 1944, then Wales, 1959–69.

MEADE, Kathleen (25 August 1899–post-1926), from Castlebelling Law, Louth; father Michael Meade, farmer. Religion Catholic. Matriculated UCD 1916/17; qualified MB BCh BAO 1921. Address but no post in Louth, 1926, then not listed.

MEENAN (later Donnellan), Annie (c.1899–post-1938), background unknown. Matriculated QCB summer 1917; qualified MB BCh BAO 1923. Jun Asst MO, District Asylum, Omagh, 1928–33, then England, address uncommunicated, 1938, then not listed.

MENARY, Vera Gladys May (c.1898–post-1932), from Armagh; father Thomas Menary, solicitor. Religion Church of Ireland. Matriculated TCD 1916/17; qualified MB BCh BAO 1922. Address but no post in Lurgan, 1927, and in Derry, 1932, then not listed.

MILLER, Mary Swan (fl. 1920–66), background unknown. Matriculated TCD 1920/21; qualified MB BCh BAO 1926. Address but no post in Derry, 1931, Sch MO, Londonderry, and Limavady Education Committee, 1936, Asst MOH and Sch MO, Leigh, 1946–66.

MITCHELL, Charlotte Eleanor (fl. 1900–12), background unknown. Matriculated QCB 1900/01; qualified MB BCh BAO 1907. Appointment at the Infirmary, Lurgan, 1912, then not listed.

MOCLAIR, Bridget Angela (8 January 1895–post-1956), from Cashel, Tipperary; father Patrick Moclair, farmer. Religion unknown. Matriculated QCB 1913/14; qualified MB BCh BAO 1921. Address but no post at Merrion Square, Dublin, 1926–56.

MOLLOY, Marie Rose Lynch (c.1884–post-1949), from ·Cork; father John Lynch, retired. Religion Catholic. Matriculated QCC 1905/06; qualified MB BCh BAO 1914. Asst MOH, Birmingham, 1919– at least 1949.

MOLONEY, Mary Frances (14 October 1894–post-1955), from Limerick; father Patrick Moloney, chemist. Religion unknown. Matriculated UCD 1915/16; qualified MB BCh BAO 1920. Address but no post in Tipperary, 1925–35, then Limerick, 1945 until at least 1955.

MOONEY, Evaline Elizabeth (fl. 1919–49), background unknown. Matriculated TCD 1919/20; qualified MB BCh BAO 1924. Address but no post in Westmeath, 1929–39, then Ophthalmic Surg, County Hospital Mullingar, 1949, then not listed.

MOORE, Marguerite Eveline (c.1887–post-1958), born in the USA; father Samuel Moore, farmer. Religion Presbyterian. Matriculated QCB 1917/18; qualified MB BCh BAO 1923. Address but no post in Derry, 1928–33, then Manchester, 1938–58.

MOORE, Marie Stella (18 January 1897–post-1927), from Dublin; father Stanley Moore, doctor. Religion Catholic. Matriculated UCD 1916/17; qualified MB BCh BAO 1922; DPH 1924. Listed at Walthamstow Sanatorium, Chingford, London, 1927, then not listed.

MORAN, Kate Agnes (4 January 1900–post-1936), from Ballintogher, Sligo; father Edward Moran, farmer. Religion unknown. Matriculated QCG 1919/20; qualified MB BCh BAO 1926; DPH 1928. Address but no post in Ballintogher, Sligo, 1931–36, then not listed.

MORRISON, Elizabeth (c.1897–1957), birthplace unknown; father farmer. Religion unknown. Matriculated QCB summer 1916; qualified MB BCh BAO 1922. Address but no post, Dervock, Antrim, 1927 until at least 1957.

MUIR, Alice Irene (c.1903–post-1933), from Belfast; father Andrew Henry Muir, accountant. Religion Congregationalist. Matriculated QCB 1921/22; qualified MB BCh BAO 1928. Listed as Ho Surg, Ethel Hedley Hospital, Windermere, England, 1933, then not listed.

MULCAHY, Aileen Mary (later Martyn) (fl. 1919–60), background unknown. Matriculated RCSI 1919/20; qualified LRCPI & LM, LRCSI & LM 1925. Address but no post in Dublin, 1930–35, and in Galway, 1940–60.

MULHERN, Annie (20 June 1898–post-1929), from Donegal; father James Mulhern, national school teacher. Religion Catholic. Matriculated UCD 1919/20; qualified MB BCh BAO 1924. Address but no post in Donegal, 1929, then not listed.

MULLIGAN, Olive Jane Elizabeth (c.1902–post-1960), from Down; father Thomas Mulligan, farmer. Religion Presbyterian. Matriculated QCB 1920/21; qualified MB BCh BAO 1925. Address but no post in Middlesex, 1930–35, then London, 1940–60.

MULLINS, Maud Marie (c.1901–post-1960), from Cork; father Jeremiah Mullins, carriage builder. Religion Catholic. Matriculated QCC 1919/20; qualified MB BCh BAO 1925; DPH 1927. Address but no post in Cork, 1930, Ho Surg, Midland Hospital, Birmingham, 1935, Sen Asst MO, Great Barr Park Colony, Birmingham, 1940, then Sen Ho MO, St Margaret's Hospital, Birmingham, 1950–60.

MURNANE (later Murnane-Power), Annie Josephine (18 August 1901–post-1961) from Killmallock, Limerick; father Richard Murnane, doctor. Religion Catholic. Matriculated UCD 1920/21; qualified MB BCh BAO 1926. Address but no post in Limerick, 1931–36, then MO, Caherconlish Dispensary District, 1951–61.

MURNANE (later Dunne), Helen Mary (c.1896–post-1955), from Dublin; father 'D.I. in R.I.B.' Religion unknown. Matriculated QCB 1914/15; qualified MB BCh BAO 1920; DPH 1923. Address but no post in Dublin, 1925, appointment at Grangegorman Mental Hospital, 1930, appointment at the Mental Hospital Sligo, 1935, address but no post in Dublin, 1945–55. Married to John Dunne, doctor.

MURPHY, Elizabeth (c.1892–post-1932), from Macroom; father John Murphy, farmer. Religion Catholic. Matriculated QCC 1911/12; qualified MB BCh BAO 1917. Address but no post in Cork, 1922, then MO, Shiveragh Dispensary District, 1927–32, then not listed.

MURPHY, Ellen (c.1897–post-1955), from Old Forge, Lissarda, Cork; father Cornelius Murphy, farmer. Religion Catholic. Matriculated QCC 1915/16; qualified MB BCh BAO 1920. Address but no post in Cork, 1925–30, then Kerry, 1935–55.

MURPHY (later Taffs), Evelyn Nora (?–28 June 1951), background unknown. Matriculated RCSI 1915/16; qualified LRCPI & LM, LRCSI & LM 1921. Address but no post in Cork, 1926, and London, 1931–46.

MURPHY, Lillie Josephine (fl. 1909–25), background unknown. Matriculated Catholic University 1909/10; qualified MB BCh BAO 1915. Address but no post in Macroom, Cork, 1920–25, then not listed.

MURPHY, Margaret (c.1901–post-1958), from Cork; father James Murphy, farmer. Religion Catholic. Matriculated QCC 1918/19; qualified MB BCh BAO 1923. Address but no post in Cork, 1928, Asst MO, Northern Hospital, London, 1933–38, then MO, Surrey Sanatorium, 1948, and MO, Milford Chest Hospital, 1958.

MURPHY, Mary (c.1887–post-1927), from Macroom, Cork; father Patrick Murphy. Religion Catholic. Matriculated QCC 1906/07; qualified MB BCh BAO 1912. Address but no post in Macroom, 1917–27, then not listed.

MURPHY, Mary John (c.1899–post-1960), from Cork; father James Murphy, vintner. Religion Catholic. Matriculated QCC 1918/19; qualified MB BCh BAO 1925; diploma in mental diseases 1930. Address but no post in Cork 1930–35, MO, Castlebar Mental Hospital, 1940–60.

MURRAY, Jeannie Rose (fl. 1898–1931), background unknown. Matriculated QCB 1898/1900; qualified MB BCh BAO 1906. Address but no post in Antrim, 1911, then Sch Med Inspector, Stoke-on-Trent, 1916–31.

NASH, Amy Florence (c.1887–post-1945), from Dublin; father William Henry Nash, GP. Religion Church of Ireland. Matriculated RCSI 1904/05; qualified LRCPI & LM, LRCSI & LM 1910. Address but no post in Dublin, 1915, and in English provinces (address uncommunicated), 1920, Temp Asst MO, County Asylum, Rainhill, 1925, later address but no post in Hants, England, 1935–45.

NEILL, Harriette Rosetta (?–2 July 1942), background unknown. Matriculated QCB 1889/90; qualified MB BCh BAO 1894. Hon Phys, Home of Rest, Bangor, 1899–1909, then address but no post in Bangor, 1919 until at least 1929.

NEILL (later Neill-Kennedy), Matilda Gertrude (c.1898–post-1956), birthplace unknown; father draper. Religion unknown. Matriculated QCB summer 1916; qualified LRCPI & LM, LRCSI & LM 1921. MOH and MO, Bellarena Dispensary District, Derry, and MO to the Post Office, 1926–46, then address but no post in Derry, 1956.

NELIS, Iris Philippine (fl. 1916–58), background unknown. Matriculated RCSI 1916/17; qualified LRCPI & LM, LRCSI & LM 1923; DPH 1924. Address but no post in London, 1928, then MO and Public Vaccinator in Flintshire, Wales, 1933, MOH, Holywell Rd, Mold, District MO and Public Vaccinator, 1938–48, then address but no post in Gloucester, England, 1958.

NELSON, Maggie Martin (c.1896–post-1957), birthplace unknown; father farmer. Religion unknown. Matriculated QCB 1915/16; qualified LRCPI & LM, LRCSI & LM 1922. Address but no post in Down, 1927, Belfast, 1932, then MO, Clogher Union Hospital, 1937–47, address but no post in Clogher, 1957.

NEVILLE, Ellen Mary (c.1897–post-1957), from Ballytrasna, Cork; father Edward Neville, farmer. Religion Catholic. Matriculated QCC 1915/16; qualified MB BCh BAO 1922. Address but no post in Cork, 1927–32, then address but no post in Manchester, 1937–57.

NEVILLE, Marie A. (c.1902–post-1951), from Cork; father Edward Neville, farmer. Religion Catholic. Matriculated QCC 1919/20; qualified MB BCh BAO 1926. Address but no post in Cork, 1931–36, then address in England provinces (uncommunicated), 1941–51.

NOLAN, Agnes Josephine (c.1892–post-1955), from Dublin; father Patrick Nolan, porter Kildare St Club, Dublin. Religion Catholic. Matriculated UCD 1915/16; qualified MB BCh BAO 1920. Address but no post in Limerick, 1925, then MOH and Dispensary MO, Shanagolden and Ballyhahill District, 1930–55.

NOLAN, Margaret Mary (11 November 1896–post-1960), from Kildare; father Edward Nolan, farmer. Religion Catholic. Matriculated UCD 1918/19; qualified MB BCh BAO 1925; diploma in tropical medicine 1927; DPH 1927. Address but no post in Dublin, 1930, then Res Surg, Eden Hospital, Calcutta, India, 1935, MO, Women's Medical Service, India, Ishwari Hospital, Benares, and Res Surg, Eden Hospital, Calcutta, 1940, Gynaecologist, St Luke's Hospital, Anna Uyo District, Nigeria, 1950–60, medical missionary with the Medical Missionaries of Mary. Published 'Short account of ten cases of eclampsia treated by intravenous injections of magnesium sulphate', *Indian Medical Gazette*, 1935.

NOLAN, Mary Rose (fl. 1916–28), birthplace unknown; father farmer. Religion unknown. Matriculated RCSI 1916/17; qualified LRCPI & LM, LRCSI & LM 1923. Address but no post in Limerick, 1928, then not listed.

NORRIS, Nanette (fl. 1916–56), birthplace unknown; father farmer. Religion unknown. Matriculated TCD 1916/17; qualified MB BCh BAO 1921. Address but no post in King's County, 1926, then Fitzwilliam Square, Dublin, 1931–56.

O'BOYLE, Sarah Bridget (15 January 1896–post-1961), from Belmullet, Mayo; father Francis O'Boyle, shopkeeper and farmer. Religion Catholic. Matriculated UCD 1917/18; qualified MB BCh BAO 1926. Address but no post in Mayo, 1931, then south-east London, 1936, MO, Etloe House Institute, London, 1941–51, address but no post in London, 1961.

O'BRIEN, Catherine (24 June 1901–post-1960), from Milltown Malbay; father Michael O'Brien, doctor. Religion Catholic. Matriculated QCG 1920/21; qualified MB BCh BAO 1925; DPH 1927. Address but no post in Galway, 1930, in London, 1935, then Chief Sch MO, Dublin Borough, 1940–50, and Asst MOH, Dublin, 1960. Published 'School Medical Service', *Irish Journal of Medical Science*, 1937.

O'BRIEN, Eveleen Josephine (3 March 1901–post-1959), from Sligo; father Thomas O'Brien, constable in the Royal Irish Constabulary. Religion unknown. Matriculated UCD 1920/21; qualified MB BCh BAO 1924. Address but no post in Dublin, 1929, Asst MO, Portrane Mental Hospital, 1934, Asst MO, Grangegorman Mental Hospital, Dublin, 1939–59. Published 'Treatment of epilepsy', *Journal of Mental Science*, 1931.

O'BRIEN, Kathleen (c.1899–post-1930), from Midleton, Cork; father Patrick O'Brien, doctor. Religion Catholic. Matriculated QCC 1915/16; qualified MB BCh BAO 1920. Address but no post in Cork, 1925, and Limerick, 1930, not listed thereafter.

O'BRIEN, Mary Catherine (fl. 1916–26), birthplace unknown; father farmer. Religion unknown. Matriculated RCSI 1916/17; qualified LRCPI & LM, LRCSI & LM 1921. Address but no post in Athlone, 1926, then not listed.

O'CALLAGHAN, Mary Ruth (c.1900–post-1927), from Cork; father Edward O'Callaghan, lieutenant. Religion Catholic. Matriculated QCC 1917/18; qualified MB BCh BAO 1922. Address but no post in Cork, 1927, then not listed.

O'CONNELL (later Fitzgerald), Nora (c.1904–post-1942), from Cork; father John O'Connell, surveyor of customs and excise. Religion Catholic. Matriculated QCC 1921/22; qualified MB BCh BAO 1927. Address but no post in Cork, 1932, then appointment at Grangegorman Mental Hospital, Dublin, 1937–42.

O'CONNER, Aileen (20 April 1901–post-1926), from Waterford; father James O'Conner, spirit merchant. Religion Catholic. Matriculated UCD 1921/22; qualified MB BCh BAO 1926. Not listed in *Medical Directory*.

O'CONNOR, Anne (7 July 1899–post-1926), from Swinford; father Thomas O'Connor, merchant. Religion unknown. Matriculated QCG 1917/18; qualified LRCPI & LM, LRCSI & LM 1921. Address but no post in Swinford, 1926, then not listed.

O'CONNOR, Annie (c.1904–post-1931), from Cork; father Michael O'Connor, first-class excise officer. Religion Catholic. Matriculated QCC 1921/22; qualified MB BCh BAO 1926; DPH 1929; BSc public health 1931. Address but no post in Cork, 1931, then not listed.

O'CONNOR, Bridget Imelda (c.1893–post-1950), from Cork; father Michael O'Connor, first-class excise officer. Religion Catholic. Matriculated QCC 1911/12; qualified MB BCh BAO 1915. Asst MOH and Asst Med Supt, Borough Hospital, Plymouth, MO, maternity and welfare centres, Plymouth, 1920–25, address but no post in London, 1930–50.

O'CONNOR (later Saunders), Elizabeth (c.1900–post-1959), from Belfast; father Michil O'Connor, Inland Revenue officer. Religion Catholic. Matriculated QCC 1918/19; qualified MB BCh BAO 1924. Address but no post in Surrey, 1929, then Kilkerran, Douglas Rd, Cork, 1934–59.

O'CONNOR, Frances Elizabeth (c.1908–post-1950), from Dublin; father Charlie O'Connor, builder. Religion Church of Ireland. Matriculated TCD 1919/20; qualified MB BCh BAO 1925; DPH 1933. Address but no post in Dublin, 1930–35, then Canterbury as MOH, 1940, then MOH in Essex, 1950.

O'CONNOR, Mary (c.1897–post-1925), from Kinsale, Cork; father Michael O'Connor, customs and excise officer. Religion Catholic. Matriculated QCC 1914/15; qualified MB BCh BAO 1915; bachelor of dental surgery 1918. Sch MO in Plymouth, 1920, then address but no post in London, 1925.

O'CONNOR, Mary Joseph (c.1887–post-1925), from Cork; father Cornelius O'Connor, worker for assurance company. Religion Catholic. Matriculated QCC 1908/09; qualified MB BCh BAO 1915. Supt, Rossclare Sanatorium, 1920 and 1925, then not listed.

O'DONOHUE, Monica A. (c.1902–post-1927), from Sligo; father Maurice O'Donohue, engineer. Religion Catholic. Matriculated QCC 1921/22; qualified MB BCh BAO 1927. Not listed in *Medical Directory*.

O'DOWD, Anne Mary (1 October 1894–post-1960), born in Hull; father John O'Dowd, MP. Religion unknown. Matriculated UCD 1915/16; qualified MB BCh BAO 1925. Address but no post in Ballymote, Sligo, 1930–40, then MO, Whittington Hospital, Preston, 1960.

O'DRISCOLL, Elizabeth Josephine (23 August 1894–post-1922), from Queenstown; father Daniel O'Driscoll, insurance superintendent. Religion Catholic. Matriculated QCC 1912/13; qualified MB BCh BAO 1917; DPH 1920. Initially Ho Surg, Hospital for Tropical Diseases, London, 1922, then not listed.

O'DWYER, Nora (22 June 1897–post-1958), from Cork; father Daniel O'Dwyer, farmer. Religion unknown. Matriculated UCD 1917/18; qualified MB BCh BAO 1923. Address but no post in Clare, 1928–58.

O'DWYER, Nora Mary (c.1900–post-1959), background unknown. Matriculated QCC 1918/19; qualified MB BCh BAO 1924. Address but no post in Cork, 1929–59.

O'FARRELL, Margaret (4 July 1898–post-1930), from Limerick; father John O'Farrell, caterer. Religion Catholic. Matriculated UCD 1919/20; qualified MB BCh BAO 1925. Address but no post in Limerick, 1930, then not listed.

O'FLANAGAN, Mary Margaret (11 January 1901–post-1928), from Dublin; father Milo O'Flanagan, commercial traveller. Religion Catholic. Matriculated UCD 1918/19; qualified MB BCh BAO 1923. Address but no post at Circular Rd, Dublin, 1928, then not listed.

O'FLANAGAN (later Hearth), Pauline Kathleen (29 June 1901–post-1959), from Dublin; father Milo O'Flanagan, commercial traveller. Religion Catholic. Matriculated UCD 1918/19; qualified MB BCh BAO 1924. Married Howard Hearth. Address but no post in Dublin, 1929, then Leicester, 1934–39, then Asst MOH, Leicester, 1949–59.

O'HANLON, Winifred M. (31 March 1899–post-1949), from Sligo; father J. O'Hanlon, teacher. Matriculated QCG 1917/18; qualified MB BCh BAO 1924. Address but no post in Riverstown, Sligo, 1929–34, address uncommunicated in Ireland, 1939–49.

O'KANE, Patricia (c.1903–post-1961), from Tyrone; father Patrick O'Kane, grocer/ spirit merchant and farmer. Religion Catholic. Matriculated TCD 1919/20; qualified LRCPI & LM, LRCSI & LM 1926. Address but no post in Drumquin, Tyrone, 1931–36, then Glasgow, 1941–61.

O'KEEFFE, Catherine (c.1901–post-1935), from Cork; father Richard O'Keeffe, farmer. Religion Catholic. Matriculated QCC 1919/20; qualified MB BCh BAO 1925. Address but no post in Cork, 1935, then not listed.

O'KEEFFE, Eileen May (c.1885–25 February 1928), from Cork; father Arthur O'Keeffe, occupation unknown. Religion Church of Ireland. Matriculated QCC 1904/05; qualified MB BCh BAO 1912. Asst Ho Surg, Royal South Hampshire and Southampton Hospital, 1917–22, then address but no post in Cork, 1927.

O'LEARY (later Morton), Mary (c.1898–post-1947), from Waterford; father Charles O'Leary, cashier, Cappoquin bacon factory. Religion Catholic. Matriculated QCC 1917/18; qualified MB BCh BAO 1922. Address but no post in Cork, 1927–32, then London, 1937, address in England uncommunicated, 1947.

O'MAHONY, Annie (later Mother M. Eiblin, a nun) (c.1901–post-1961), from Cork; father John O'Mahony, farmer. Religion Catholic. Matriculated QCC 1920/21; qualified MB BCh BAO 1926. Address but no post in Cork, 1931–36, then St Gabriel's Convent, Berkshire, 1941. Working in Pakistan at St Raphael's Hospital, Punjab, 1961.

O'MAHONY, Marguerite Sylvia (22 December 1899–post-1931), from Limerick; father John O'Mahony, bookseller. Religion Catholic. Matriculated UCD 1920/21; qualified MB BCh BAO 1926. Address but no post in Limerick, 1931, then not listed.

O'MAHONY, Nora (c.1896–post-1929), from Letterlowes; father Florence O'Mahony, farmer. Religion Catholic. Matriculated QCC 1916/17; qualified MB BCh BAO 1924. Address but no post in Letterlowes, 1929, then not listed.

O'NEILL, Eileen Mary (28 December 1897–post-1936), born in Baugaloe, India; father Richard O'Neill, army captain. Religion unknown. Matriculated UCD 1918/19; qualified MB BCh BAO 1926. Address but no post in Dublin, 1931–36, then not listed.

O'REILLY, Anna Josephine (fl. 1917–27), background unknown. Matriculated RCSI 1917/18; qualified LRCPI & LM, LRCSI & LM 1922; DPH 1926. In 1927 listed as Asst to Professor of Bacteriology, RCSI, and MOH, Swanlinbar, then not listed again. Published 'Notes on *Brit. machilidae*, with descriptions of two new species', *Annals and Magazine of Natural History*, 1915.

O'RIORDAN, Teresa (c.1888–post-1959), from Cork; father Michael O'Riordan, occupation unknown. Religion Catholic. Matriculated QCC 1918/19; qualified MB BCh BAO 1924; DPH 1925. Address but no post in Cork, 1929, then Newport, Wales, 1934–49, then Cork, 1959.

O'SHEA (later O'Connell), Mary Esther (c.1900–post-1948), from Cork; father Patrick O'Shea, farmer. Religion Catholic. Matriculated QCC 1918/19; qualified MB BCh BAO 1923; BSc 1922. Address but no post in Cork, 1928–38, then listed as MO, Millstreet Hospital, Cork, 1948.

O'SULLIVAN, Eileen A. (c.1901–post-1935), from Cork; father Cornelius O'Sullivan, occupation unknown. Religion Catholic. Matriculated QCC 1919/20; qualified MB BCh BAO 1925; DPH 1927. Address but no post in Patrick Street, Cork, 1930–35, then not listed.

O'SULLIVAN (later Morrogh), Maev Attracta (c.1898–post-1921), from Cork; father Robert O'Sullivan, draper. Religion Catholic. Matriculated QCC 1915/16; qualified MB BCh BAO 1921. Not listed in *Medical Directory*.

O'SULLIVAN (later Lahiff), Maureen Margaret (c.1901–post-1957), from Cork; father P. J. O'Sullivan, doctor. Religion Catholic. Matriculated QCC 1917/18; qualified MB BCh BAO 1922. Address but no post in Mitcham, Surrey, 1927–37, then Wexford, 1947, Waterford, 1957.

OVENDEN, Ella (later Webb) (fl. 1904–1934); father rector. Religion Church of Ireland. Year of matriculation unknown; qualified MB BCh BAO Catholic University 1904. Listed as Anatomy Demonstrator at TCD, 1909, Examiner to the Department of Agriculture, Visiting Phys, Baggstrath Female Prison, 1914, Anaesthetist and Phys, Out-patient Department, Children's Adelaide Hospital, and External Examiner, Department of Agriculture, 1919, and Phys, St Ultan's Hospital, Dublin, 1934, then not listed.

PARK (later Moon), Anna Rebecca (c.1905–post-1961), from Tyrone; father Reverend W. Park, Presbyterian clergyman. Religion Presbyterian. Matriculated TCD 1921/22; qualified MB BCh BAO 1926; DPH 1930. Address but no post in Derry, 1931, London, 1936, Dublin, 1941–51, then Asst MO, Surrey County Council, 1961. Married Reginald Moon.

PEDLOW, Margaret Ethel (fl. 1920–60), background unknown. Matriculated TCD 1920/21; qualified MB BCh BAO 1925. Address but no post in Dublin, 1930–60.

PHILLIPPS, Cecilia (16 November 1900–post-1938), born in Queensland; father William Phillipps, victualler. Religion unknown. Matriculated UCD 1918/19; qualified MB BCh BAO 1923. Address but no post in Sydney, Australia, 1933–38, then not listed.

PIGOTT, Lucy Elizabeth Rainsford (c.1900–post-1936), from Dublin; father William Frederick Pigott, doctor. Matriculated TCD 1918/19; qualified MB BCh BAO 1926. Listed at Persia Church Missionary Society Mission Hospital, 1936, then not listed.

POLLOCK (later Moffatt), Grace Kathleen (c.1901–post-1941), from Antrim; father James Pollock, jeweller. Matriculated QCB 1919/20; qualified MB BCh BAO 1926; DPH 1931. Clin Asst, Hospital for Sick Children, Belfast, 1931, then Maternity and Child Welfare Officer in Belfast, 1936–41.

POMEROY, Helena (c.1896–post-1924), from Cork; father Richard Pomeroy, clerk of petty sessions. Religion Catholic. Matriculated QCC 1913/14; qualified MB BCh BAO 1919. Address but no post in Cork, 1924, then not listed.

POMEROY (later O'Brien), Mary (c.1899–post-1957), from Cork; father Richard Pomeroy, farmer and clerk to petty sessions. Religion Catholic. Matriculated QCC 1916/17; qualified MB BCh BAO 1922. Address but no post in Cork, 1927, then London, 1932 until at least 1957.

PORTER, Rachel Elizabeth (c.1901–post-1950), from Tyrone; father David Porter, farmer. Religion Presbyterian. Matriculated QCB 1917/18 and some training at TCD; qualified MB BCh BAO 1925. Address but no post in Castlederg, Tyrone, 1930–35, then GP (Kelly and Porter), Gillingham, Kent, 1940–50.

PORTLEY, Catherine (20 October 1900–post-1929), from Limerick; father John Portley, accountant. Religion Catholic. Matriculated UCD 1918/19; qualified MB BCh BAO 1924. Address but no post in Limerick, 1929, then not listed.

POWELL, Lilian Anna (fl. 1889–1930), birthplace unknown; father minister. Religion unknown. Matriculated QCB 1889/90; qualified MB BCh BAO 1895. Address but no post in Kent, 1900–10, listed as retired in Cornwall, 1920–30.

POWELL, May Evelyn (fl. 1917–57), background unknown. Matriculated TCD 1917/18; qualified MB BCh BAO 1922. Address but no post in Cheltenham, 1927, then Dohnavur Tinnevelly District, India, possibly medical missionary, 1932 until at least 1957.

POWER (later Whelan), Mary Pauline (28 June 1901–post-1960), from Dublin; father Thomas Power, grocer. Religion Catholic. Matriculated UCD 1919/20; qualified MB BCh BAO 1925; DPH 1927. Address in Dublin, 1930–35, then Stradbally, Leix, 1940 until at least 1960.

PRENTICE, Muriel Victoria (fl. 1918–29), background unknown. Matriculated RCSI 1918/19; qualified LRCPI & LM, LRSI & LM 1924. Listed address but no post in Dublin, 1929, then not listed.

PRICE, Muriel Grace (c.1900–post-1938), from Belfast; father James Price, draper. Religion Presbyterian. Matriculated QCB 1917/18; qualified MB BCh BAO 1923. Address but no post in Belfast, 1928 and 1933, then part-time MO, Belfast Corporation Maternal and Child Welfare Department, 1938, then not listed.

PURCE, Agnes Mary (1898–post-1957), from Antrim; father James Purce, station master. Religion Presbyterian. Matriculated QCB 1915/16; qualified MB BCh BAO

1922; DPH 1929. Tuberculosis Officer in Wigan, 1932, Sen Ho Surg (obstetrics and gynaecology), St Mary's Hospital, Manchester, 1937, Asst MO, Metropolitan Borough of Bethnal Green, London, 1947, then address but no post in Yorkshire, 1957.

PURCE, Margaret Sloan (c.1894–post-1926), from Antrim; father James Purce, station master. Religion Presbyterian. Matriculated QCB 1911/12; qualified MB BCh BAO 1916. Ho Surg, Royal Victoria Hospital, Belfast, Sen Demonstrator in Anatomy, QCB, 1921, Hon Surgical Registrar, Eye, Ear, Throat Department, North Staffs Infirmary, Stoke on Trent, 1926, then aurist for Derbyshire, 1931, then not listed.

PURCELL, Catherine (1 April 1899–post-1962), from Thurles, Tipperary; father W. J. Purcell, clerk of unions. Religion unknown. Matriculated UCD 1921/22; qualified MB BCh BAO 1927. MO, Kildare County Fever Hospital, Naas, 1937, then Naas, Kildare, address but no post, 1942 until at least 1962.

PURCELL, Margaret Mary (23 November 1900–post-1960), from Thurles, Tipperary; father W. J. Purcell, gentleman. Religion unknown. Matriculated UCD 1921/22; qualified MB BCh BAO 1925; DPH 1928. Address but no post in Kildare, 1930, MO, Moone Dispensary District, 1935, then MO, Rathmore Dispensary, 1940–60.

PURDY (later Sloan), Kathleen Ismenia (?–2 January 1949), background unknown. Matriculated TCD 1921/22; qualified MB BCh BAO 1926. Address but no post in Enniscorthy, Wexford, 1931–41, then not listed.

QUILLINAN, Mary (c.1900–post-1960), from Tipperary; father Michael Quillinan, pensioned officer. Religion Catholic. Matriculated UCC 1919/20; qualified MB BCh BAO 1925; DPH 1927. Address but no post in Cork, 1930–35, Asst MOH, Cork, 1940 until at least 1960.

QUIN, Emily Isabel May (c.1898–post-1957), birthplace unknown; father clergyman. Religion unknown. Matriculated QCB summer 1916; qualified MB BCh BAO 1922. Address but no post in Antrim, 1927, then Anaesthetist, County Antrim Infirmary, Lisburn, 1932–47. Listed address but no post in Surrey, 1957.

QUINLAN, Catherine (c.1901–post-1959), from Cork; father John Quinlan, insurance agent. Religion Catholic. Matriculated QCC 1918/19; qualified MB BCh BAO 1924. Address but no post in Tralee, 1929–49, then listed at address in California, 1959.

QUINN, Catherine Anne (fl. 1921–61), background unknown. Matriculated RCSI 1921/22; qualified LRCPI & LM, LRCSI & LM 1926. Address but no post in Longford, 1931, Ho Phys, Richmond Hospital, Dublin, 1936, address but no post in Dublin, 1941, then Asst Ophthalmic Surg, Jervis Street Hospital, Dublin, 1951 until at least 1961.

QUINN, Mary Patricia (c.1900–post-1938), background unknown. Matriculated QCB summer 1918; qualified MB BCh BAO 1923; DPH 1926. Address in Belfast, 1928–38, then not listed.

RAMSAY, Mary Frances (c.1899–post-1958), from Tyrone; father William Ramsay, farmer. Religion Methodist. Matriculated QCB 1917/18; qualified MB BCh BAO 1923. Address but no post in Newtownstewart, 1928, Tyrone, 1933, Asst Tuberculosis Officer, Antrim, 1938–48, then listed as Chest Phys, North Ireland Tuberculosis Authority, 1958.

RANKIN, Grace Jessica (fl. 1920–60), background unknown. Matriculated TCD 1920/21; qualified MB BCh BAO 1925. Address but no post in Brighton, 1930, then

GP (Sugden and Rankin), London, 1935–40, then address but no post in Somerset, 1950, and Dorset, 1960.

REA, Helen Gladys (c.1896–post-1933), from Dublin; father James Condell Rea, professor of mathematics. Religion Church of Ireland. Matriculated RCSI 1913/14; qualified LRCPI & LM, LRCSI & LM 1918. Address c/o Dr Williamson, Ipswich, 1923, address but no post in Surrey, 1928–33.

REID, Martha (fl. 1918–28), background unknown. Matriculated TCD 1918/19; qualified MB BCh BAO 1923. Address but no post in Derry, 1928, then not listed.

REVINGTON (later Fisher), Georgina (c.1889–post-1957), from Dublin; father unknown. Religion unknown. Matriculated TCD 1907/08; qualified MB BCh BAO 1912; DPH 1915; MD 1917. Worked abroad Kalene Hill, N. Rhodesia, via Lusaka, until at least 1957.

REYNOLDS, Jane Elizabeth (c.1876–5 January 1951), from Cork; father William Reynolds, occupation unknown. Religion Church of Ireland. Matriculated QCC 1895/96; qualified MB BCh BAO 1905. Address but no post in Dublin, 1910–15, Res MO, Poor Law Institution, Derby, 1920, then retired in London, 1930, retired in English provinces (address uncommunicated), 1940.

RICHARDS, Flora Jane (c.1889–post-1959), born in London; father Richard Evans, shirt and collar manufacturer. Religion Presbyterian. Matriculated QCB summer 1917; qualified MB BCh BAO 1924. Address but no post at Northland Road, Derry, 1929 until at least 1959.

ROBB, Elizabeth ('Lilla') (22 October 1889–fl. 1962), born in Lisburn, Antrim; father linen merchant. Year of matriculation unknown; qualified MB BCh BAO from QUB 1914. Worked in India, 1915–21, at Hassan Hospital, Mysore State, South India. Married Robert Wallace Harland upon her return to the north of Ireland in July 1922. Med Supt, Malone Place Maternity Home, 1922–55, in addition to general practice at 44 Ulsterville Avenue, Belfast. (Information courtesy of Dr Jennifer Fitzgerald.)

ROBINSON (later Magill), Edith (Mrs Magill) (fl. 1908–49), birthplace unknown; father managing director, Banbridge. Religion unknown. Matriculated QCB 1908/09; qualified MB BCh BAO 1914; MD 1920. Asst Sch MO, London County Council, 1924–39, address uncommunicated, 1949.

ROBINSON, Margaret Mary Frances (1901–post-1963), unknown; father engineer and surveyor. Religion unknown. Matriculated QCB 1921/22; qualified MB BCh BAO 1928; DPH 1935. Ho Surg, Ulster Hospital Women and Children, 1933, address but no post in Belfast, 1938, Asst MOH, Liverpool, 1943, then Asst MOH, Derby, 1953 and 1963. Published 'Breech presentation', *British Medical Journal*, 1932.

ROBSON, Mary Martha McConnell (c.1903–post-1962), birthplace unknown; father Presbyterian minister. Religion Presbyterian. Matriculated QCB summer 1920; qualified MB BCh BAO 1927. Address but no post in Belfast, 1932 and 1937, then Asst MO, Antrim Mental Hospital, 1942 and 1952, then Sen MO, Holywell Hospital, Antrim, 1962.

RODGERS, Martha Winifred (c.1903–post-1962), from Armagh; father James Rodgers, national school teacher. Religion Presbyterian. Matriculated QCB 1921/22; qualified MB BCh BAO 1927. Address but no post in Belfast, 1932 and 1937, then Sunderland, 1942, MOH, Sedgefield and Darlington, 1952 and 1962.

ROHAN, Mary Teresa (c.1898–post-1947), from Cork; father James Rohan, manager to shipping firm. Religion Catholic. Matriculated QCC 1916/17; qualified MB BCh BAO 1922; DPH 1923. Address but no post in Cork, 1927 and 1932, then Nottingham, 1937 and 1947.

ROWAN, Maria (fl. 1901–6), birthplace unknown; father doctor. Religion unknown. Matriculated QCB 1901/02; qualified MB BCh BAO 1906. Not listed in *Medical Directory*.

RUSSELL, Eveline Maggie (c.1898–post-1956), birthplace unknown; father merchant. Religion unknown. Matriculated QCB summer 1916; qualified MB BCh BAO 1921. MO, Moira Dispensary District, 1926–46, address but no post in Moira, 1956.

RUSSELL, Margaret Heath (c.1896–post-1924), birthplace unknown; father missionary. Religion unknown. Matriculated QCB 1914/15; qualified MB BCh BAO 1919. Listed at CP Mission, Banswara, South Rajputana, India, 1924, then not listed.

RYAN, Annie (27 October 1896–post-1927), from Smithstown, Clare; father John Ryan, teacher. Religion unknown. Matriculated UCD 1916/17; qualified MB BCh BAO 1922. Address but no post at Abbeyleix, Clare, 1927, then not listed.

RYAN, Eileen (12 October 1895–post-1925), from Tipperary; father James F. Ryan, solicitor. Religion unknown. Matriculated UCD 1914/15; qualified MB BCh BAO 1920. Address but no post in Thurles, 1925, then not listed.

RYAN, Ellen (c.1901–post-1940), from Cork; father Michael Ryan, doctor. Religion Catholic. Matriculated QCC 1919/20; qualified MB BCh BAO 1925. Address but no post in Mallow, 1935 and 1940, then not listed.

RYAN, Ellen Mary (1 July 1894–post-1925), from Tipperary; father James Ryan, farmer. Religion unknown. Matriculated UCD 1916/17; qualified MB BCh BAO 1925. Not listed in *Medical Directory*.

RYAN, Ita (12 April 1901–post-1960), from Loughrea; father John Ryan, doctor. Religion Catholic. Matriculated UCD 1919/20; qualified MB BCh BAO 1925. Address in Loughrea, 1930 and 1935, then MO, County Home, Loughrea, 1950 and 1960.

RYAN, Mary (fl. 1917–58), background unknown. Matriculated UCD 1917/18; qualified MB BCh BAO 1923. Address but no post in Thurles, Tipperary, 1928 and 1933, then MO and MOH, Nenagh, 1948 and 1958.

RYAN, Mary (Mrs) (fl. 1921–61), background unknown. Matriculated RCSI 1921/22; qualified LRCPI & LM, LRCSI & LM 1926. Address but no post in Portumna, 1931, MO, Terryglass Dispensary, 1936, then address but no post in Sussex, 1941 and 1951, and Kent, 1961.

RYAN, Mary Agnes (later Sister M. Therese) (fl. 1917–38), birthplace unknown; father unknown. Religion Catholic. Matriculated UCD 1917/18; qualified LRCPI & LM, LRCSI & LM 1923. Became a nun in the Convent of the Holy Rosary, Killeshandra, Cavan. Listed as medical missionary in Nigeria, 1928–38, then not listed.

SCALLY, Clara Lucia Mary (13 December 1897–post-1956), from Tullamore; father Malachy Scally, draper. Religion unknown. Matriculated UCD 1916/17; qualified MB BCh BAO 1921; DPH 1934. Listed as late MOH, Killoughly, 1931, then Asst MOH, Barnsley, England, 1936–56. Published 'Atropine poisoning', *British Medical Journal*, 1936.

SCOTT, Teresa Mary (28 September 1899–post-1958), from Corofin; father Stephen Scott, insurance agent. Religion Catholic. Matriculated UCD 1917/18; qualified MB BCh BAO 1923. Address but no post in Dublin, 1928 and 1933, then Asst Sch MO, London County Council, 1938 and 1948, then address but no post in London, 1958.

SCULLY, Annie (12 June 1897–post-1947), from Dublin; father Daniel Scully, telegraphist. Religion Catholic. Matriculated UCD 1915/16; qualified MB BCh BAO 1922. Address but no post in Dublin, 1927–47.

SHEPPARD, Mary Christina (fl. 1913–59), background unknown. Matriculated TCD 1913/14; qualified MB BCh BAO 1919; DPH 1922. Address but no post in Clontarf, 1924 and 1929, then Asst MOH, and Asst Sch MO, Education Committee, Walthamstow, London, 1934. Listed as barrister-at-law, Gray's Inn, and Sen MO, Essex, 1949 and 1959.

SHILLINGTON, Elizabeth Graham (c.1899–post-1957), from Armagh; father major in the Royal Irish Fusiliers. Religion Methodist. Matriculated QCB 1917/18; qualified MB BCh BAO 1922; DPH 1925. Listed as Ho Surg, Royal Victoria Hospital, Belfast, and Belfast Hospital for Sick Children, 1927 and 1932, then address but no post in Belfast, 1937. Listed as Clin Asst, Belfast Ophthalmology Hospital, 1947 and 1957.

SIMMS, Mary Evelyn (fl. 1898–1909), birthplace unknown; father grocer and draper. Religion unknown. Matriculated QCB 1898/99; qualified MB BCh BAO 1904. Listed as MO, Mission Hospital, Canning Town, 1909, then not listed.

SINCLAIR, Frances Elizabeth (fl. 1894–1903), birthplace unknown; father 'consult' to Belgium. Religion unknown. Matriculated QCB 1894/95; qualified MB BCh BAO 1898; MD 1903. Not listed in *Medical Directory*.

SMITH, Isobel Gillespie (fl. 1918–59), birthplace unknown; father unknown. Religion unknown. Matriculated TCD 1918/19; qualified MB BCh BAO 1924. Address but no post in Templeogue, Dublin, 1929–34, then London, 1939. Not listed, 1949, but then listed in South Africa, 1959.

SMITH, Lucy Eleanor (c.1870–1929), from Midleton, Cork; father Reverend John Smith, Presbyterian clergyman. Religion Presbyterian. Matriculated QCC 1890/91; qualified MB BCh BAO 1898. Address but no post in Cork, 1903, Phys, Erinville Lying-In Hospital, Cork, 1908, Phys, County and Cork Lying-In Hospital, 1913, and Visiting Phys, HM Fem Prison, Cork, Phys, Lying-In Hospital, Cork, 1923.

SMITH, Mabel Marion (fl. 1920–60), birthplace unknown; father unknown. Religion unknown. Matriculated RCSI 1920/21; qualified LRCPI & LM, LRCSI & LM 1925. Address but no post in Dublin, 1930, then Oakbridge, Peekskill, New York, USA, 1935 until at least 1960.

SMITH, Sarah Ethel (20 May 1899–post-1926), from Galway; father Richard Smith, headmaster at model school. Religion Church of Ireland. Matriculated QCG 1916/17; qualified MB BCh BAO 1921. Listed as MO, Jane Furze Memorial Hospital, South Africa, 1926, then not listed.

SNODGRASS, Kathleen Rebecca (c.1896–post-1956), from Tyrone; father Andrew Snodgrass, merchant. Religion Presbyterian. Matriculated QCB 1915/16; qualified MB BCh BAO 1921. Address but no post in Strabane, 1926, Carlisle, 1931, Strabane, 1936, Lancashire, 1946, and Donegal, 1956.

SPEEDY, Isabella Hogg (c.1900–post-1933), from Dublin; father Thomas Speedy, insurance manager. Matriculated TCD 1918/19; qualified MB BCh BAO 1923. Address but no post at Iona Rd, Dublin, 1928 and 1933, then not listed.

STACK, Mary Josephine (fl. 1915–32), background unknown. Matriculated UCD 1915/16; qualified MB BCh BAO 1922. Address but no post in Tralee, 1927, then Australia, 1932, then not listed.

STAFFORD, Anne Mary (24 June 1900–post-1959), from Wexford; father James Stafford, merchant. Religion unknown. Matriculated UCD 1919/20; qualified MB BCh BAO 1924; DPH 1926. Address but no post in Wexford, 1929, then MO, County Fever and District Hospital, New Ross, 1934, until at least 1959.

STANTON (later Magan), Sybil Catherine (c.1896–post-1956), from Cork; father John Stanton, solicitor. Religion Catholic. Matriculated QCC 1915/16; qualified MB BCh BAO 1921. Address but no post in Essex, 1926, then MO, Post Office, Granard, 1931–46, then listed as working in Medical Missionaries of Mary Hospital in Singida, Tanzania, 1956.

STEPHENSON, Kathleen Evelyn (c.1905–post-1926), from Down; father George Alexander Stephenson, Church of Ireland clerk in holy orders. Religion Church of Ireland. Matriculated QCB 1921/22; qualified MB BCh BAO 1926. Not listed in *Medical Directory*.

STEWART, Martha (fl. 1889–1905), birthplace unknown; father fish curer. Religion unknown. Matriculated QCB 1889/90; qualified LRCP LRCS Edin 1895. Address but no post in Newry, 1900 and 1905, then not listed.

STRANGMAN (later Fitzgerald), Lucia Frances (c.1872–1958), from Waterford; father unknown. Religion Church of Ireland. Matriculated RCSI 1891/92; qualified LRCPI & LM, LRCSI & LM 1896. Worked as Sen MO, District Lunatic Asylum, later Cork Mental Hospital, 1901 until at least 1931.

STRANGMAN, Mary Somerville Parker (c.1876–30 January 1943), from Waterford; father unknown. Religion unknown. Matriculated RCSI 1891/92; qualified LRCPI & LM, LRCSI & LM 1896; FRCSI 1902. Address but no post in Waterford, 1901, Hon Phys, Maternity Hospital and Burchall Asylum Waterford, 1906 until at least 1931. Published 'Morphinomania treated successfully with atropine', *British Medical Journal*, 1907.

STRITCH, Mary Agnes (c.1899–post-1957), from Cork; father John Henry Stritch, draper. Religion Catholic. Matriculated QCC 1916/17; qualified MB BCh BAO 1922; DPH 1923. Address but no post in Nottingham, 1927–37, then Cork, 1947 and 1957.

STUART, Charlotte Annie (fl. 1917–57), background unknown. Matriculated TCD 1917/18; qualified MB BCh BAO 1922. Address but no post in Wicklow, 1927, then listed at Church Mission Society Hospital, Old Cairo, Egypt, 1932–57.

SULLIVAN, Anne (7 June 1900–post-1958), from Fenmore, Cavan; father Thomas Sullivan, farmer. Religion unknown. Matriculated TCD 1918/19; qualified MB BCh BAO 1923; DPH 1925. Address but no post in Fenmore, 1928, then not listed again until 1958, when address but no post in Nigeria given.

SULLIVAN, Annie Monica (c.1894–post-1957), from Bantry, Cork; father John Sullivan, farmer. Religion Catholic. Matriculated QCC 1916/17; qualified MB BCh BAO 1922; DPH 1924. Address but no post in Cork, 1927, then Sch MO, Cork, 1932 until at least 1957.

SULLIVAN, Evelyn Mary (c.1899–post-1942), from Cork; father D. J. Sullivan, merchant. Religion Catholic. Matriculated QCC 1917/18; qualified MB BCh BAO 1927. Address but no post in Sunday's Well, Cork, 1932, after which address uncommunicated, 1937 and 1942, but located in Ireland.

TATE, Isobel Addey (?–28 January 1917), birthplace unknown; father merchant. Religion unknown. Matriculated QCB 1893/94; qualified MB BCh BAO 1899; MD 1902; DPH 1904. Res MO, Burnley Union Infirmary, 1904–9, Medical Inspector of School Children, Lancashire Education Committee, 1914.

TAYLOR, Eleanor (c.1886–post-1913), from Armagh; father Henry Taylor, chaplain guide of orphan house. Religion Church of Ireland. Matriculated TCD 1908/09; qualified MB BCh BAO 1913. Not listed in *Medical Directory*.

TEEVAN, Ellen Mary Teresa (fl. 1915–25), background unknown. Matriculated UCD 1915/16; qualified MB BCh BAO 1920. Address but no post in Dundalk, 1925, then not listed.

TENNANT, Elizabeth Alysia (c.1867–1938), from Carlow; father unknown. Religion Church of Ireland. Matriculated RCSI 1889/90; qualified LRCPI & LM, LRCSI & LM 1894. Worked as MO, St Catherine's School and Orphanage, 1899 until at least 1909, then not listed.

THOMPSON, Frances C. (c.1898–post-1931), birthplace unknown; father doctor. Religion unknown. Matriculated QCB 1915/16; qualified MB BCh BAO 1921. Address but no post in Derry, 1926, then listed as MO, Bellaghy Dispensary District, Derry, 1931, then not listed.

THOMPSON, Mary Georgina (fl. 1917–45), birthplace unknown; father doctor and farmer. Year of matriculation unknown; qualified MB BCh BAO from QUB 1917. Married Professor Donald Breadlbane Blacklock, 1922, and moved to Sierra Leone with him to collaborate on his work on human parasitology. Returned to England, 1929, but continued to travel extensively. Won Leverhulme Fellowship to travel to China, Malaya, Burma, India and Ceylon, 1935, to study the health of women and children. (Information courtesy of Dr Jennifer Fitzgerald.)

TIMON, Ethel Margaret (26 August 1895–post-1957), from Roscommon; father Patrick Timon, national school teacher. Religion unknown. Matriculated UCD 1915/16; qualified MB BCh BAO 1922. Address but no post in Mayo, 1927 and 1932, then Surrey, 1937, and Asst MO, Public Health Department, Central Administrative Staff, London County Council, 1947 and 1957.

TIMONY, Maude Florence (19 February 1901–post-1943), from Mayo; father John Timony, merchant. Religion Catholic. Matriculated UCD 1919/20; qualified MB BCh BAO 1928. Address but no post in Mayo, 1933–43, then not listed.

TWOMEY, Mary (c.1898–post-1947), from Macroom, Cork; father T. J. Twomey, draper. Religion Catholic. Matriculated QCG 1916/17; qualified MB BCh BAO 1922. Address but no post in Cork, 1927–47, then not listed.

TWOMEY, Nora (c.1900–post-1923), from Cork; father John Twomey, farmer, vintner and flour merchant. Religion Catholic. Matriculated QCC 1918/19; qualified MB BCh BAO 1923. Not listed in *Medical Directory*.

VANCE (later Knox), Alice (fl. 1889–1929), background unknown. Matriculated Catholic University 1899/1900; qualified MB BCh BAO 1904. Husband Knox, doctor.

Address but no post in Hamilton, Scotland, 1909, in London, 1914, MO, Maternal Centre, North Islington School for Mothers, 1919–29. Published 'General practice and X-rays'.

WALKER, Elizabeth Stephenson (c.1891–post-1930), from Donaghdee, Down; father Samuel Walker, Presbyterian minister. Religion Presbyterian. Matriculated QCB 1910/11; qualified MB BCh BAO 1915. Attendant, Royal Army Medical Corps, 1918, then MO, Women's Medical Service for India, 1925 and 1930, then not listed.

WALKER, Jane Sproull (c.1901–post-1930), birthplace unknown; father doctor of music. Religion unknown. Matriculated QCB summer 1919; qualified MB BCh BAO 1925. Address but no post in Belfast, 1930, then not listed.

WALSH, Margaret (c.1897–post-1957), from Cork; father John Walsh, farmer. Religion Catholic. Matriculated QCC 1918/19; qualified MB BCh BAO 1922. Address but no post in Mayo, 1927 and 1932, then MO, Dispensary, Ballina, 1937 until at least 1957.

WALSH, Margaret Ellen (13 December 1892–post-1922), from Mayo; father Patrick Walsh, teacher. Religion unknown. Matriculated UCD 1917/18; qualified MB BCh BAO 1922. Career unknown.

WALSH, Mary (8 September 1898–post-1938), from Wexford; father John Walsh, merchant. Religion unknown. Matriculated UCD 1918/19; qualified MB BCh BAO 1928. Address but no post in Kiltimagh, Mayo, 1933–38, then not listed.

WALSH, Sarah Josephine (27 November 1901–post-1936) from Thurles; father John Walsh, engineer. Religion unknown. Matriculated UCD 1921/22; qualified MB BCh BAO 1926. Address but no post in Thurles, 1931–36, then not listed.

WALSH, Teresa J. (c.1891–post-1956), birthplace unknown; father Martin Walsh, merchant. Religion Catholic. Matriculated QCG 1910/11; qualified MB BCh BAO 1916. Address but no post in Tuam, 1921, then MO, Abbey Dispensary District, Galway, 1926 until at least 1956.

WEATHERILL, Gladys (c.1899–post-1928), from Dublin; father John Weatherill, ship-owner. Religion Presbyterian. Matriculated TCD 1918/19; qualified MB BCh BAO 1923. Address but no post in Dublin, 1928, then not listed.

WELPLY, Mary Frances (c.1891–post-1925), from Cork; father unknown. Religion Catholic. Matriculated Catholic University 1909/10; qualified LRCPI & LM, LRCSI & LM 1915. Address but no post, 1920, then Consultant Phys, Medical Board, Ministry of Pensions, Dublin, 1925, then not listed.

WHELAN (later O'Sullivan), Hilda M. G. (21 June 1898–post-1961), from Williamsgate St, Galway; father John Whelan, chemist. Religion Catholic. Matriculated QCG 1919/20; qualified MB BCh BAO 1926; DPH 1931. Address but no post in Galway, 1931 and 1936, then London, 1941, and Galway, 1951–61.

WHELTON, Hannah (c.1900–post-1928), from Cork; father M. J. Whelton, occupation unknown. Religion Catholic. Matriculated QCC 1918/19; qualified MB BCh BAO 1923; DPH 1925. Address but no post in Cork, 1928, then not listed.

WIGODER, Sylvia Beatrix (c.1901–post-1949), from Dublin; father George Wigoder, doctor. Religion Jewish. Matriculated TCD 1917/18; qualified MB BCh BAO 1924; MD 1925. Clin Asst, Dublin Skin and Cancer Hospital, 1929, Clin X-ray Asst, Waterloo

Hospital and Cancer Hospital, 1934, Radium Officer, Bristol Royal Infirmary, 1939, Radiotherapist, North England Cancer Committee, 1949, Consultant Radiotherapist, Newcastle Regional Hospital, 1959. Published 'Familial abdominal lesions', *Lancet*, 1925; 'Appendicitis', *Lancet*, 1925; 'Use of morphine in skin bleeding', *British Medical Journal*, 1927; 'Preliminary notes on x-ray dosage with specific reference to animal experiments', *Irish Journal of Medical Science*, 1929.

WILLIAMSON, Cecilia Florence (?–1964), birthplace unknown; father unknown. Religion Brethren. Matriculated RCSI 1904/05; qualified LRCPI & LM, LRCSI & LM 1909; FRSCI 1910. Address but no post in Ipswich, 1914 and 1919, then Asst Phys and Anaesthetist, Ipswich and East Suffolk Hospital, 1924 until at least 1944.

WILLOCK, Edith Florence (fl. 1916–26), background unknown. Matriculated TCD 1916/17; qualified MB BCh BAO 1921. Address but no post in Dublin, 1926, then not listed.

WISEMAN (later O'Connell), Nora (c.1901–post-1926), background unknown. Matriculated QCC 1920/21; qualified MB BCh BAO 1926. Not listed in *Medical Directory*.

WOLFE, Sarah Christine (c.1886–post-1938), from Skibbereen; father J. J. Wolfe, warehouseman. Religion Methodist. Matriculated QCC 1907/08; qualified MB BCh BAO 1913. Listed in Ireland but address uncommunicated, 1918 and 1923, then listed in China at Women's Hospital, Wesleyan Mission, Hankow, 1928, and General Hospital Wesleyan Mission, Chungslang, Hupeh, China, 1938.

YORKE (later Pettit), Victorine (24 April 1899–post-1958), from Longford; father John Yorke, doctor. Religion Catholic. Matriculated QCG 1918/19; qualified MB BCh BAO 1923. Address but no post in Galway, 1928, and Longford, 1933 and 1938, then listed as Anaesthetist, Longford Hospital, 1948 and 1958.

YOUNG, Augusta Maud (fl. 1920–60), background unknown. Matriculated TCD 1920/21; qualified MB BCh BAO 1925. Address but no post in Wicklow, 1930, Asst in Skin and Children's Departments, Adelaide Hospital, Hon Dermatologist, Children's Sunshine Home, Stillorgan, 1935, Dermatologist, Meath Hospital and Children's Sunshine Home, Stillorgan, 1940–60.

YOUNG, Brenda Mary (c.1901–post-1935), from Dublin; father Henry Young. Religion Catholic. Matriculated RCSI 1920/21; qualified LRCPI & LM, LRCSI & LM 1925; DPH 1927. Address but no post in Sandycove, Dublin, 1930 and 1935, then not listed.

Bibliography

Archival sources

Church Body Representative Library, Dublin
Bishop Kenneth Kennedy, *Fifty Years in Chota Nagpur: An Account of the Dublin University Mission from Its Beginnings* (Dublin: Church of Ireland Printing and Publishing, 1939).

National Archives of Ireland, Dublin
1911 census (online at www.census.nationalarchives.ie, accessed March 2010).

National University of Ireland Archives, Dublin
Matriculation albums of students matriculating through the Royal/National University of Ireland from 1890 to 1922.

National University of Ireland Galway (Registrar's Office)
Matriculation albums for students at Queen's College Galway, 1902–22.
Queen's College Galway council minutes.
Queen's College Galway governing body minutes.

Presbyterian Women's Association, Belfast
Woman's Work magazine.

Private collection of Niall Martin, Edinburgh
Letter dated October 1892, signed by twenty-two lecturers from the Dublin teaching hospitals, the King and Queen's College of Physicians and the Royal College of Surgeons.
Emily Winifred Dickson papers.

Private collection of Brian O'Connor, Sligo
J. D. O'Connor, 'Doctor in the dales', *Yorkshire Dalesman*, December 1983, pp. 750–1.

Public Record Office of Northern Ireland, Belfast
Florence Stewart papers (D3612/3/1).
Forty Years of the Kirin Manchuria Hospital, 1896–1936 (D2332/2).
Irish Presbyterian Mission Hospital, Kirin, Manchuria, Report 1937 (D2332/3).
Letter from Emma M. Crooks, Presbyterian Mission, Kirin, Manchuria, to 'Ned' (nickname for a female friend), dated 9 February 1904 (D1727/2/1).

Letter from Emma M. Crooks to Ned, dated 15 November 1907, Sunshine Cottage, Irish Presbyterian Mission, Kirin, Manchuria, N. China (D1727/2/2).

Queen's University Belfast Archives
Belfast Medical Students' Association, Minutes, 1898–1907.
Belfast Medical Students' Association, Minute book (internal committee meetings), 1899–1925.
Matriculation albums for students at Queen's College Belfast, 1888–1922.
Minute book of the medical faculty, Queen's College Belfast, 1891–1907.

Royal College of Physicians Archives, Dublin
Kirkpatrick Archive. This is a collection of biographical information on 10,000 doctors in the form of notes, news cuttings and obituaries, compiled by T. P. C. Kirkpatrick.
Letter from Sophia Jex-Blake to Dr Duffey, dated 26 March 1879.
Minutes of the KQCPI, vols 15 and 16, 1874–77.
Register of fellows of the KQCPI 1667–1985.
Register of licentiates of Apothecaries' Hall, AH/5/5/1/1 and AH/5/5/1/4.
Register of midwifery licentiates of the KQCPI.
Roll of licentiates, 1877–1910.

Royal College of Surgeons Archives, Dublin
RCSI minutes of council, vol. 7, 1882–84.
Register of fellows of the Royal College of Surgeons in Ireland.

Royal Free Hospital Archives, London
Scrapbooks relating to the Royal Free Hospital and the medical education of women.

Royal Victoria Hospital, Belfast
Belfast Medical Students' Association, Minute book (internal committee meetings), 1899–1925.
Belfast Medical Students' Association, Minute book (general meetings), 1907–32.
Medical staff minutes, 1875–1905.
Medical staff minutes, 1905–37.
Medical staff reports, 1881–99.
Medical staff reports, 1899–1936.

University College Cork Archives
Matriculation albums for students at Queen's College Cork, 1890–1922.
Queen's College Cork governing body minutes, 1883.
Undated letter from Janie Reynolds to the members of council, Queen's College Cork (UC/Council/19/51).

University College Dublin Archives
Catholic University School of Medicine, Governing body minute book, vol. 1, 1892–1911 (CU/14).
Undated letter (from period 1902–13) from the Munster Branch of the Irish Association of Women Graduates and Candidate Graduates to the Board of Management of Victoria Hospital, Cork (NUWGA1/3).

Wellcome Library, London
Letter from Kathleen Lynn to Medical Women's Federation secretary, dated 1915, Medical Women's Federation Archives (SA/MWF/C.80).
Letter giving dates of first women medical students at UK institutions, Medical Women's Federation Archives (SA/MWF/C.10).

Women's Library, London
Billington-Greig, T. 'Why we need women doctors', in *Woman's Wider World* (weekly syndicated article), 28 February 1913 (7/TBG2/G7).

Unpublished dissertations
Cullen, C. 'The Museum of Irish Industry (1845–1867): research environment, popular museum and community of learning in mid-Victorian Ireland' (PhD thesis, University College Dublin, 2008).
Kelly, L. 'Irish medical students at the University of Glasgow, 1859–1900' (MLitt thesis, University of Glasgow, 2007).

Government publications
Royal Commission on University Education in Ireland. *Final Report of the Commissioners* (London: HM Stationery Office, 1903).

Contemporary periodicals
General periodicals
Catholic Bulletin and Book Review, Common Cause of Humanity, Daily Graphic, Economic Journal, Englishwoman's Review, Fortnightly Review, Freeman's Journal, Irish Citizen, Irish Times, Morning Chronicle, North American Review, Queen, Standard, Times, Votes for Women: Official Organ of the United Suffragists, Weekly Irish Times, Woman's Work, Woman's World, Yorkshire Dalesman.

Medical periodicals
British Medical Journal, Dublin Journal of Medical Science, Dublin Medical Press, Lancet, Medical Times and Gazette.

Student periodicals
Alexandra College Magazine, Magazine of the London School of Medicine for Women and Royal Free Hospital, National Student, QCB, QCC, QCG, Quarryman, RCSI Student Quarterly, St Stephen's, TCD: A College Miscellany, UCG: A College Annual, Women Students' Medical Magazine.

Contemporary publications
Adams, E. K. *Women Professional Workers: A Study Made for the Women's Educational and Industrial Union* (New York: Macmillan, 1924).
Ashe, I. *Medical Education and Medical Interests.* Carmichael prize essay (Dublin: Fannin, 1868).
Bewley, H. 'Medical education: a criticism and a scheme', *Dublin Journal of Medical Science*, 129 (1910), pp. 81–97.
Bradshaw, M. (ed.) *Open Doors for Irishwomen: A Guide to the Professions Open to Educated Women in Ireland* (Dublin: Irish Central Bureau for the Employment of Women, 1907).
Cameron, C. A. *History of the Royal College of Surgeons in Ireland and of the Irish Schools of Medicine Including Numerous Biographical Sketches; Also a Medical Bibliography* (Dublin: Fannin, 1886).
Countess of Aberdeen (ed.) *Ireland's Crusade Against Tuberculosis. Vol. 1: The Plan of Campaign: Being a Series of Lectures Delivered at the Tuberculosis Exhibition, 1907, Under the Auspices of the Women's National Health Association of Ireland* (Dublin: Maunsel, 1908).
Davies, E., *Thoughts on Some Questions Relating to Women, 1860–1908* (Cambridge: Bowes and Bowes, 1910).
Dickson, E. W. 'The distribution of weight in clothing', *Aglaia: The Journal of the Healthy and Artistic Dress Union*, no. 1 (1893), pp. 9–13b.

Dickson, E. W. 'Women as workhouse doctors', *BMJ*, 14 April 1894, p. 839.

Dickson, E. W. *The Need for Women as Poor Law Guardians* (Dublin: John Falconer, 1895).

Dickson, E. W. 'Medicine as a profession for women', *Alexandra College Magazine*, 14 (June 1899), pp. 368–75.

Fairfield, L. 'Women and the public health service', *Magazine of the London School of Medicine for Women and Royal Free Hospital*, 19:87 (1924), p. 14.

Fawcett, M. G. 'Equal pay for equal work', *Economic Journal*, 28:109 (1918), pp. 1–6.

Garrett Anderson, E. 'A special chapter for ladies who propose to study medicine', in C. B. Keetley, *The Student's Guide to the Medical Profession* (London: Macmillan, 1878).

Garrett Anderson, L. 'Why medical women are suffragists', *Votes for Women*, 6:273 (1913), p. 509.

General Medical Council. *Medical Directory*, issues from 1891 to 1969 consulted.

General Medical Council. *Medical Students' Register*, issues from 1885 to 1922 consulted.

Griscom, M. 'Obituary for Winifred Dickson Martin', *Medical Women's Federation Quarterly Review*, July 1944.

Guide for Medical Students, More Especially for Those About to Commence Their Medical Studies, by the Registrar of the Catholic University Medical School (Dublin: Browne and Nolan, 1892).

Hardy, N. *The State of the Medical Profession in Great Britain and Ireland in 1900* (Dublin: Fannin, 1902).

Haslam, T. 'Letter to the editor', *Freeman's Journal*, 2 February 1871, p. 3.

Henry, L. 'Medical women and public health work', *Medical Women's Federation Quarterly Newsletter*, February 1922, p. 18.

Hun, H. *A Guide to American Medical Students in Europe* (New York: William Wood, 1883).

Hutchinson, J. 'A review of current topics of medical and social interest', *BMJ*, 19 August 1876, p. 233.

Iles, M. 'Notes on two centres of post-graduate work', *Magazine of the London School of Medicine for Women and Royal Free Hospital*, no. 18 (1901), p. 730.

Irish Medical Student's Guide (Dublin: Dublin Medical Press, 1877).

Jacobi, M. P. 'Shall women practice medicine?', *North American Review*, 134:302 (1882), pp. 69–70.

Jex-Blake, S. *Medical Women: Two Essays* (Edinburgh: William Oliphant, 1872).

Jex-Blake, S. 'The medical education of women', a paper read at the Social Science Congress, Norwich, October 1873 (London: no publisher given, 1874).

Jex-Blake, S. *Medical Women: A Thesis and a History* (Edinburgh: Oliphant, Anderson and Ferrier, 1886).

Jex-Blake, S. *Medical Education of Women: A Comprehensive Summary of Present Facilities for Education, Examination and Registration* (Edinburgh: National Association for Promoting the Medical Education of Women, 1888).

Keetley, C. B. *The Student's Guide to the Medical Profession* (London: Macmillan, 1878).

Kirkpatrick, T. P. C. *History of the Medical Teaching in Trinity College Dublin and of the School of Physic in Ireland* (Dublin: Hanna and Neale, 1912).

Kirkpatrick, T. P. C. *The History of Doctor Steevens' Hospital Dublin, 1720–1920* (Dublin: Ponsonby and Gibbs, 1924).

Lamport, E. F. 'Medicine as a profession for women', in *Education and Professions*, The Women's Library, vol. 1 (London: Chapman and Hall, 1903).

Lowry, E. 'Some side paths in the medical inspection of school children', *Magazine of the London School of Medicine for Women and Royal Free Hospital*, 7:48 (1911), p. 362.

Mapother, E. D. 'The medical profession and its work', *Dublin Journal of Medical Science*, 82 (1886), pp. 177–206.

Marsh, H. 'Women doctors and the war', *Times* (London), 8 December 1914, p. 9.

Marshall, M. A. 'Medicine as profession for women', *Woman's World*, January 1888, p. 108.

'Mater', 'A lady on lady doctors', *Lancet*, 7 May 1870, p. 680.

Maudsley, H. 'Sex in mind and education', *Fortnightly Review*, 15 (1874), pp. 466–83.

McGrigor Allan, J. 'On the real differences in the minds of men and women', *Journal of the Anthropological Society of London*, 7:212 (1869).

Molloy, G. *Progress of the Catholic University Medical School: Extract from the Evidence of the Right Rev. Monsignor Molloy, D.D. D.Sc., Given Before the Royal Commission on University Education in Ireland, 1901* (Dublin: Humphrey and Armour Printers, 1907).

Morley, E. J. 'The medical profession', in *Women Workers in Seven Professions: A Survey of Their Economic Conditions and Prospects* (London: Routledge, 1914).

Ovenden, E. 'Medicine', in M. Bradshaw (ed.), *Open Doors for Irishwomen: A Guide to the Professions Open to Educated Women in Ireland* (Dublin: Irish Central Bureau for the Employment of Women, 1907).

Pringle, J. 'Coombe Lying-In Hospital and Guinness Dispensary', *Women Students' Medical Magazine*, 1:1 (1902), p. 42.

Reaney, M. F. *The Medical Profession: The Carmichael Prize Essay for 1904* (Dublin: Browne and Nolan, 1905).

Rivington, W. *The Medical Profession of the United Kingdom, Being the Essay to Which Was Awarded the First Carmichael Prize by the Council of the Royal College of Surgeons in Ireland, 1887* (Dublin: Fannin, 1888).

Rolleston, H. 'An address on the problem of success for medical women', *BMJ*, 6 October 1923, pp. 591–4.

Royal College of Surgeons in Ireland. *Calendar, October 1923 to September 1924* (Dublin: Dublin University Press, 1923–24).

Scott, C. M. 'Rotunda Hospital', *Women Students' Medical Magazine*, 1:1 (1902), p. 44.

Skeffington, F. S. 'The position of women', *St Stephen's*, 1:12 (1903), pp. 252–3.

Thompson, W. J. 'Medical inspection of school children', *Dublin Journal of Medical Science*, 136:3 (1913), pp. 161–73.

Todd, M. *The Life of Sophia Jex-Blake* (London: Macmillan, 1918).

'Tommie', 'The editor's letter box', *Irish Times*, 2 February 1895, p. 1.

West, C. *Medical Women: A Statement and an Argument* (London: J. and A. Churchill, 1878).

Williams, C. L. 'A short account of the school of medicine for men and women, RCSI', *Magazine of the London School of Medicine for Women and Royal Free Hospital*, no. 3 (January 1896), pp. 91–132.

Wilson, R., *Aesculapia Vitrix* (London: Chapman and Hall, 1886).

Woodhouse, S. 'To students', *Dublin Journal of Medical Science*, 68:4 (1879), p. 351.

Secondary sources

Alexander, W. *First Ladies of Medicine: The Origins, Education and Destination of Early Women Medical Graduates of Glasgow University* (Glasgow: Wellcome Unit for the History of Medicine, 1988).

Baker, R. 'The history of medical ethics', in W. F. Bynum and R. Porter (eds), *Companion Encyclopedia of the History of Medicine* (London: Routledge, 1993), vol. 2, pp. 852–87.

Ball, A. *Faces of Holiness: Modern Saints in Photos and Words* (Huntington, IN: Our Sunday Visitor Publishing, 1998).

Barrington, R. *Health, Medicine and Politics in Ireland 1900–1970* (Dublin: Institute of Public Administration, 1987).

Bashford, A. *Purity and Pollution: Gender, Embodiment and Victorian Medicine* (London: Macmillan, 1998).

Bates, A. W. 'Dr Kahn's museum: obscene anatomy in Victorian London', *Journal of the Royal Society of Medicine*, 99:12 (2006), pp. 618–24.

Bates, A. W. '"Indecent and demoralising representations": public anatomy museums in mid-Victorian England', *Medical History*, 52:1 (2008), pp. 1–22.

Bittel, C. *Mary Putnam Jacobi and the Politics of Medicine in Nineteenth-Century America* (Chapel Hill, NC: University of North Carolina Press, 2009).

Blake, C. *Charge of the Parasols: Women's Entry into the Medical Profession* (London: Women's Press, 1990).

Bonner, T. N. *To the Ends of the Earth: Women's Search for Education in Medicine* (Cambridge, MA: Harvard University Press, 1992).

Bonner, T. N. *Becoming a Physician: Medical Education in Britain, France, Germany and the United States, 1750–1945* (Oxford: Oxford University Press, 1996).

Bourke, J. *Husbandry to Housewifery: Women, Economic Change and Housework in Ireland, 1890–1914* (Wotton-under-Edge: Clarendon Press, 1993).

Braybon, G. 'Women, war and work', in H. Strachan (ed.), *The Oxford Illustrated History of the First World War* (Oxford: Oxford University Press, 1998), pp. 149–63.

Breathnach, E. 'Women and higher education in Ireland (1879–1914)', *Crane Bag*, 4:1 (1980), pp. 47–54.

Breathnach, E. 'Charting new waters: women's experience in higher education, 1879–1908', in M. Cullen (ed.), *Girls Don't Do Honours: Irish Women in Education in the 19th and 20th Centuries* (Dublin: Women's Education Bureau, 1987).

Brookes, B. 'A corresponding community: Dr Agnes Bennett and her friends from the Edinburgh Medical College for Women of the 1890s', *Medical History*, 52:2 (2008), pp. 237–56.

Browne, A. (ed.) *Masters, Midwives and Ladies-in-Waiting: The Rotunda Hospital, 1745–1995* (Dublin: A. and A. Farmar, 1995).

Browne, J. 'Squibs and snobs: science in humorous British undergraduate magazines around 1830', *History of Science*, 30 (June 1992), pp. 165–97.

Bryant, M. *The Unexpected Revolution: A Study in the History of the Education of Women and Girls in the Nineteenth Century* (London: University of London Institute of Education, 1979).

Burstyn, J. 'Education and sex: the medical case against higher education for women in England, 1870–1900', *Proceedings of the American Philosophical Society*, 117:2 (1973), pp. 79–89.

Bynum, W. F. and Porter, R. (eds) *Companion Encyclopedia of the History of Medicine* (London: Routledge, 1993).

Clarke, R. *The Royal Victoria Hospital Belfast: A History, 1797–1997* (Belfast: Blackstaff Press, 1997).

Clear, C. *Social Change and Everyday Life in Ireland, 1850–1922* (Manchester: Manchester University Press, 2007).

Coakley, D. *The Irish School of Medicine: Outstanding Practitioners of the 19th Century* (Dublin: Town House, 1988).

Coakley, D. *Irish Masters of Medicine* (Dublin: Town House, 1992).

Coleman, M. 'A terrible danger to the morals of the country: the Irish hospitals' sweepstake in Great Britain', *Proceedings of the Royal Irish Academy*, 105:5 (2005), pp. 197–220.

Collins, A. *St Vincent's Hospital, Fairview: Celebrating 150 Years of Service* (Dublin: Albertine Kennedy Publishing, 2007).

Condell, D. and Liddiard, J. (eds) *Working for Victory? Images of Women in the First World War, 1914–18* (London: Butler and Tanner, 1987).

Connolly, S. *Religion and Society in Nineteenth-Century Ireland* (Dundalk: Economic and Social History Society of Ireland, 1985).

Cooke, A. M. 'Queen Victoria's medical household', *Medical History*, 26:3 (1982), pp. 307–20.

Cooke, A. M. *My First 75 Years of Medicine* (London: Royal College of Physicians, 1994).

Cowell, J. *A Noontide Blazing. Brigid Lyons Thornton: Rebel, Soldier, Doctor* (Dublin: Currach Press, 2005).

Creese, M. R. S. 'British women of the nineteenth and early twentieth centuries who contributed to research in the chemical sciences', *British Journal for the History of Science*, 24:3 (1991), pp. 275–305.

Crookes, G. *Dublin's Eye and Ear: The Making of a Monument* (Dublin: Town House, 1993).

Croskery, S. *Whilst I Remember* (Belfast: Blackstaff Press, 1983).

Crowther, A. and Dupree, M. 'The invisible general practitioner: the careers of Scottish medical students in the late nineteenth century', *Bulletin of the History of Medicine*, 70:3 (1996), pp. 387–413.

Crowther, A. and Dupree, M. *Medical Lives in the Age of Surgical Revolution* (Cambridge: Cambridge University Press, 2007).

Cullen, C. 'The Museum of Irish Industry, Robert Kane and education for all in the Dublin of the 1850s and 1860s', *History of Education*, 38:1 (2009), pp. 99–113.

Cullen, M. (ed.) *Girls Don't Do Honours: Irish Women in Education in the 19th and 20th Centuries* (Dublin: Women's Education Bureau, 1987).

Cullen, M. (ed.) *Stars, Shells and Bluebells: Women Scientists and Pioneers* (Dublin: Women in Technology and Science, 1997).

Daly, M. E. 'An atmosphere of sturdy independence: the state and the Dublin hospitals in the 1930s', in G. Jones and E. Malcolm (eds), *Medicine, Disease and the State in Ireland, 1650–1914* (Cork: Cork University Press, 1999), pp. 234–52.

Delaney, J. *No Starch in My Coat: An Irish Doctor's Progress* (London: P. Davies, 1971).

Digby, A. *Making a Medical Living: Doctors and Patients in the English Market for Medicine, 1720–1911* (Cambridge: Cambridge University Press, 1994).

Digby, A. *The Evolution of British General Practice, 1850–1948* (Oxford: Oxford University Press, 1999).

Donnelly, D. 'Catholic medical missions', *Studies: An Irish Quarterly Review*, 19:76 (December 1930), pp. 661–70.

Dowling, J. *An Irish Doctor Remembers* (Dublin: Clonmore and Reynolds, 1955).

Drachman, V. G. 'The limits of progress: the professional lives of women doctors, 1881–1926', *Bulletin of the History of Medicine*, 60:1 (1986), pp. 58–72.

Dries, A. 'Fire and flame: Anna Dengel and the medical mission to women and children', *Missology*, 27:4 (1999), pp. 495–502.

Dyhouse, C. *No Distinction of Sex? Women in British Universities 1870–1939* (London: University College London Press, 1993).

Dyhouse, C. 'Driving ambitions: women in pursuit of a medical education, 1890–1939', *Women's History Review*, 7:3 (1998), pp. 321–43.

Dyhouse, C. *Students: A Gendered History* (London: Routledge, 2006).

Elston, M. A. '"Run by women (mainly) for women": medical women's hospitals in Britain, 1866–1948', in L. Conrad and A. Hardy (eds), *Women and Modern Medicine*, Clio Medica Series (Amsterdam: Rodopi, 2001), pp. 73–108.

Fealy, G. M. *A History of Apprenticeship Nurse Training in Ireland* (London: Routledge, 2006).

Finn, I. 'Councillor Mary Strangman and the "health of the city", 1912–20', *Decies: Journal of the Waterford Archaeological and Historical Society*, 56 (2000), pp. 189–203.

Finn, I. 'From case-study to life: Mary Strangman (1872–1943)', in M. Clancy, C. Clear and T. Nic Giolla Choille (eds), *Women's Studies Review Vol. 7: Oral History and Biography* (Galway: Women's Studies Centre, NUI, Galway, 2000), pp. 81–98.

Finn, I. 'Women in the medical profession in Ireland, 1876–1919', in B. Whelan (ed.), *Women and Paid Work in Ireland, 1500–1930* (Dublin: Four Courts Press, 2000), pp. 102–19.

Forbes, G. 'Medical careers and health care for Indian women: patterns of control', *Women's History Review*, 3:4 (1994), pp. 515–30.

Froggatt, P. 'The distinctiveness of Belfast medicine and its medical school', *Ulster Medical Journal*, 54:2 (1985), pp. 89–108.

Garner, J. S. 'The great experiment: the admission of women students to St Mary's Hospital Medical School, 1916–1925', *Medical History*, 42:1 (1998), pp. 68–88.

Garry, T. *African Doctor* (London: John Gifford, 1939).

Gatenby, P. *Dublin's Meath Hospital: 1753–1996* (Dublin: Town House, 1996).

Geddes, J. F. 'The doctors' dilemma: medical women and the British suffrage movement', *Women's History Review*, 18:2 (2009), pp. 203–18.

Gelfand, T. 'The history of the medical profession', in R. Porter and W. F. Bynum (eds), *Companion Encyclopedia of the History of Medicine* (London: Routledge, 1993), vol. 2, pp. 1119–50.

Gillie, A. 'Elizabeth Blackwell and the "Medical Register" from 1858', *BMJ*, 22 November 1958, pp. 1253–7.

Godfrey, C. M. 'The origins of medical education of women in Ontario', *Medical History*, 17:1 (1973), pp. 89–94.

Goldman, L. (ed.), *The Oxford Dictionary of Biography* (online resource, 2010).

Gorham, D. *The Victorian Girl and the Feminine Ideal* (London: Croom Helm, 1982).

Hamilton, C. S. P. *East, West: An Irish Doctor's Memories* (London: Christopher Johnson, 1955).

Hardy, A., 'Public health and the expert: the London medical officers of health, 1856–1900', in R. MacLeod (ed.), *Government and Expertise: Specialists, Administrators and Professionals, 1860–1919* (Cambridge: Cambridge University Press, 2003), pp. 128–42.

Harford, J. 'The movement for the higher education of women in Ireland: gender equality or denominational rivalry?', *History of Education*, 34:5 (September 2005), pp. 497–516.

Harford, J. *The Opening of University Education to Women in Ireland* (Dublin: Irish Academic Press, 2008).

Harrison, R. F. 'Medical education at the Rotunda Hospital 1745–1995', in A. Browne (ed.), *Masters, Midwives and Ladies-in-Waiting: The Rotunda Hospital, 1745–1995* (Dublin: A. and A. Farmar, 1995).

Harte, N. *The University of London 1836–1986* (London: Athlone Press, 1986).

Hawkins, S. *Nursing and Women's Labour in the Nineteenth Century: The Quest for Independence* (London: Routledge, 2010).

Healy, T. M. *From Sanatorium to Hospital: A Social and Medical Account of Peamount 1912–1997* (Dublin: A. and A. Farmar, 2002).

Heffernan, P. *An Irish Doctor's Memories* (Dublin: Clonmore and Reynolds, 1958).

Henry, H. M. *Our Lady's Hospital, Cork: History of the Mental Hospital Spanning 200 Years* (Cork: Haven Books, 1989).

Hill, M. 'Gender, culture and "the spiritual empire": the Irish Protestant female missionary experience', *Women's History Review*, 16:2 (2007), pp. 203–26.

Hilton, M. F. *Dr. Emma Crooks*, Highway series no. 5 (Belfast: Presbyterian Church in Ireland Foreign Mission, c.1937).

Hogan, E. M. *The Irish Missionary Movement: A Historical Survey 1830–1980* (Dublin: Gill and Macmillan, 1990).

Hunter, R. H. 'A history of the Ulster Medical Society', *Ulster Medical Journal*, 5:3 (1936), pp. 178–95.

Jacyna, L. S. 'The laboratory and the clinic: the impact of pathology on surgical diagnosis in the Glasgow Western Infirmary, 1875–1910', *Bulletin of the History of Medicine*, 62:3 (1988), pp. 384–406.

Jalland, P. (ed.) *Octavia Wilberforce: The Autobiography of a Pioneer Woman Doctor* (London: Cassell, 1994).

Jones, G. 'Marie Stopes in Ireland: the Mother's Clinic in Belfast, 1936–47', *Social History of Medicine*, 5:2 (1992), pp. 255–77.

Jones, G. *'Captain of All These Men of Death': The History of Tuberculosis in Nineteenth and Twentieth Century Ireland* (Amsterdam: Rodopi, 2001).

Jones, G. '"Strike out boldly for the prizes that are available to you": medical emigration from Ireland, 1860–1905', *Medical History*, 54:1 (2010), pp. 55–74.

Jones, G. and Malcolm, E. (eds) *Medicine, Disease and the State in Ireland, 1650–1940* (Cork: Cork University Press, 1999).

Jordan, A. *Margaret Byers: A Pioneer of Women's Education and Founder of Victoria College, Belfast* (Belfast: Institute of Irish Studies, Queen's University Belfast, 1987).

Jordanova, L. 'Has the social history of medicine come of age?', *Historical Journal*, 36:2 (1993), pp. 437–49.

Kelham, B. B. 'The Royal College of Science for Ireland (1867–1926)', *Studies: An Irish Quarterly Review*, 56:223 (1967), pp. 297–309.

Kennedy, F. *Family, Economy and Government in Ireland* (Dublin: Economic and Social Research Institute, 1989).

Kinsella, A. 'Some medical aspects of Easter 1916', *Dublin Historical Record*, 50:2 (autumn 1997), pp. 137–70.

Lamont, T. 'The Amazons within: women in the BMA 100 years ago', *BMJ*, 19–26 December 1992, pp. 1529–32.

Lefkowitz Horowitz, H. *Campus Life: Undergraduate Cultures from the End of the Eighteenth Century to the Present* (New York: Alfred A. Knopf, 1987).

Loudon, I. *Medical Care and the General Practitioner, 1750–1850* (Oxford: Oxford University Press, 1986).

Luddy, M. *Women in Ireland, 1800–1918: A Documentary History* (Cork: Cork University Press, 1995).

Luddy, M. *Women and Philanthropy in Nineteenth-Century Ireland* (Cambridge: Cambridge University Press, 1995).

Lutzker, E. 'Edith Pechey-Phipson: the untold story', *Medical History*, 11:1 (1967), pp. 41–5.

Lutzker, E. *Women Gain a Place in Medicine* (New York: McGraw-Hill, 1969).

Lyons, J. B. *The Irresistible Rise of the RCSI* (Dublin: Royal College of Surgeons, 1984).

Lyons, J. B. *The Quality of Mercer's: The Story of Mercer's Hospital, 1734–1991* (Dublin: Glendale, 1991)

McClelland, G. *Pioneering Women: Riddel Hall and Queen's University Belfast* (Belfast: Ulster Historical Foundation, 2005).

McDermid, J. 'Women and education', in J. Purvis (ed.), *Women's History: Britain, 1850–1945* (London: Routledge, 1995), pp. 107–30.

Macdona, A. *From Newman to New Woman: The Women of UCD Remember* (Dublin: New Island, 2001).

McGregor Hellstedt, L. (ed.) *Women Physicians of the World: Autobiographies of Medical Pioneers* (Washington, DC, and London: Medical Women's International Federation, Hemisphere Publishing Corporation, 1978).

MacLeod, R. (ed.) *Government and Expertise: Specialists, Administrators and Professionals, 1860–1919* (Cambridge: Cambridge University Press, 2003).

Malcolm, E. *Swift's Hospital: A History of St Patrick's Hospital, Dublin, 1746–1989* (Dublin: Gill and Macmillan, 1989).

Meenan, F. O. C. *Cecilia Street: The Catholic University School of Medicine, 1855–1931* (Dublin: Gill and Macmillan, 1987).

Meenan, F. O. C. *St Vincent's Hospital, 1834–1994: An Historical and Social Portrait* (Dublin: Gill and Macmillan, 1994).

Moody, T. W. and Beckett, J. C. *Queen's Belfast 1849–1945: The History of a University* (London: Faber and Faber, 1959).

Morantz-Sanchez, R. M. *Sympathy and Science: Women Physicians in American Medicine* (Chapel Hill, NC: University of North Carolina Press, 1985).

Morantz-Sanchez, R. M. *Conduct Unbecoming a Woman: Medicine on Trial in Turn-of-the-Century Brooklyn* (Oxford: Oxford University Press, 2000).

More, E. S. *Restoring the Balance: Women Physicians and the Practice of Medicine, 1850–1995* (Cambridge, MA: Harvard University Press, 1999).

Mullin, J. *The Story of a Toiler's Life* (Dublin: Maunsel and Roberts, 1921).

Mulvihill, M. (ed.) *Lab Coats and Lace: The Lives and Legacies of Inspiring Irish Women Scientists and Pioneers* (Dublin: Women in Technology and Science, 2009).

Murray, J. *Galway: A Medico-Social History* (Galway: Kenny's Bookshop and Art Gallery, 1994).

O'Brien, E. *The Royal College of Surgeons in Ireland: 1784–1984* (Dublin: Eason, 1984).

Ó hÓgartaigh, M. *Kathleen Lynn: Irishwoman, Patriot, Doctor* (Dublin: Irish Academic Press, 2006).

O'Rahilly, R. *Benjamin Alcock: The First Professor of Anatomy and Physiology in Queen's College Cork* (Cork: Cork University Press, 1948).

O'Rahilly, R. *A History of the Cork Medical School, 1849–1949* (Cork: Cork University Press, 1949).

O'Sullivan, D. J. *The Cork School of Medicine: A History* (Cork: UCC Medical Alumni Association, University College Cork, 2007).

Parkes, S. M. 'Higher education, 1793–1908', in W. E. Vaughan (ed.), *A New History of Ireland. Vol. 6: Ireland Under the Union II 1870–1921* (Oxford: Clarendon Press, 1996), pp. 539–70.

Parkes, S. M. *A Danger to the Men: A History of Women in Trinity College Dublin, 1904–2004* (Dublin: Lilliput Press, 2004).

Parry, J. and Parry, N. *The Rise of the Medical Profession: A Study of Collective Social Mobility* (London: Croom Helm, 1976).

Perkin, J. *Victorian Women* (New York: New York University Press, 1993).

Peterson, M. J. *The Medical Profession in Mid-Victorian London* (Berkeley, CA: University of California Press, 1978).

Poovey, M. *Uneven Developments: The Ideological Work of Gender in Mid-Victorian England* (Chicago, IL: University of Chicago Press, 1986).

Purvis, J. (ed.) *Women's History: Britain, 1850–1945* (London: Routledge, 1995).

Raftery, D. *Female Education in Ireland 1700–1900: Minerva or Madonna* (Dublin: Irish Academic Press, 2007).

Reinarz, J. 'Unearthing and dissecting the records of English provincial medical education, c.1825–1948', *Social History of Medicine*, 21:2 (2008), pp. 381–92.

Reinarz, J. *Health Care in Birmingham: The Birmingham Teaching Hospitals 1779–1939* (Woodbridge: Boydell Press, 2009).

Richards, E. 'Huxley and woman's place in science: the "woman question" and the control of Victorian anthropology', in J. R. Moore (ed.), *History, Humanity and Evolution: Essays for John C. Greene* (Cambridge: Cambridge University Press, 1989), pp. 253–85.

Roberts, S. *Sophia Jex-Blake: A Woman Pioneer in Nineteenth Century Medical Reform* (London: Routledge, 1993).

Rowold, K. *Gender and Science: Late Nineteenth-Century Debates on the Female Mind and Body* (Bristol: Thoemmes Press, 1996).

Russett, C. E. *Sexual Science: The Victorian Construction of Womanhood* (Cambridge, MA: Harvard University Press, 1989).

Ryan, L. and Ward, M. *Irish Women and Nationalism: Soldiers, New Women and Wicked Hags* (Dublin: Irish Academic Press, 2004).

Sappol, M. *A Traffic of Dead Bodies: Anatomy and Embodied Social Identity in Nineteenth-Century America* (Princeton, MA: Princeton University Press, 2001).

Scott, J. M. 'Women and the GMC', *BMJ*, 22–29 December 1984, pp. 1764–7.

Showalter, E. *The Female Malady: Women, Madness and English Culture, 1830–1980* (London: Virago Press, 1987).

Smith, D. *Dissecting Room Ballads from the Dublin Schools of Medicine Fifty Years Ago* (Dublin: Black Cat Press, 1984).

Smith-Rosenberg, C. and Rosenberg, C. 'The female animal: medical and biological views of woman and her role in nineteenth-century America', *Journal of American History*, 60:2 (1973), pp. 332–56.

Solomons, B. *One Doctor in His Time* (London: Christopher Johnson, 1956).

Summerfield, P. 'Women and war in the twentieth century', in J. Purvis (ed.), *Women's History: Britain, 1850–1945* (London: Routledge, 1995), pp. 307–32.

Summerfield, P. 'Gender and war in the twentieth century', *International History Review*, 19:1 (1997), pp. 2–15.

Thom, D. *Nice Girls and Rude Girls: Women Workers in World War I* (London: I. B. Tauris, 1998).

Usborne, C. 'Women doctors and gender identity in Weimar Germany (1918–1933)', in L. Conrad and A. Hardy (eds), *Women and Modern Medicine*, Clio Medica Series (Amsterdam, Rodopi, 2001), pp. 109–26.

Waddington, K. 'Mayhem and medical students: image, conduct and control in the Victorian and Edwardian London teaching hospital', *Social History of Medicine*, 15:1 (2002), pp. 45–64.

Walsh, O. *Anglican Women in Dublin: Philanthropy, Politics and Education in the Early Twentieth Century* (Dublin: University College Dublin Press, 2005).

Warner, J. H. and Rizzolo, L. J. 'Anatomical instruction and training for professionalism from the 19th to the 21st centuries', *Clinical Anatomy*, 19:5 (2006), pp. 403–14.

Warwick, A. *Masters of Theory: Cambridge and the Rise of Mathematical Physics* (Chicago, IL: University of Chicago Press, 2003).

Waterloo Directory of English Periodicals and Newspapers, 1800–1900 (Waterloo, Ontario: North Waterloo Academic Press, 2003).

Weatherall, M. 'Making medicine scientific: empiricism, rationality and quackery in mid-Victorian Britain', *Social History of Medicine*, 9:2 (1996), pp. 175–94.

Whelan, B. (ed.) *Women and Paid Work in Ireland, 1500–1930* (Dublin: Four Courts Press, 2000).

Widdess, J. D. H. *A History of the Royal College of Physicians of Ireland, 1654–1963* (Edinburgh: E. and S. Livingstone, 1964).

Widdess, J. D. H. *The Royal College of Surgeons in Ireland and Its Medical School* (Edinburgh: E. and S. Livingstone, 1967).

Wilkinson, D. M. 'Winifred Dickson Martin', *Medical Women's Federation Quarterly Review*, July 1944.

Wilson, T. G. *Victorian Doctor: Being the Life of William Wilde* (London: Methuen, 1946).

Witz, A. '"Colonising women": female medical practice in colonial India, 1880–1890', in L. Conrad and A. Hardy (eds), *Women and Modern Medicine*, Clio Medica Series (Amsterdam: Rodopi, 2001), pp. 23–52.

Wyman, A. L. 'The surgeoness: the female practitioner of surgery, 1400–1800', *Medical History*, 28:1 (1984), pp. 22–41.

Index

Lightning Source UK Ltd.
Milton Keynes UK
UKOW06f0829240515

252165UK00007B/81/P